Depression and Physical Illness

Edited by

Andrew Steptoe

Department of Epidemiology and Public Health
University College London
London, UK

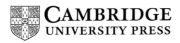

CAMBRIDGE
UNIVERSITY PRESS

CAMBRIDGE UNIVERSITY PRESS
Cambridge, New York, Melbourne, Madrid, Cape Town, Singapore, São Paulo

Cambridge University Press
The Edinburgh Building, Cambridge CB2 2RU, UK

Published in the United States of America by Cambridge University Press, New York

www.cambridge.org
Information on this title: www.cambridge.org/9780521603607

© Cambridge University Press 2007

First published 2007

Printed in the United Kingdom at the University Press, Cambridge

A catalogue record for this publication is available from the British Library

ISBN-13 978-0-521-60360-7 paperback
ISBN-10 0-521-60360-9 paperback

Contents

Contributors

Ephi Betan
Georgia School of Professional
  Psychology
Atlanta, GA
USA

James A. Blumenthal
Department of Psychiatry and
  Behavioral Sciences
Duke University Medical Center
Durham, NC
USA

Angela Bowling
Department of Psychiatry and
  Behavioral Sciences
Emory University School of
  Medicine
Atlanta, GA
USA

Lucile Capuron
Department of Psychiatry and
  Behavioral Sciences
Emory University School of
  Medicine
Atlanta, GA
USA

Robert M. Carney
Behavioral Medicine Center
  Department of Psychiatry
Washington University School of
  Medicine
St Louis, MO
USA

Nathalie Castanon
Integrative Neurobiology
Université Victor Segalen Bordeaux 2
Bordeaux
France

Lucy Cooke
Health Behaviour Unit
  Department of Epidemiology and
  Public Health
University College London
London, UK

James C. Coyne
Department of Psychiatry
University of Pennsylvania School of
  Medicine
Philadephia, PA
USA

Francis Creed
Department of Psychiatry
University of Manchester
Manchester, UK

Robert Dantzer
Integrative Neurobiology
Université Victor Segalen
    Bordeaux 2
Bordeaux
France

Chris Dickens
Department of Psychiatry
University of Manchester
Manchester, UK

Kenneth E. Freedland
Behavioral Medicine Center,
    Department of Psychiatry
Washington University School of
    Medicine
St Louis, MO
USA

Natalie Gilles
Department of Psychiatry and
    Behavioral Sciences
Emory University School of
    Medicine
Atlanta, GA
USA

Ian M. Goodyer
Developmental Psychiatry
    Section
Department of Psychiatry
Cambridge University
Cambridge, UK

Benjamin L. Hankin
Department of Psychology
University of South Carolina
Barnwell College
Columbia, SC
USA

Peter-Panagioti Harakas
Department of Psychology
Arizona State University
Tempe, AZ
USA

Michael Irwin
Cousins Center for
    Psychoneuroimmunology
UCLA Neuropsychiatric Institute
University of California, Los Angeles
Los Angeles, CA
USA

Jon D. Kassel
Department of Psychology
University of Illinois at Chicago
Chicago, IL
USA

Hannah Larsen
Department of Psychiatry and
    Behavioral Sciences
Emory University School of Medicine
Atlanta, GA
USA

Jacques Lestage
Integrative Neurobiology
Université Victor Segalen Bordeaux 2
Bordeaux
France

Heather S. Lett
Department of Psychiatry and
　Behavioral Sciences
Duke University Medical Center
Durham, NC
USA

Maite Moreau
Integrative Neurobiology
Université Victor Segalen Bordeaux 2
Bordeaux
France

Dominique L. Musselman
Department of Psychiatry and
　Behavioral Sciences
Emory University School of
　Medicine
Atlanta, GA
USA

Steven C. Palmer
Department of Psychiatry
University of Pennsylvania School of
　Medicine
Philadephia, PA
USA

Brenda W. J. H. Penninx
Department of Psychiatry
VU University Medical Centre
Amsterdam
The Netherlands

Suzanne Phelan
Department of Psychiatry and Human
　Behavior
Brown Medical School
Providence, RI
USA

Lawrence S. Phillips
Department of Medicine, Division of
　Endocrinology
Emory University School of Medicine
Atlanta, GA
USA

Farhat Rasul
Centre for Psychiatry, Wolfson Institute
　of Preventive Medicine
Queen Mary's School of Medicine and
　Dentistry
London, UK

Douglas A. Raynor
Department of Psychology, State
　University of New York
Geneseo, NY
USA

Andrew Sherwood
Department of Psychiatry and
　Behavioral Sciences
Duke University Medical Center
Durham, NC
USA

Alice E. Simon
Health Behaviour Unit
Department of Epidemiology and
　Public Health
University College London
London, UK

Stephen Stansfeld
Centre for Psychiatry, Wolfson Institute
　of Preventive Medicine
Barts and the London
Queen Mary's School of Medicine and
　Dentistry
London, UK

Andrew Steptoe
Department of Epidemiology and
    Public Health
University College London
London, UK

Christina M. Van Puymbroeck
Department of Psychology
Arizona State University
Tempe, AZ
USA

Jane Wardle
Health Behaviour Unit
Department of Epidemiology and
    Public Health
University College London
London, UK

Lana Watkins
Department of Psychiatry and
    Behavioral Sciences
Duke University Medical Center
Durham, NC
USA

Peter D. White
Department of Psychological
    Medicine
Barts and the London
Queen Mary's School of Medicine and
    Dentistry
London, UK

Rena R. Wing
Department of Psychiatry and Human
    Behavior
Brown Medical School
Providence, RI
USA

Alex J. Zautra
Department of Psychology
Arizona State University
Tempe, AZ
USA

Preface

The past few years have witnessed an upsurge in work on depression and physical illness. This has been coupled with renewed interest in the biological processes underpinning depression and exhortation of physicians to recognise and treat depression in their patients. There are many reasons why the study of depression and physical illness is important. First, there is growing evidence that depression and depressive symptoms are determinants of some types of physical pathology. The investigation of depression therefore contributes to knowledge about factors promoting disease development and illness progression in people with existing disorders. Second, depression is crucial to the everyday functioning and healthcare utilisation of people suffering from physical illnesses. Severe depression is a good indicator of whether daily functioning is likely to be impaired and whether there is an increased risk of suicide. Third, self-management is a central feature of many clinical conditions and disabilities. If depression impairs people's engagement in appropriate self-care, then the burden of distress and disability will be increased and the effectiveness of medical management may be compromised. Fourth, treating comorbid depression is likely to improve the wellbeing and quality of life of patients with physical illnesses, and this may have an impact on the severity and progression of underlying pathology. Bearing in mind the global burden of disease and predictions concerning the future high demands on healthcare systems attributable to depression [1], there is a pressing need to understand the relationship of depression with physical illness and disability.

This book addresses the issue of depression and physical illness from a number of perspectives, including disease aetiology, patient care, adaptation to illness, underlying biology, and behavioural and lifestyle factors. The wealth of scholarship presented attests to the vigour with which the topic is being addressed by researchers and clinicians. The book is divided into four parts. Part 1 sets the scene, with discussion of the occurrence of depression in medically ill patients and the influence of sociodemographic and psychosocial factors on clinical depression and subclinical depressive symptoms. Part 2 is devoted to chapters that assess the relationship between depression and a number of health problems. Coronary heart disease is given the greatest emphasis in view of the extensive work that has been carried out on this topic, but other chapters concern disability, diabetes, chronic pain, cancer, chronic fatigue and obesity. Part 3 addresses the biological and behavioural processes that may link depression with physical health outcomes. From the perspective of biology, there are discussions of inflammatory, neuroendocrine and immunological processes, while the behavioural factors addressed include smoking, physical activity and adherence to medical advice. In Part 4, a final chapter by the editor brings together a number of the themes that have been presented in earlier contributions.

I am grateful to all the contributors who have made working on this volume such a pleasure, to Lorna Gibson and Saskia Dijk for their assistance, and to the staff of Cambridge University Press for their professionalism and courtesy.

Andrew Steptoe

REFERENCE

1. C. J. Murray, A. D. Lopez, Alternative projections of mortality and disability by cause 1990–2020: Global Burden of Disease Study. *Lancet* **349** (1997), 1498–504.

Part 1

Introduction to depression and its determinants

Depression in the medically ill

Francis Creed and Chris Dickens

Introduction

Psychiatric disorders of all types are more common in people with physical illness compared with the general population. Depression is the most common disorder, accounting for approximately 50% of psychopathology in the medically ill, with the remainder made up of various anxiety disorders and mixed subsyndromal symptoms of anxiety and depression. The importance of depression in the medically ill lies in its adverse effect on outcome, most notably health-related quality of life, combined with the fact that it is rarely detected and treated adequately in people who have physical illness.

The prevalence of depression in medically ill populations varies greatly according to the definition of depression and the type of measure used [1–4]. Variation in the definition and measuring instrument are the main reasons for the large variation in the prevalence figures quoted in the literature [5]. A higher prevalence of depression has been reported by studies that have used a self-administered questionnaire compared with those that used standardised research interviews administered by a trained interviewer [6]. The prevalence of depression also varies according to sociodemographic characteristics of the sample and the location of the survey (out-patient, in-patient, community) [3]. Only after all of these factors have been taken into account is it possible to assess whether the prevalence of depression varies according to type of medical disorder, its chronicity or severity [2,3].

In this chapter we indicate the ways in which different definitions and different modes of measurement used in previous research can affect the prevalence of depression. We examine the prevalence of depression in different groups (in-patients, out-patients, population-based samples) and review briefly the few studies that have examined the incidence of depression in the medically ill. Finally, we mention the effect of depression on outcome – assessed in terms of health-related

Depression and Physical Illness, ed. A. Steptoe.
Published by Cambridge University Press. © Cambridge University Press 2006.

quality of life and healthcare costs. This topic is discussed more fully in later chapters.

'Depressive disorder' or 'depression' in the medically ill

In published studies, the prevalence of depression in the medically ill ranges between 15% and 61% [7]. The first figure comes from a study that used a standardised research interview, the latter figure from a study that used self-administered questionnaires with cut-off points indicating probable depression. This variation cannot be attributed to a variation in disorders, as the same phenomenon can be observed in a single disorder – rheumatoid arthritis – where the prevalence of depression was reported as being between 19% and 53% in studies using self-administered questionnaires compared with a narrower variation of 17% and 27% in studies that used a standardised research interview [6].

These types of measure reflect, in part, a conceptual difference regarding depression. Questionnaires usually measure depression as a continuous variable – more symptoms indicate more marked depression, and this is regarded as a continuum, like blood pressure or heart rate. The concept of a 'case' of depression, however, implies that a certain number of symptoms, present for a certain duration, amount to a threshold, above which depressive disorder is diagnosed. The idea of the threshold is that it identifies the point beyond which depression carries complications, mostly an increased risk of impaired daily function and increased suicide risk. When a questionnaire is used, the results are expressed as a mean score for the medically ill population; e.g. the mean depression score on the Hamilton rating scale for depression was 11.8 for stroke patients two months after the stroke [8]. When the concept of a case is used, the results are expressed as the proportion of the population that has been classified as depressed, e.g. 27% of stroke patients classified as having a depressive disorder after a research interview, or 29% scored greater than 17 on the Hamilton rating scale for depression [8].

These two methods of measuring depression merge into one if a cut-off score on a self-administered questionnaire is used to determine the proportion of the population who are probably cases of depressive disorder. Such data are frequently reported in the literature, but it is important to be aware that such a translation from one method to another may lead to misleading results. The sensitivity and specificity of a self-administered questionnaire refer to the ability of the questionnaire to detect cases (determined by research interview) and its accuracy in doing so, when a particular cut-off score is used. It is necessary to consider these parameters because many patients are misclassified as having depressive disorder that is not confirmed by interview (false positives), and vice versa (false negatives) [1,9]. There is no clear consensus as to which method is preferable in physically ill people. This is not so different from the measurement of blood pressure – although there is an upper limit of normal blood pressure, above which treatment is recommended, not everyone with raised blood pressure will develop complications.

In general, the two methods of assessment can reach broad agreement as long as the cut-off score on self-administered questionnaires is adjusted for the physically ill population being screened (see below) [10,11]. In practice, the choice of method may reflect the purpose for the study. A self-administered questionnaire is required to screen a large population of physically ill patients [12] and may be used as the first stage of a two-phase survey, which includes research interviews to determine the actual cases of depressive disorder [13]. The latter method is also required to identify cases for inclusion in a treatment trial.

Standardised research interviews

The standardised interview method of ascertaining depressive disorder tends to be the approach used most often by psychiatrists. In epidemiological research, the identification of cases of depressive disorder within a given population of physically ill patients allows (a) the comparison of the prevalence of depressive disorder between physically ill and healthy controls and (b) the comparison between cases and non-cases within the physically ill group, which is an essential step to identifying risk factors. This approach forms the bulk of the research presented in this chapter; the tables below provide data indicating the prevalence of depressive disorder in different groups of medically ill populations.

Although used widely, there are problems with this approach. The main problem is that the threshold for depressive disorder, established in research performed in the general population or psychiatric patients, may not be that associated most closely with impairment in the physically ill; subthreshold disorders may also lead to impairment [3,9,14–16]. Further studies are required to identify the threshold of depression that is associated with impaired daily functioning, increased suicide risk and increased healthcare use [9,12]. There are also several different but related psychiatric diagnoses that may be relevant. These include major and minor depressive disorder, dysthymia and depressive adjustment disorder; it is not clear whether all or only some of these diagnoses correlate closely with impairment in the physically ill.

Self-administered questionnaires

The alternative approach views depression as a continuum without any clear cut-off separating depressed and non-depressed populations. This approach is probably a more accurate representation of the true picture [12].

Most studies using this approach have employed self-rated questionnaires that were originally designed for use in the general population, or in psychiatric populations, but not for use in the medically ill. These assessments (e.g. Beck Depression

Table 1.1 Endicott criteria: symptoms of depression in the medically ill

Fearful or depressed appearance
Social withdrawal or decreased talkativeness
Psychomotor retardation
Depressed mood
Mood that is non-reactive to environmental events
Markedly diminished interest or pleasure in most activities
Brooding, self-pity or pessimism
Feelings of worthlessness or excessive or inappropriate guilt
Recurrent thoughts of suicide or death

Inventory (BDI), Centre for Epidemiological Studies Depression Scale) contain a number of questions relating to physical (bodily) symptoms of depression, such as fatigue, weight loss, pain and anorexia. Since these physical symptoms may be a direct result of physical illnesses, such as renal failure or rheumatoid arthritis, it is inappropriate to include them as contributors to a diagnosis of depression. Doing so inflates the depression score simply because a physical illness is present. This phenomenon has been termed 'criterion contamination' and is responsible for some studies finding extremely high rates of depression in medically ill populations. For example, early studies that used the Minnesota Multiphase Personality Inventory in rheumatoid arthritis reported a high prevalence of depression until the following items were excluded from the definition of depression: inability to work as usual, failure to be in as good health as previously, easy fatigability, and presence of pain [17]. All of these symptoms could be attributable directly to the rheumatoid arthritis, and it is misleading to use them as symptoms of depression.

A number of strategies have been used to overcome this problem of criterion contamination. First, Endicott [18] suggested alternative criteria to diagnose depression in cancer patients, whereby biological symptoms of depression were replaced by cognitive and emotional symptoms and signs of depression (see Table 1.1). This may be done with other questionnaires (e.g. BDI), but doing so alters the psychometric properties of the questionnaires, and the validity of the measures used in this way cannot be assumed without formal testing against a gold-standard measure. Studies suggest removing some of the BDI items (weight loss, sleep disturbance, work inhibition) to increase its validity in chronic patients with back pain [19] and with headache [20], but the full BDI has been found to be satisfactory in patients with diabetes and multiple sclerosis [21,22].

Second, some questionnaires have been designed for, and validated in, medical patients, such as the Hospital Anxiety and Depression Scale (HADS) [23], or for use in populations where physical health problems are common, such as the Geriatric

Depression Scale (GDS) [24,25]. The HADS is probably the most commonly used, as it excludes many of the physical symptoms of depression (loss of appetite and weight, sleep disturbance, fatigue, decreased sexual drive, poor concentration, psychomotor changes) included in more conventional depression questionnaires [26–28]. Cut-off scores were determined that best identified possible cases (scores of 8 or above) or probable cases (scores of 11 or above) on the depression and anxiety subscales, although these may need to be revalidated for the population in question [27]. Finally, it is possible to use a well-known self-administered questionnaire but with a modified cut-off score. When the General Health Questionnaire (GHQ) (28-item version) score was used in neurological patients, the cut-off score had to be raised from the usual 4/5 to 11/12 [10].

Standardised observer-rated research interviews

Use of observer-rated interview assessments carries the advantage that such assessments allow a trained interviewer to ask clarifying questions to determine whether a symptom has arisen directly as the result of a comorbid medical illness. Semi-standardised research interviews, such as the Schedule for Clinical Assessment in Neuropsychiatry (SCAN) interview [29], enable researchers to ask follow-up questions to ascertain whether a bodily symptom is likely to arise as the result of a medical illness as opposed to a psychological disorder. Such interview-based measures are considered to be the most reliable method of diagnosing depression; in general, studies using such rigorous assessments provide the most conservative estimates of the prevalence of depressive disorder in medically ill populations. The disadvantages of such interview assessments are that interpretation of any follow-up questions relating to the cause of a physical symptom relies on the judgement of the interviewer. Since it is not always possible to determine whether a bodily symptom is attributable to depression or to a comorbid medical illness, the diagnosis of depression may rest on the interviewer's judgement. This subjectivity could undermine the value of delivering a standardised interview, however. The other main disadvantage of semi-standardised interview assessments is the long time taken to perform the assessment, which makes them acceptable for research purposes but too unwieldy for clinical use.

Depressive disorders in medical in-patients

The prevalence of depressive disorders in medical in-patients is shown in Table 1.2. There are differences between studies in the prevalence rates, which can be explained partly by the different diagnostic schema employed in different studies. Arolt and colleagues [30] state that their findings (16.4% had depressive disorder) are essentially similar to those of Feldman and colleagues [31] (14% with depressive

Table 1.2 Prevalence of depressive disorders in medical in-patients

Study	Instrument	No. of patients	Prevalence of depressive disorder	Associated features of depressive disorder	Comment
Feldman et al. [31]	PSE	453	All depressive disorders = 14%	Younger women Unrelated to severity of medical illness	
Silverstone et al. [34]	SCAN/DSM-IV	186	Depressive disorder = 9.7%	Young age, female Unrelated severity of illness or medical diagnosis	Nurses (33%) than doctors (22%) better at recognising depression
Silverstone [32]	SCAN/DSM-IV	313	Major depressive disorder = 5.1%; adjustment disorder = 13.7%	Young age Unrelated to sex, severity of illness or medical diagnosis	Endicott criteria used Low prevalence, as depression present before admission often resolved after hospital admission
Arolt et al. [30]	CIDI/ICD-10	250	Depressive episode = 4.8%; dysthymia = 4%; depressive adjustment disorder = 7.6%; Total depression = 16.4%	Divorced/widowed status	Worst social functioning associated with dysthymia, young age, depression preceding medical illness and chronic disease
Martucci et al. [7]	CIDI/ICD-10 diagnoses	1039 (298 interviewed)	Depressive disorder = 12.8%	Female sex Recent life events, low family support	Disability days increased in cases and subthreshold cases
Creed et al. [9]	SCAN	263	Depressive disorder = 20%	Female sex, severity and number of medical illnesses	Impaired functioning associated in dose–response relationship with cases/subthreshold cases and controls.
Hansen et al. [42]	SCAN	294	Depressive disorders (including dysthymia) = 8.3%	Young age, female sex and life-threatening illness but not chronic illness	Of depressed patients only 18% recognised by physicians
Nair and Pillay [33]	SCID	230	Depressive disorders = 7%	Females Unrelated to severity of medical illness	

CIDI, Composite International Diagnostic Interview; DSM-IV, *Diagnostic and Statistical Manual of Mental Disorders*, 4th edn; ICD-10, *International Classification of Diseases*, 10th revision; PSE, Present State Examination; SCAN, Schedule for Clinical Assessment in Neuropsychiatry; SCID, Structured Clinical Interview for the revised version of the Diagnostic and Statistical Manual of Mental Disorders.

disorder), assuming, apparently, that dysthymia and depressive adjustment disorder in the Composite International Diagnostic Interview (CIDI) are similar to the depressive disorder diagnosis of the Present State Examination (PSE). This may be reasonable as the difference between these categories might be a single symptom and depression in those with physical illness tends to be chronic, making a diagnosis of dysthymia (fluctuating depression present for two years or more) a common form of depression in this population. The more recent SCAN interview [29] provides diagnoses of, according to the 10th revision of the International Classification of Diseases (ICD-10), mild, moderate and severe depression. Mild depression is the most common form of the disorder in physically ill patients and is likely to overlap with depressive adjustment disorder.

The studies that used a diagnosis of major depressive disorder reported prevalence figures of 5.1%, 4.8%, and 7.0% [32–34], whereas those that used the ICD-10 diagnosis of depressive disorder (all ranges of severity) reported figures of 4.8%, 12.8%, and 20% [7,9,30]. The latter of these may be particularly high because of the selection of patients from a deprived inner-city area [9], but the figures have been summarised as mostly being in the range 5–14%, which is clearly higher than that in the general population (2–5%) [35]. The prevalence rate is generally higher among younger patients, and there is the expected excess in females. Typically in people with chronic physical diseases there is an absence of the other usual risk factors for depression, such as age and marital status [9,31] (see below).

Depressive disorders in medical out-patients and primary care

Table 1.3 shows that the prevalence of depressive disorder in medical out-patients varies with the reason for the clinical presentation. For patients whose symptoms are explained by organic disease, the prevalence is 4–12%, not dissimilar from that in medical in-patients. The prevalence of depressive disorders is higher (10–24%) in patients whose symptoms are not explained by organic disease.

One study indicates the particularly high prevalence (26%) of major depressive disorder in patients attending a neurology clinic [36] compared with the more usual figure (13%) for general medical clinics [37]. The study also found that minor depression (8%) and dysthymia (15%) were common among new out-patients at a neurology clinic. These prevalences can be explained in part by the high proportion of patients with medically unexplained symptoms attending a neurology clinic but also by the high prevalence of depressive disorders associated with chronic and disabling neurological diseases. The high prevalence of depression in patients with medically unexplained symptoms is often associated also with a large number of bodily symptoms (somatisation), which may lead to medical help-seeking and increased healthcare use [38].

Table 1.3 Prevalence of depressive disorders in medical out-patients

Study	Instrument	Sample	Prevalence of depressive disorder		Comments
			Organic disease explains symptoms	MUS	
Van Hemert et al. [65]	PSE	Randomly selected new patients at general medicine clinic	4% (n = 91)	24% (n = 100)	High prevalence of anxiety, somatisation and hypochondriacal disorders in MUS patients
Nimnuan et al. [66]	HADS (depression score >10)	Consecutive new patients at 7 out-patient clinics	12.6% (n = 254)	10% (n = 278)	
Feder et al. [67]	CIDI	Inner-city primary care	9% (n = 130)	22% (n = 42)	
Kooiman et al. [68]	HADS (depression score >10)	New general medical out-patients clinic	7% (n = 152)	15% (n = 169)	
Strik et al. [69]	ICDL/DSM-IV	Consecutive first myocardial infarction patients	11.1% MDD; 7.8% minor depression (n = 206)		Total HADS gave better results than the separate subscales
Lowe et al. [37]	ICDL/ICD-10	Out-patients at university hospital clinic and few GPs	15.8% depressive episode (mild = 5.4%, moderate = 5.6%, severe = 4.8%; MDD = 13.2%; any depressive disorder = 25.1% (n = 501)		PHQ, HADS and WBI-5 all distinguished satisfactorily the 3 types of depressive disorder
Escobar et al. [70;71]	CIDI	Out-patients at a university-affiliated primary care clinic	19% major depressive disorder (n = 1455)	13.6% of non-somatisers and 37.5% of somatisers had depressive disorder	
Carson et al. [36]	PRIME-MD, DSM-IV	Consecutive new patients at 5 neurology clinics	Major depression 26%; minor depression 8%; dysthymia 5% (n = 300)	38% of organic group and 60% of patients with MUS had some form of psychiatric disorder	

CIDI, Composite International Diagnostic Interview; DSM-IV, *Diagnostic and Statistical Manual of Mental Disorders*, 4th edn; HADS, Hospital Anxiety and Depression Scale; ICD-10, *International Classification of Diseases*, 10th revisions; ICDL, International Diagnostic Checklist for ICD-10; MDD, Major depressive disorder; MUS, medically unexplained symptoms; PHQ, Patient Health Questionnaire; PSE, Present State Examination; WBI-S, Well-Being Index, version 5.

Depressive disorder is the most common psychiatric disorder among patients attending primary care worldwide [39]. Of the 25 916 patients attending primary care in a study by the World Health Organization (WHO), the estimated prevalence of depressive disorder was 10.4%, with generalised anxiety disorder (7.9%) and neurasthenia (chronic fatigue; 5.4%) being the next most common psychiatric disorders [39]. In the UK centre of the WHO study, the estimated prevalence of depressive disorder was 18.3% of attenders; approximately half of the patients with a psychiatric disorder also had a concurrent physical illness compared with one-third of patients without a psychiatric disorder.

Population-based studies

Cross-sectional studies demonstrate a close association between depressive disorders and physical illness in population-based studies. In the first large study, people with cancer, heart disease, neurological disorder or physical handicap were found to have a significantly higher prevalence of anxiety and depressive disorders (30.3%–37.5%) than people without a chronic physical illness (17.5%) [16]. In another population-based study, chronic disabling physical illness emerged together with lack of a close confidant as the two predictors of depression and anxiety [40]. The nature of the association between physical and psychiatric disorders cannot be discerned from cross-sectional studies, but evidence from a large ($n = 7076$) population-based study suggests that some common generic factors (low educational attainment, high neuroticism) may be associated independently with psychiatric and physical disorders [41].

The traditional view has tended towards seeing depression in physically ill people as an understandable reaction to the symptoms and disabling effects of physical illness. There is only limited evidence to support this notion, however, and some studies show little or no association between depression and the severity of physical illness [31,35]. Hansen and colleagues [42] found that life-threatening, but not chronic, physical illness was associated with increased risk of depression.

Prospective studies are required to assess causality. Several studies have shown, especially in older people, that physical illness is a risk factor for later development of depression [43–45] and for continuing depression [46]; a long-term physical illness can double the chance of subsequent depression [47]. There is evidence, however, that psychiatric disorders, notably depressive disorder, are a predictor of later physical illness [48,49]. This is especially so for coronary heart disease [50]. Thus, there are probably numerous ways in which physical and psychiatric disorders may coexist.

Prospective studies in clinical samples have shown the importance of separating depressive disorders that precede and follow the onset of the physical illness. For example, when depressive disorder precedes a myocardial infarction, the usual risk factors for depression apply: younger age, female sex, social isolation, past history of depression, separation from parent during childhood and experience of marked social difficulties [51,52]. When depression occurs after heart attack, however, these risk factors do not apply – the presence of one or more serious concurrent physical illness (e.g. arthritis, chest disease) was associated with later depression [51]. Depression that precedes the onset of physical illness has the greatest effect on social functioning [29].

Consequences of depressive disorder in people with physical illness

Most of the studies listed in Table 1.2 have shown that impaired functioning is greatly increased when a physical illness is accompanied by depressive disorder. In the large WHO study of primary-care patients, current depressive disorder was associated with the presence of one or more chronic physical illness, but there was clear evidence that both the physical illness (odds ratio [OR] = 1.67) and the number of psychiatric disorders (OR = 2.29) independently contributed to disability [39]. In this study, there was a clear dose–response relationship between increasing depressive symptoms and impaired functioning. A similar relationship has been reported in other studies, where subthreshold disorders are associated with a level of disability in between patients with definite depressive disorders and non-cases after adjustment for sociodemographic features and measures of severity and number of medical illnesses [7,9].

Population-based studies have shown clearly how depressive disorders exert a powerful effect on functioning, and this is superimposed on any decrement on functioning resulting from the concurrent physical illness. In the USA National Comorbidity survey of 5877 respondents, major depressive disorder occurred in 10% of the whole sample, but the prevalence was increased two to three times in those who reported that they also suffered from hypertension, asthma, arthritis or ulcers [53]. The number of days of impairment, over the past month, was 0–0.6 for people with one of these medical conditions if they did not have concurrent major depression, but this increased to 3–4.7 if they had one of the medical conditions and concurrent major depression. Since accurate measures were used in this study, the results indicate that depressive disorders are responsible for much of the impairment in daily-role functioning found in people with chronic physical disorders. Another large study of employees ($n = 15\,153$) found similar results [54]. People with diabetes, heart disease, hypertension or back problems, and who did not also have depression, were absent on sick leave for an average of 6.6 days per annum. The corresponding figure for people with depression but no physical illness was

8.8 days. For people who had both one of the physical illnesses and depression, the mean figure was 13.5 days [54].

In another study, the effect of depressive or anxiety disorders on subjective health-related quality of life in the physical domain was considerable. The presence of a chronic physical illness led to a mean reduction of four points on the physical component summary score of the Short Form 36 (SF36) compared with healthy controls [55–57]. The presence of a mood disorder alone led to a similar reduction of four points, but if both a chronic physical illness and a mood disorder were present then the SF36 physical component score was reduced by 11 points compared with healthy controls [58]. Similar findings have been reported in clinical samples. For example, in gastroenterology patients, whether the disorder is organic (inflammatory bowel disease) or functional (irritable bowel syndrome), the SF36 physical component score is reduced greatly when a concurrent depressive disorder is present [59,60].

Four causal processes have been suggested to account for the marked deterioration of role daily-functioning when depressive disorders accompany physical illness: depressive disorders may (a) amplify subjective reactions to somatic symptoms, (b) reduce motivation to care for physical illness, (c) lead to maladaptive direct physiological effects on bodily symptoms and (d) reduce the capacity to cope with physical illnesses through limitation of energy, cognitive capacity, affect regulation, perception of shame or social stigma [53].

As well as leading to poor health-related quality of life, depressive disorder that accompanies physical illness may lead to a number of other poor outcomes, including increased mortality and increased healthcare use. In a large sample of medical in-patients followed up over two years, and after adjustment for a number of confounders, depressive symptoms were related to subsequent mortality. The adjusted relative risk of death for depressed versus non-depressed patients was 1.9 (95% confidence interval [CI] 1.2–3.1) [61]. This effect has been shown in coronary artery disease (see Chapter 4) and stroke [11,62].

In medical in-patients, subsequent high utilisation and costs have been shown to be associated with psychiatric disorder (mostly depressive disorders and sub-threshold disorders) [9]. In medical out-patients, the best predictors of outpatient utilisation were number of medical diagnoses, number of somatic symptoms, hypochondriacal attitudes and depressive disorder [63]. In primary care, healthcare costs are higher in people who have depression, even after controlling for the effect of physical illness [64].

The most important implication of these results concerning the effect of depression on outcome is the fact that physicians caring for people with these chronic physical disorders often fail to detect and treat the co-occurring depression and miss the opportunity to have maximum impact on impairment. This is a situation that reflects the dualistic nature of medical services, and a more holistic approach that theoretically pertains in primary care can help overcome this problem.

REFERENCES

1. C. J. Meakin, Screening for depression in the medically ill: the future of paper and pencil tests. *Br. J. Psychiatry* **160** (1992), 212–16.

2. G. Rodin, K. Voshart, Depression in the medically ill: an overview. *Am. J. Psychiatry* **143** (1986), 696–705.

3. R. Mayou, K. Hawton, Psychiatric disorder in the general hospital. *Br. J. Psychiatry* **149** (1986), 172–90.

4. J. S. McDaniel, D. L. Musselman, M. R. Porter, D. A. Reed, C. B. Nemeroff, Depression in patients with cancer: diagnosis, biology, and treatment. *Arch. Gen. Psychiatry* **52** (1995), 89–99.

5. F. H. Creed, Assessing depression in the context of physical illness. In M. M. Robinson, C. L. E. Katon, *Depression and Physical Illness*, ed. (Chichester: John Wiley & Sons, 1997), pp. 3–19.

6. F. Creed, Psychological disorders in rheumatoid arthritis: a growing consensus? *Ann. Rheum. Dis.* **49** (1990), 808–12.

7. M. Martucci, M. Balestrieri, G. Bisoffi, *et al.*, Evaluating psychiatric morbidity in a general hospital: a two-phase epidemiological survey. *Psychol. Med.* **29** (1999), 823–32.

8. G. Gainotti, A. Azzoni, C. Marra, Frequency, phenomenology and anatomical-clinical correlates of major post-stroke depression. *Br. J. Psychiatry* **175** (1999), 163–7.

9. F. Creed, R. Morgan, M. Fiddler, *et al.*, Depression and anxiety impair health-related quality of life and are associated with increased costs in general medical inpatients. *Psychosomatics* **43** (2002), 302–9.

10. K. W. Bridges, D. P. Goldberg, The validation of the GHQ-28 and the use of the MMSE in neurological in-patients. *Br. J. Psychiatry* **148** (1986), 548–53.

11. A. House, P. Knapp, J. Bamford, A. Vail, Mortality at 12 and 24 months after stroke may be associated with depressive symptoms at 1 month. *Stroke* **32** (2001), 696–701.

12. A. House, Mood disorders in the physically ill: problems of definition and measurement. *J. Psychosom. Res* **32** (1988), 345–53.

13. G. Dunn, A. Pickles, M. Tansella, J. L. Vazquez-Barquero, Two-phase epidemiological surveys in psychiatric research. *Br. J. Psychiatry* **174** (1999), 95–100.

14. A. Solomon, D. A. Haaga, B. A. Arnow, Is clinical depression distinct from subthreshold depressive symptoms? A review of the continuity issue in depression research. *J. Nerv. Ment. Dis.* **189** (2001), 498–506.

15. P. Rucci, S. Gherardi, M. Tansella, *et al.*, Subthreshold psychiatric disorders in primary care: prevalence and associated characteristics. *J. Affect. Dis.* **76** (2003), 171–81.

16. K. B. Wells, J. M. Golding, M. A. Burnam, Psychiatric disorder in a sample of the general population with and without chronic medical conditions. *Am. J. Psychiatry* **145** (1988), 976–81.

17. T. Pincus, L. F. Callahan, L. A. Bradley, W. K. Vaughn, F. Wolfe, Elevated MMPI scores for hypochondriasis, depression, and hysteria in patients with rheumatoid arthritis reflect disease rather than psychological status. *Arth. Rheum.* **29** (1986), 1456–66.

18. J. Endicott, Measurement of depression in patients with cancer. *Cancer* **53** (1984), 2243–9.

19. A. L. Wesley, R. J. Gatchel, J. P. Garofalo, P. B. Polatin, Toward more accurate use of the Beck Depression Inventory with chronic back pain patients. *Clin. J. Pain* **15** (1999), 117–21.

20. J. E. Holm, D. B. Penzien, K. A. Holroyd, T. A. Brown, Headache and depression: confounding effects of transdiagnostic symptoms. *Headache* **34** (1994), 418–23.

21. P. J. Lustman, R. E. Clouse, L. S. Griffith, R. M. Carney, K. E. Freedland, Screening for depression in diabetes using the Beck Depression Inventory. *Psychosom. Med.* **59** (1997), 24–31.

22. J. E. Aikens, M. A. Reinecke, N. H. Pliskin, *et al.*, Assessing depressive symptoms in multiple sclerosis: is it necessary to omit items from the original Beck Depression Inventory? *J. Behav. Med.* **22** (1999), 127–42.

23. A. S. Zigmond, R. P. Snaith, The hospital anxiety and depression scale. *Acta Psychiatr. Scand.* **67** (1983), 361–70.

24. J. S. Lyons, J. J. Strain, J. S. Hammer, A. D. Ackerman, G. Fulop, Reliability, validity, and temporal stability of the geriatric depression scale in hospitalized elderly. *Int. J. Psychiatr. Med.* **19** (1989), 203–9.

25. R. A. Incalzi, M. Cesari, C. Pedone, P. U. Carbonin, Construct validity of the 15-item geriatric depression scale in older medical inpatients. *J. Geriatr. Psychiatr. Neurol.* **16** (2003), 23–8.

26. C. Herrmann, International experiences with the Hospital Anxiety and Depression Scale: a review of validation data and clinical results. *J. Psychosom. Res.* **42** (1997), 17–41.

27. I. Bjelland, A. A. Dahl, T. T. Haug, D. Neckelmann, The validity of the Hospital Anxiety and Depression Scale: an updated literature review. *J. Psychosom. Res.* **52** (2002), 69–77.

28. M. Johnston, B. Pollard, P. Hennessey, Construct validation of the hospital anxiety and depression scale with clinical populations. *J. Psychosom. Res.* **48** (2000), 579–84.

29. World Health Organization. *Schedules for Clinical Assessment in Neuropsychiatry.* Washington, DC: American Psychiatric Press, 1994.

30. V. Arolt, A. Fein, M. Driessen, L. Dorlochter, C. Maintz, Depression and social functioning in general hospital in-patients. *J. Psychosom. Res.* **45** (1998), 117–26.

31. E. Feldman, R. Mayou, K. Hawton, M. Ardern, E. B. Smith, Psychiatric disorder in medical in-patients. *Q. J. Med.* **63** (1987), 405–12.

32. P. H. Silverstone, Prevalence of psychiatric disorders in medical inpatients. *J. Nerv. Ment. Dis.* **184** (1996), 43–51.

33. M. G. Nair, S. S. Pillay, Psychiatric disorder in a South African general hospital: prevalence in medical, surgical, and gynecological wards. *Gen. Hosp. Psychiatry* **19** (1997), 144–8.

34. P. H. Silverstone, T. Lemay, J. Elliott, V. Hsu, R. Starko, The prevalence of major depressive disorder and low self-esteem in medical inpatients. *Can. J. Psychiatry* **41** (1996), 67–74.

35. W. Katon, P. Ciechanowski, Impact of major depression on chronic medical illness. *J. Psychosom. Res.* **53** (2002), 859–63.

36. A. J. Carson, B. Ringbauer, L. MacKenzie, C. Warlow, M. Sharpe, Neurological disease, emotional disorder, and disability: they are related – a study of 300 consecutive new referrals to a neurology outpatient department. *J. Neurol. Neurosurg. Psychiatry* **68** (2000), 202–6.

37. B. Lowe, K. Grafe, S. Zipfel, *et al.*, Diagnosing ICD-10 depressive episodes: superior criterion validity of the Patient Health Questionnaire. *Psychother. Psychosom.* **73** (2004), 386–90.

38. S. Kisely, D. Goldberg, G. Simon, A comparison between somatic symptoms with and without clear organic cause: results of an international study. *Psychol. Med.* **27** (1997), 1011–19.

39. T. B. Üstün, N. Sartorius, *Mental Illness in General Health Care. An International Study.* Chichester: John Wiley & Sons 1995.

40. J. Harrison, S. Barrow, L. Gask, F. Creed, Social determinants of GHQ score by postal survey. *J. Public. Health. Med.* **21** (1999), 283–8.

41. J. Neeleman, J. Ormel, R. V. Bijl, The distribution of psychiatric and somatic III health: associations with personality and socioeconomic status. *Psychosom. Med.* **63** (2001), 239–47.

42. M. S. Hansen, P. Fink, M. Frydenberg, *et al.*, Mental disorders among internal medical inpatients: prevalence, detection, and treatment status. *J. Psychosom. Res.* **50** (2001), 199–204.

43. G. Livingston, V. Watkin, B. Milne, M. V. Manela, C. Katona, Who becomes depressed? The Islington community study of older people. *J. Affect. Dis.* **58** (2000), 125–33.

44. R. Finlay-Jones, G. W. Brown, Types of stressful life event and the onset of anxiety and depressive disorders. *Psychol. Med.* **11** (1981), 803–15.

45. E. Murphy, Social origins of depression in old age. *Br. J. Psychiatry* **141** (1982), 135–42.

46. M. G. Cole, F. Bellavance, A. Mansour, Prognosis of depression in elderly community and primary care populations: a systematic review and meta-analysis. *Am. J. Psychiatry* **156** (1999), 1182–9.

47. S. B. Patten, Long-term medical conditions and major depression in a Canadian population study at waves 1 and 2. *J. Affect. Dis.* **63** (2001), 35–41.

48. M. Hotopf, R. Mayou, M. Wadsworth, S. Wessely, Temporal relationships between physical symptoms and psychiatric disorder: results from a national birth cohort. *Br. J. Psychiatry* **173** (1998), 255–61.

49. E. Murphy, G. W. Brown, Life events, psychiatric disturbance and physical illness. *Br. J. Psychiatry* **136** (1980), 326–38.

50. H. Hemingway, M. Marmot, Evidence based cardiology: psychosocial factors in the aetiology and prognosis of coronary heart disease. Systematic review of prospective cohort studies. *Br. Med. J.* **318** (1999), 1460–67.

51. C. M. Dickens, C. Percival, L. McGowan, *et al.*, The risk factors for depression in first myocardial infarction patients. *Psychol. Med.* **34** (2004), 1083–92.

52. G. G. Lloyd, R. H. Cawley, Distress or illness? A study of psychological symptoms after myocardial infarction. *Br. J. Psychiatry* **142** (1983), 120–25.

53. R. C. Kessler, J. Ormel, O. Demler, P. E. Stang, Comorbid mental disorders account for the role impairment of commonly occurring chronic physical disorders: results from the National Comorbidity Survey. *J. Occup. Environ. Med.* **45** (2003), 1257–66.

54. B. G. Druss, R. A. Rosenheck, W. H. Sledge, Health and disability costs of depressive illness in a major US corporation. *Am. J. Psychiatry* **157** (2000), 1274–8.

55. J. E. Ware, Jr, C. D. Sherbourne, The MOS 36-item short-form health survey (SF-36). I. Conceptual framework and item selection. *Med. Care* **30** (1992), 473–83.

56. C. A. McHorney, J. E. Ware, Jr, A. E. Raczek, The MOS 36-Item Short-Form Health Survey (SF-36): II. Psychometric and clinical tests of validity in measuring physical and mental health constructs. *Med. Care* **31** (1993), 247–63.

57. J. E. Ware, Jr, M. Kosinski, M. S. Bayliss, *et al.*, Comparison of methods for the scoring and statistical analysis of SF-36 health profile and summary measures: summary of results from the Medical Outcomes Study. *Med. Care* **33** (1995), AS264–79.

58. P. G. Surtees, N. W. Wainwright, K. T. Khaw, N. E. Day, Functional health status, chronic medical conditions and disorders of mood. *Br. J. Psychiatry* **183** (2003), 299–303.

59. F. Creed, J. Ratcliffe, L. Fernandez, *et al.*, Health-related quality of life and health care costs in severe, refractory irritable bowel syndrome. *Ann. Intern. Med.* **134** (2001), 860–68.

60. E. Guthrie, J. Jackson, J. Shaffer, *et al.*, Psychological disorder and severity of inflammatory bowel disease predict health-related quality of life in ulcerative colitis and Crohn's disease. *Am. J. Gastroenterol.* **97** (2002), 1994–9.

61. C. Herrmann, S. Brand-Driehorst, B. Kaminsky, *et al.*, Diagnostic groups and depressed mood as predictors of 22-month mortality in medical inpatients. *Psychosom. Med.* **60** (1998), 570–77.

62. L. S. Williams, S. S. Ghose, R. W. Swindle, Depression and other mental health diagnoses increase mortality risk after ischemic stroke. *Am. J. Psychiatry* **161** (2004), 1090–95.

63. A. J. Barsky, G. Wyshak, G. L. Klerman, Medical and psychiatric determinants of outpatient medical utilization. *Med. Care* **24** (1986), 548–60.

64. G. E. Simon, M. VonKorff, W. Barlow, Health care costs of primary care patients with recognized depression. *Arch. Gen. Psychiatry* **52** (1995), 850–56.

65. A. M. Van Hemert, M. W. Hengeveld, J. H. Bolk, H. G. Rooijmans, J. P. Vandenbroucke, Psychiatric disorders in relation to medical illness among patients of a general medical outpatient clinic. *Psychol. Med.* **23** (1993), 167–73.

66. C. Nimnuan, M. Hotopf, S. Wessely, Medically unexplained symptoms: an epidemiological study in seven specialities. *J. Psychosom. Res.* **51** (2001), 361–7.

67. A. Feder, M. Olfson, M. Gameroff, *et al.*, Medically unexplained symptoms in an urban general medicine practice. *Psychosomatics* **42** (2001), 261–8.

68. C. G. Kooiman, J. H. Bolk, R. Brand, R. W. Trijsburg, H. G. Rooijmans, Is alexithymia a risk factor for unexplained physical symptoms in general medical outpatients? *Psychosom. Med.* **62** (2000), 768–78.

69. J. J. Strik, A. Honig, R. Lousberg, J. Denollet, Sensitivity and specificity of observer and self-report questionnaires in major and minor depression following myocardial infarction. *Psychosomatics* **42** (2001), 423–8.

70. J. I. Escobar, M. Gara, R. C. Silver, H. Waitzkin, A. Holman, W. Compton, Somatisation disorder in primary care. *Br. J. Psychiatry* **173** (1998), 262–6.

71. J. I. Escobar, H. Waitzkin, R. C. Silver, M. Gara, A. Holman, Abridged somatization: a study in primary care. *Psychosom. Med.* **60** (1998), 466–72.

2

Psychosocial factors, depression and illness

Stephen Stansfeld and Farhat Rasul

Introduction

Depression, including the full range of minor to major depressive disorders, is a common and disabling condition. As with most psychological disorders, the aetiology of depression is multifactorial, but social and psychological factors play a more prominent role in its aetiology than in most other conditions in medicine. This has importance both in understanding the aetiology and in finding opportunities for prevention and devising psychological and social treatments.

This chapter describes the evidence for social and psychological factors playing a role in the aetiology of depression. Social factors include general factors at the level of human society concerned with social structure and social processes that impinge on the individual. Psychological factors include individual-level processes and meanings that influence mental states. Sometimes these words are combined as 'psychosocial'. This is a shorthand term for the combination of psychological and social, but it also implies that the effect of social processes is sometimes mediated through psychological understanding. Hence, it has been said that the impact of social inequality on health may be mediated partly through perceptions of shame.

Much of the data on psychosocial factors and mental health deal with broader categories than depression, such as common mental disorder, of which depression is a prominent component. This chapter focuses on depressive disorders but also includes landmark studies that have used the broader categories that illustrate the role of psychosocial variables.

Sociodemographic factors

Gender differences in depression

Both major and minor depressive disorders are more common in women than men [1,2]. The evidence suggests that psychosocial factors play a more important role

Depression and Physical Illness, ed. A. Steptoe.
Published by Cambridge University Press. © Cambridge University Press 2006.

in these differences than do biological or genetic factors [3]. Females seem more sensitive than males to adverse experiences in childhood and are at greater risk of sexual abuse, which may have long-term mental health consequences [4]. Women have onset of depression at an earlier age than men; early-onset depression predicts more and longer episodes of depression in adulthood [5]. Anxiety disorders, which are more common in women, often predict early-onset depression and, hence, partly explain the gender difference in rates of depression [6]. In adulthood, women do not consistently experience more life events than men, but the reaction of women to life events, particularly salient events related to children and relationships, may have more meaning and subsequently more impact for women than men [7].

There are several hypotheses about the impact of different social roles on health. Multiple roles, including work, domestic roles and leisure activities, are generally thought to be beneficial for health as these spread an individual's commitments and sources of support and have different domains of satisfaction, resources and esteem [8]. Conversely, the role overload hypothesis suggests that coping with too many roles may be a risk factor for depression and that conflict and spill-over between roles, for instance between home and work, may be a risk factor for mental ill-health [9,10]. What seems to be crucial is the quality of each of the roles [11]. Undervalued roles, such as that of the housewife or lowly paid employment, may contribute to higher rates of depression in women [12,13], although differences in roles are only a partial explanation for gender differences [14]. Indeed, in studies where psychosocial differences are controlled, such as in Jenkin's [15] study of executive officers in the civil service, the rates of mental ill-health were the same in both sexes. There are probably multiple causes for gender differences in rates of depression; suffice to say these causes are largely psychosocial.

Marital status and depression

Married people typically display better health than unmarried people [16], but marriage in women is related to higher rates of depression than in men [17]. Explanations for this link have generally been supportive of the causal notion that marital experience determines health, and that marriage has a protective effect on health that is more evident for men than women, whose role in marriage tends to be less rewarding. There is also some support for a selection account in which health determines marital experience: in this case, depressed individuals are less likely to be selected into marriage in the first instance [18]. An additional complication is that in major depression, there may be assortative mating of individuals with depression [19]. By contrast, separated people and divorced people experience higher levels of depression than married people and single people [20]. Separation, divorce and widowhood can be seen as stressful life events putting individuals at greater risk of depression. Alternatively, a selection hypothesis would suggest that healthier individuals may be more likely to remain in a marriage, whereas ill-health may contribute to marital strain, thereby increasing the risk of divorce or separation.

Depression and socioeconomic position

Apart from gender differences, the most fundamental association between social factors and depression is the relationship with socioeconomic position (SEP) and the level of social disadvantage this connotes [21]. A number of studies have shown that depression, particularly severe depressive illnesses, are more frequent in people of less advantaged SEP [22]. A meta-analysis of 51 prevalence studies, 5 incidence studies and 4 persistence studies found that low-SEP individuals had a higher risk of being depressed than high-SEP individuals (odds ratio [OR] = 1.81, $p < 0.001$) [23].

The predominance of illness among people of lower SEP has been explained by two competing theories: social selection and social causation. In psychiatric disorders, such as schizophrenia, it seems most likely that individuals, either in the early stages of the illness or having developed this disabling condition, drift down the social scale, being less able to work and maintain social relationships. In this case, the social decline is secondary to the illness. Conversely, for depression, it seems that the social factors are part of the causation of depression, and thus exposure to the different aspects of lower SEP such as poverty and adverse environmental conditions contributes to the social causation of depression. Despite the evidence being largely for social causation, some downward drift in social status over time, due largely to unemployment, has also been observed in patients with major depressive disorder [24].

The picture in minor depressive disorder and common mental disorder is less clear cut, since the social gradient in common mental disorder is shallow and inconsistent across many studies [20]. This may partly represent different social gradients for different types of common mental disorder. It also seems that SEP, usually measured by occupational social class, is only a distal determinant of depression and, as has been shown by Weich and Lewis [25,26] and a systematic review of nine large community surveys carried out since 1980 [27], the more important factors are financial disadvantage, unemployment, low income, low education and low material standard of living, which have a more proximal effect on risk of depression.

Social causation plays a role in several different types of psychiatric disorder, including major affective disorders, personality disorders and substance misuse [28]. If the aetiology of depression is related to environmental stressors, then it may be, as some authors have suggested [29], that stressors such as life events and chronic difficulties, which are more common in individuals of lower SEP, explain the predominance of these disorders in people in less advantaged social positions. In addition, individuals of lower SEP have less access to material resources; as measured by income, this is an important contributor to social-class differences and psychiatric disorder [30]. It has also been demonstrated that low-income women are at greater risk of depressive symptoms in areas of high income inequality than in areas of low income inequality [31]. It seems possible that income inequality confers additional risk to having a low income. This might be explained by perceptions of relative deprivation being more powerful a risk in areas of high inequality, although these relationships with income inequality have not been shown in all studies.

Exposure to lower SEP across the life course may carry greater risk of depression [32]. In the Amsterdam Longitudinal Aging Study, older adults with high lifetime SEP had a lower risk for depression than older adults with a low lifetime level of SEP [33]. This is in keeping with findings that long-term income is more important for health than current income, and that persistent poverty has more effect than occasional episodes of poverty [34]. Low SEP in childhood is also associated with a higher risk of major depression in adulthood, after adjusting for childhood sociodemographic factors, family history of mental illness and adult SEP [35], although in some studies adult SEP has been shown to have a stronger effect than childhood SEP [36]. Social gradients in depression have also been found in adolescents in US studies [37]. A study of adults and their offspring suggests that although parental SEP is a risk factor for depression, there is no evidence of the reverse process of health selection, i.e. that parental depression influenced offspring social position [38]. Thus, social inequalities in depression are likely to have their origins in childhood as well as long-term low SEP carrying a greater risk of depressive onset.

Less access to material resources may also be accompanied by fewer psychosocial resources. There is evidence for this in that greater perceived support, measured by a global score of support from spouse, relations, friends and co-workers, was found in higher-SEP groups [39]. Moreover, the inverse association between social support and depression was stronger among those with low incomes than in those with high incomes in an adult US sample [40]. This suggests that low support may have a more powerful effect on the risk of depression in individuals with few financial resources; conversely, there is perhaps less of a need for the protective effects of support against developing depression in higher-income groups. The availability of mastery and self-esteem has been put forward as an explanation for the SEP gradient in depression [41]. As discussed below, self-esteem may be on the pathway to depression. Control at work, similar to mastery, provides a powerful statistical explanation for the gradient in depressive symptoms in male civil servants [42]. There remains, however, the question of how much mastery or control is merely an indicator of higher social position.

There is some evidence that low SEP, and factors related to it such as poverty, may have stronger effects on maintaining depression than on onset of depression. In Lorant's meta-analysis, the OR for onset (OR = 1.24) was lower than that for persistent depression (OR = 2.06) [23]. Poverty, financial difficulties and low income may prevent an individual getting better once he or she is depressed [26].

Life events, chronic strain and major difficulties

In a study of social causation of psychiatric disorders, Dohrenwend [43] suggests that the likelihood of the onset of these disorders is increased by two factors: '(1) the proportion of the individual's usual activities in which uncontrollable negative changes take place following a major negative event; and (2) how central the uncontrollable changes are to the individual's important goals and values.'

Life events have been studied as the classical social risk factor for depression. In the psychoanalytic literature, depression has traditionally been viewed as a response to loss. So-called 'loss events', such as loss of a loved one by death or the break-up of a relationship, job loss or a symbolic loss such as loss of trust as a result of infidelity, are powerfully related to the onset of depression. There is some suggestion that different types of life event precede depression and anxiety. In a general practice sample, loss events were found before depression, while danger or threat events preceded anxiety [44].

Most early studies of life events were cross-sectional, and the question arose as to the direction of causation. For instance, becoming unemployed might lead to depression; alternatively, becoming depressed and functioning less well at work might subsequently lead to unemployment. Concern about this issue led to the development of the elaborate Life Events and Difficulties Schedule by Brown and Harris [45], which gathered contextual details of an individual's life around the life event and assessed these objectively for the presence of severe threat. In order to avoid contamination of life events by existing illness, independent life events were conceptualised as 'apparently imposed upon the subject and which were, for all practical purposes, outside his or her control' [45].

Of these events, only 'severe' events, connoting marked or moderate long-term threat, were four times more common among depressed patients than among controls [45]. Sixty-one per cent of female patients had a severe event compared with 20% of non-depressed women. Paykel [46] estimated that the increased risk of developing depression in the six months after the most stressful classes of life event was approximately six-fold, falling off rapidly with time after the event. Most of the events involved in depression, unlike those involved, for example, in the precipitation of schizophrenia, included loss and disappointment, e.g. separation, death of a parent and life-threatening illness of someone close. In general, there was a time limit to the impact of life events on depression: most depressive onsets occurred within nine weeks and to a lesser extent within six months of the event. A review of life events and depression found that 17 of 29 retrospective comparisons of psychiatrically treated depressed patients and general population control samples reported more life events before depressive onset than in the control sample [47]. In 11 studies, depressed patients reported more separations than a control group. Life events are important in aetiology in both minor and major depressive disorder [48].

In a further study of women in Islington, London, almost all (41/58) of the severe events that provoked depressive onset involved the individual feeling humiliated or trapped [49]. Feeling trapped included being trapped in a punishing situation or feeling that any escape from an unrewarding setting was blocked. Humiliation meant being devalued in relation to others or the self. Entrapment events were defined as arising from an ongoing marked difficulty of at least six months' duration that served at the same time to underline that the situation would persist or get worse [49]. Events rated as severe losses played a relatively minor role after losses that involved humiliation, entrapment and death had been taken into account. Perceptions of lack of control, instilling feelings of helplessness and powerlessness, may be critical in depressive risk in keeping with Seligman's theory of learned helplessness [50]. Two other themes that were associated with increased depressive risk were marginalisation – being made to feel unwanted – and the reawakening of unresolved conflict.

Do multiple life events carry a greater risk of depression? This did not seem to be the case when seemingly separate events were part of the same overall chain of events. However, additive effects on risk of depression were observed for the co-occurrence of unrelated life events; 29% of depressed patients and 9% of non-depressed women had two or more life events. In assessing the effects of multiple life events, Brown and Harris [45] give particular weight to the meaning of the events. Simple additivity of unrelated events had little effect, but where they were seen as yet more issues to be dealt with, or were more threatening because of the social context (e.g. pregnancy following a separation) or had symbolic meaning (e.g. death of a parent following the birth of a baby), the impact was likely to be greater.

Major difficulties and chronic strains

As well as life events, chronic strains – termed by Brown and Harris [45] 'major difficulties' – are important in both the aetiology and the maintenance of depression. Chronic marital problems, poor housing conditions and continued financial difficulties all may initiate and then maintain depression. It may be that socio-economic disadvantage, as shown by Weich and Lewis [26], for common mental disorder has more effects on maintaining than initiating depression. In this study, a composite poverty index of low income, low car ownership and poor housing was associated with the duration but not the onset of disorder [26]. Financial disadvantage by contrast was associated with both onset and maintenance of common mental disorder.

Resolution events

Life events are not always negative in their impact; for instance, so-called 'resolution events' that remove prolonged negative circumstances, such as re-employment after prolonged unemployment, may lead to resolution of depression [51,52], and even when difficulties remain in one domain a fresh start in another domain can begin the process of remission [53].

Gender differences in response to life events

In a community study of 100 couples who had recently experienced a threatening life event, women were found to have a greater risk of depression than men. This greater risk seemed to be restricted to depression that followed events involving children, housing and reproductive problems. Moreover, the depression was confined to those women in which the couples showed strictly differentiated roles and there was no sharing of the responsibility for the event between man and woman. Nazroo and colleagues [7] invoke this as an explanation of gender differences in rates of depression. In this case, women were holding themselves responsible for such events and thus were more at risk for depression, while men, who distanced themselves from the events, were protected against depression. Conversely, some studies have shown that men are at greater risk of depression than women following marital separation or divorce [54,55], which may represent the greater reliance of men for social support on their spouse [56].

Life events, marital status and depression

In the Islington study, the risk of depressive onset among single mothers was double that of married mothers (16% vs. 7.9%) [57]. Risk of onset was related to financial hardship, which was more common in single mothers than married mothers. Risk of onset, however, was high among single mothers irrespective of financial hardship. What might explain the difference between single mothers and married mothers in rates of depressive onset? First, the level of humiliation and entrapment events was much higher among single mothers than married mothers. Second, full-time work was an important risk factor for single mothers, of whom 38% of the employed women compared with 14% of the rest of the single mothers experienced depressive onset; this was not found for the married group. Many single mothers working full time suffered from marked work overload or strain compared with those in part-time work. The two background risk factors of financial hardship and full-time work seem to make these women more prone to the development of humiliation or entrapment events. The bulk of these events involved delinquent or disruptive behaviour on the part of a child, lover or close relative. Part of the impact of full-time work might be through reduced contact with the child, although negative interaction with the child was found to be related highly to marked financial hardship but not to full-time work. At the time, a major reason for choosing to work full time rather than part time was in order to avoid poverty, and thus these women were especially at risk [57].

Predisposition to life events

Life events tend to cluster in certain people. In part, one life event leads to another, which may explain the clustering of life events in people of lower SEP and without adequate material resources to resist or cope with events. Life events have also shown a familial tendency, which might be related either to learned family patterns of maladaptive coping or to genetic predispositions to behave in ways that might lead to major life events. Non-independent events seem to be more susceptible to genetic influence in twin studies [58]. High neuroticism scores, earlier episodes of depression and teenage behaviour problems all increase the incidence of adult life events [5,59,60].

Another genetic aspect of vulnerability has been discovered: a gene for a chemical transporter called 5-hydroxytryptamine transporter (5-HTT) that fine-tunes transmission of serotonin has been identified in the Dunedin adolescent cohort study [61]. Being homozygous on this gene increases the risk of developing depression when exposed to a life event. This is a convincing example of a gene – environment interaction in depression and raises the possibility of further refining the contribution of environmental factors to the aetiology of depression.

Social vulnerability to depression

Life events lead to depression in less than a quarter of people exposed: 20% of women exposed to severely threatening events developed a depressive illness. This suggested that some people might be more vulnerable to depression than others and led to an investigation of a broader range of factors that might make people more prone to depression when exposed to a life event. In their original study of working-class women in Camberwell, London, Brown and Harris [45] identified four vulnerability factors that made women more prone to develop depression when exposed to a life event: (i) the absence of a close confiding relationship, (ii) unemployment, (iii) looking after three or more children at home and (iv) death of the individual's mother before the age of 11 years. In summary, these vulnerability factors seem to signify social and emotional isolation. In a further study carried out among women in Islington, London, a slightly different pattern of vulnerability factors was found; these factors included low self-esteem and complex aspects of social support [62]. This suggests that vulnerability factors are not entirely fixed but vary according to social circumstances. Low self-esteem has not only been shown to be a significant risk factor for developing clinical depression [62] but has also been related to other psychosocial risk factors, such as the quality of close relationships and early adverse experience [63]. Over time, negative evaluation of self improved for about half of those who had negative evaluation of self at baseline. Although negative evaluation of self was associated with current depressive symptoms, the improvement could not always be associated with recovery from depression [64].

Early lack of care, abuse, neglect and risk of depression

Further research on the effect of loss of the mother during childhood on risk of adulthood depression has suggested that it is not the loss itself but the quality of the care of the child subsequent to the loss that relates to increased risk [65]. Parental divorce seemed to carry higher risk for adulthood depression than parental death [66]. Parental indifference and physical and sexual abuse predict adult depression [67–69]. The effect of early loss of the mother is eliminated after adjustment for childhood adversity, implying that the childhood adversity is critical and the loss of mother is an important risk factor for adult disorder only because it increases the chance of these negative experiences in childhood. By contrast, loss of the father was unrelated to depression once loss of the mother had been taken into account.

In a prospective study of 105 working-class mothers with vulnerability factors but without baseline depression, the majority of those who developed depression during follow-up had experienced a severe life event. Risk was only a little less among those with only one of two vulnerability factors. The greatest risk was among those who had experienced an episode of depression before the age of 20 years. The relationship between childhood neglect and abuse and adult onset of depression was accounted for entirely by such early depression [70]. Childhood adversity has been related to an increased likelihood of recurrence of depression and a decreased rate of remission [71,72]. Abuse and neglect of one's children is related to inadequate parenting in the woman's own childhood and subsequent maternal depression [73]. Hence, there is a potential pathway for intergenerational transmission of depression involving long-term damage to self-esteem and attachment and inability to access emotional support [53,73].

Life events and outcome of depressive disorder

In short-term studies of four to six weeks, life events at onset seemed to have little effect on the outcome of depression [47]. However, in longer follow-ups of six to nine months, break-up of an intimate relationship in the year preceding milder depression has been found to be associated with good outcome [74].

Social support

Social support has been defined as 'resources provided by other persons' [75]. It has been seen as 'information leading the subject to believe that he is cared for and loved, is esteemed and valued and belongs to a social network of communication and mutual obligation' [76]. One of the most important distinctions is between social networks and the functional aspects of support, i.e. the quality and type of support that is provided by the network member. Social networks refer to the social contacts of a group of individuals. Such contacts can be described in terms of number of contacts and frequency of contacts.

Two psychological mechanisms have been postulated for the beneficial effect of social relations on mental health: (i) support has a direct effect on wellbeing, and (ii) the buffering hypothesis, whereby support moderates the impact of stressors on the risk of depression [77]. Kessler and McLeod [78] proposed that network size has a direct effect on mental wellbeing, such that larger networks are associated with better health. In contrast, they suggest that emotional support has a buffering effect in the face of stressors. They cited three cross-sectional studies [45,79,80] and two panel studies [81,82] in support of a pervasive buffering effect on mental health across all types of event. However, some authors dispute that these vulnerability factors really increase the risk of depression in a multiplicative fashion. Although it seems plausible that the opportunities for sharing and diffusing negative emotions, provision of reassurance and active emotional support alleviate the negative impact of a life event, many studies suggest that the effects of life events and social support on the risk of depressive illness are merely additive [83]. In a large panel study of adult female twins, Kessler *et al.* [84] found a buffering effect for perceived support on major depression. They found no evidence to support an underlying genetic factor influencing perception of support and accommodation to stress. Neither did they find evidence that buffering was attributable to any improvement in coping promoted by social support. They also rejected the possibility that stress-moderating effects of perceived support are mediated by received support. Kessler and colleagues suggested the possibility that perceived availability of support may lead to cognitive appraisals that are less threatening to mental health.

There have been a few longitudinal studies of social support where questions of causation can be better addressed. Some community studies have been completely prospective, identifying deficiencies in social support before the onset of depression and relating this to the onset of depression. Two studies found a buffering or interactive effect [62,85]. The study by Brown *et al.* [62] found little predictive effect on mental health of 17 measures of emotional support measured at baseline in an inner-city sample of married mothers. However, Brown and colleagues did find a greater risk of depression in women who received little crisis support, i.e. little support when it was needed in order to cope with a life event. A negative response from a partner in a crisis was also associated with a subsequent risk of depression. Among single mothers, the report of a close relationship at baseline was protective against the development of depression following a subsequent life event. The onset of postnatal depression in 507 women was predicted by lack of social support from the primary group and lack of support in relation to becoming pregnant, adjusting for antenatal depression, neuroticism, family and personal psychiatric history, and adversity [86].

A longitudinal study of British middle-aged civil servants (the Whitehall II study) showed in relation to psychological distress rather than depressive illness a protective effect on mental health of emotional support from the closest person in men [87] and from the primary group in women [56]. These were not abolished by adjusting for either hostility as a measure of personality or psychiatric disorder at baseline. This is relevant because measures of personality often confound associations between social support and mental illness. Moreover, this study showed prospectively that negative aspects of close relationships were associated with greater risk of future psychiatric disorder up to five years later. Negative aspects of close relationships were associated consistently with worse mental health in both men and women. Negative aspects of close relationships have a negative effect on mental health both directly [88–90] and in the presence of life events.

Emotional support is what the respondent receives from the close person and is associated with better mental health [62]. Perceived emotional support has a larger effect than tangible or practical aspects of support, as has also been found in elderly people [91]. Emotional support is distinct from confiding, which requires the respondent to actively disclose information to the close person, although in adaptive relationships these occur reciprocally. Some studies suggest that ill-advised confiding, asking for support from sources unable to provide it, and confiding without active emotional support may be risk factors for depression, and this may explain why confiding in and receiving emotional support from a spouse does not show a direct effect in women [92].

Social support in adulthood may help to buffer the persistent effects of early childhood abuse and neglect. A study of women who had been in care during childhood shows how social support in adulthood may exert a beneficial effect on parenting problems, marital difficulties and psychiatric disorder [93]. Many of these women returned from care to a discordant home environment, from which they then tried to escape by early marriage. However, the women's marital relationships often turned out badly and resulted in the women becoming more vulnerable to further difficulties. Nevertheless, a third of those women showed good parenting ability. This seemed to relate to positive school experiences, including examination success, good relationships with peers and the later presence of a supportive marital relationship, which prevented subsequent parenting difficulties and depression from occurring.

Health selection and social support

There are methodological difficulties in studying social support and health. Illness itself may result in social withdrawal and thus lower support may encourage supporters to rally round and increase levels of contact and support. Kessler and Magee [84] found that individuals with weak social support networks were significantly at risk for major depression. They also noted that the majority of individuals diagnosed with depression are likely to be experiencing a recurrent episode rather than a first episode. When they controlled for a history of depression, they found that the effect of social support on current depression was significantly reduced. Thus, it is likely that a previous history of depression has had a negative influence on the provision of social support and social networks [84].

Social support and outcome of depressive disorder

A few studies have followed up clinical samples of depressed patients in order to assess the effect of social support on outcome of depression. A longitudinal study of 130 male and female patients with depression showed that the types of social relationship and support assessed at interview that predicted subsequent recovery from depression differed according to gender [94]. Living as a married couple was related to recovery in men, but having a larger number of close relatives and good friends was related to recovery in women after adjustment for clinical predictors of recovery. In this study, social support was related to a better outcome for individuals in a relapse as distinct from an initial first onset episode of depression [94]. Low levels of social support and social participation also predicted maintenance of depression in an elderly urban sample [95]. Thus, the continuity of support may influence the course of depression.

However, the pattern of associations is unlikely to be simple. Veiel and Kuhner [96] found that supportive kin networks after discharge from hospital were related to development of further depressive symptoms, whereas contact with friends at a slightly later stage seemed to have a more positive effect. Thus, returning to a home environment that may have been implicated in the onset of the depression does not necessarily have a positive effect. Considerable strain may be imposed on individuals caring for depressed patients; Fadden *et al.* [97] found that caring for a depressed spouse was a risk factor for depression in the carer. Alternatively, high expressed emotion, i.e. a high level of critical comments and overinvolvement, may be a risk factor for depressive relapse as well as relapse in schizophrenia.

Ethnicity and depression

Ethnicity is considered to be a key explanatory concept within the context of health variations in mental illness. It is clear from many surveys that the prevalence of mental illness varies across ethnic groups. For example, two key findings have been the apparently high rates of schizophrenia among Afro-Caribbean people and low rates of depression in South Asian people in the UK [98]. Evidence suggests that some of the variation in reported psychiatric disorder might be explained in terms of ethnic density – the degree of geographical clustering of ethnic minority groups at a local level. Different levels of social support in ethnic minority groups may in part mediate the effect of ethnic density on psychiatric disorder.

Data from the British 2001 census estimated that ethnic minorities make up 7.9% of the total UK population, or about 4.6 million people. Indians were the largest minority group (22.7%), followed by Pakistanis (16.1%), people of mixed ethnic backgrounds (14.6%), black Caribbeans (12.2%), black Africans (10.5%), Bangladeshis (6.1%) and Chinese (5.3%). As in previous censuses, the 2001 census also highlighted marked variation in geographical location and socioeconomic position of ethnic minorities. Within such variation, there are vast socioeconomic disparities in the 'lived experience' of ethnic minority groups.

Estimates of psychiatric disorder within ethnic minority groups have been problematic. Previous research into such estimates has relied on psychiatric admission rates as a measure of mental health, e.g. Cochrane and Bal's study [99]. However, psychiatric admission rates for people of ethnic minority groups may not reflect accurately psychiatric disorder. Psychiatric admission rates are subject to systematic biases, for example differences in treatment by clinicians or access to services [100].

More recent research into the mental health of people of ethnic minority groups has used community survey data assessing mental health more directly with well-validated psychiatric assessment instruments. It is only relatively recently that large-scale epidemiological surveys of ethnic minority mental health have been carried out to assess the prevalence of psychiatric disorder across groups. Using the Clinical Interview Schedule (CIS) in a community sample, Nazroo [98] found that the weekly rate of depressive neurosis was 2.7% for British white males and 4.8% for British white females. For Irish people, the respective rates were 5.8% and 6.8%, and for Afro-Caribbeans 5.6% and 6.4%. However, the respectives rates for Indians were 2.5% and 3.2%, for Pakistanis 3.8% and 2.9%, for Bangladeshis 1.6% and 2.2%, and for Chinese people 1.6% and 1.7%. In age- and gender-standardised analyses, Irish people and Afro-Caribbean people had much higher rates of depression than white British people. However, except for the Pakistani group, age- and gender-standardised rates of neurotic depression were much lower in other groups compared with the white British group, the low prevalence being particularly marked in Chinese and Bangladeshi people. The Ethnic Minority Psychiatric Illness Rates in the Community (EMPIRIC) study [101] showed that among women, current depressive episodes were most common in Indian and Pakistani women and least common in Bangladeshi and Afro-Caribbean women. In North America, research examining ethnic differences in depression has revealed inconsistent findings [102]. Despite these inconsistencies, the question remains about what underlies such variation in depression in different ethnic minority groups.

There has been much interest in ethnic density as an explanation for variation in psychiatric disorder. Halpern [103] suggests that the general patterns of between group differences in psychiatric admissions in Britain and elsewhere could be explained by a group density effect, whereby groups that tend to cluster together tend to show lower levels of psychiatric admissions [62]. The earliest evidence for the group density effect came from a study by Faris and Dunham [104], who showed an inverse association between ethnic density and psychiatric admission rates for black people; in other words, the higher the concentration of black people in an area, the lower the admission rates. Even more surprisingly, they found that black people who had moved to more affluent, predominantly white neighbourhoods of Chicago had higher psychiatric admission rates. Such an ethnic density effect has been replicated in other studies [105–107].

In a more recent test of the ethnic density effect on psychiatric disorder, Halpern and Nazroo [108] assessed psychiatric disorder in a community survey rather than using psychiatric admission rates. Initial examination of the pattern of neurotic symptoms levels between minority groups showed that in general, the more clustered the ethnic minority, the lower the neurotic symptom levels. Thus, South Asians – Indian, Pakistani, Bangladeshi and African Asian people – all showed high levels of clustering and lower average neurotic symptom scores compared with the less clustered Chinese and Caribbean groups. Further analyses taking into account age, sex and hardship strengthened the relationship between ethnic density and average neurotic symptom scores for people of ethnic minorities. Additional adjustment for age at migration did not weaken the inverse association, but fluency in English did. However, the latter did not account totally for the inverse association between ethnic density and average neurotic symptom levels, as the association remained statistically significant. Examination of the ethnic density effect within each ethnic minority group showed that there was a modest but significant inverse association between ethnic density and neurotic symptom levels in only the Indian and Caribbean groups. These analyses broadly confirmed the existence of an ethnic density effect on neurotic symptoms. People of ethnic minority groups living in more clustered areas tend to report lower neurotic symptom levels. This begs the question: why should ethnic minority individuals have lower reported neurotic symptom levels in areas of high concentration?

Ethnicity and social support

One explanation for the ethnic density effect on reported psychiatric morbidity is that the differences in neurotic symptom levels result from the benefits of group concentration, namely increased social support. It has been suggested that one reason for individuals having better mental health in areas of high group concentration is that this increases social support, which may then protect against psychiatric morbidity [108]. Halpern and Nazroo [108] tested this in their study by developing three indicators of mutual social support: providing (i) 'regular help or service to a friend, relative or neighbour', (ii) 'receiving money from a person outside the household' and (iii) 'sending money to dependants not living in the household'. In multivariate analyses, higher ethnic density was associated with significantly more provision of help to people outside the household, more giving of money to dependants outside the household, and receiving of money from people outside the household. This finding reinforced previous work showing that ethnic minority individuals receive more support from members of their own ethnic group [109,110]. Additionally, Halpern and Nazroo [108] examined whether ethnic minority clustering had an effect on protection from social stress – essentially, having been physically attacked or having their property damaged in the past 12 months. The results showed that individuals from ethnic minority groups reported significantly lower levels of property damage when living in areas of high own-group density. This was true across all ethnic groups. Halpern and Nazroo interpreted this as strong evidence for a protective effect of group clustering. This evidence reinforces the view that the ethnic density effect on psychiatric disorder in people from ethnic minorities may in part be moderated by greater instrumental support and reduced exposure to direct prejudice.

Given that higher rates of depression are not always found in ethnic minority groups and that social support acts as a buffer in moderating the relationship between ethnicity and depression, it could be expected that the types and quality of social support vary between ethnic groups. The quality of social support has been identified as an important factor in predicting relapse in depressive episodes and future levels of depressive moods and symptoms [111–114]. Further, it has been argued that social support networks among minority groups are qualitatively different and stronger than social support networks in white people. This may be because ethnic minority group members originate from cultures that tend to emphasise the importance of relationships, viewing the self as inherently interconnected to family and friends. In contrast, white people in the USA have roots in European countries with cultures that are focused on individual goals and tend to emphasise the achievement of the individual rather than group goals [115]. A person's cultural heritage may influence whether the individual tends to be individualistic or collectivist in nature; for example, Hispanic Americans tend to be more collectivist than non-Hispanic Americans [116]. It may also be that ethnic minority group members seek more affiliation as a way of coping with greater hardship than white people. Ethnic minority group members coming from a collectivist cultural heritage or having been exposed to greater hardship may have a greater tendency than white people to develop stronger social support networks. This in turn may afford protection against psychiatric disorder.

In a study of 4700 participants, Plant and Sachs-Ericsson [117] examined whether there was any qualitative difference in social support between ethnic minorities and white people and whether the quality of social support protected minority group members from depression. The sample consisted of 85% white, 10% Hispanic, 4% black and 1% Native American people of both sexes. The quality of social support was measured using an interpersonal functioning scale. Overall, ethnic minority groups tended to report better interpersonal functioning than white participants. Black and Hispanic participants had lower scores on interpersonal functioning than white participants; Native American participants' scores fell between the two. Further analysis indicated that more problems in interpersonal functioning were related to both more depressive symptoms and prevalence of depression. Taken together, these results pointed to the possibility that the quality of social support may moderate the relationship between ethnicity and depression. When interpersonal functioning was controlled for in the prediction of depressive symptoms and major depression, differences between ethnic minority groups and the white group increased. People from ethnic minority groups reported even higher levels of depressive symptoms and significantly higher risk of major depression compared with white people. These findings suggested that social support, as measured by interpersonal functioning, suppresses group differences in depressive symptoms and prevalence of major depression [117].

Can this be taken as evidence that social support moderates the relationship between ethnicity and depression? There are some problems with this study. First, although physical functioning was measured and was clearly associated with depression, it is not clear from the analyses whether this was controlled for. Second, ethnic groups were combined into one group, labelled 'minority group members'. There are similarities among ethnic minority groups (e.g. low SEP), but there are also many differences between them. Third, this was a cross-sectional study and therefore the temporal relationship between these factors and depression cannot be determined definitely. Only a longitudinal approach could track changes in risk and protective factors for depression in ethnic minority and other groups.

There is some evidence that black and Hispanic ethnic minority people in the USA have more supportive family and social networks, tend to have larger households and are more likely to have extended family members living together compared with white people [110,118–120]. Such close supportive networks may moderate the effects of adverse circumstances and protect members of ethnic minority groups from stress and depression. Holahan and Moos [121] showed that having high social resources lessened the effects of stress through their association with active coping strategies. Ennis *et al.* [122] showed that black women with acute economic problems had lower levels of depressive symptoms if they had a strong social support system than if they did not have such a strong support system.

Other social factors, such as religion, may also play an important role in mental health for both minority group and white people. Religious activity may be especially protective for members of ethnic minority groups; it is thought that this protects against suicide in black and Hispanic people. Increased opportunities for social support through engaging in religious activities may be the mechanism by which religious activities confer a protective effect on mental health of ethnic minorities [123–125].

Many factors may be associated with ethnic minority mental health variation, including pre- and post-migratory factors (e.g. biological factors, forced migration, culture conflict, acculturation) and factors associated with the process of migration itself. People from ethnic minorities also tend to experience more difficulties in terms of racism, discrimination, economic difficulties and decreased opportunities than people from non-ethnic minorities. Some of these factors may be causal or simply associated with poor mental health in ethnic groups [126]. An additional difficulty is that tools developed for Western psychiatric practice may be inappropriate for use in psychiatric surveys of people from ethnic minority populations, who experience and express mental illness within culturally bound norms [127]. Nevertheless, as the vast literature on social capital and wellbeing shows, it is not unreasonable to suppose that the protective effect of clustering on depression might in part be mediated by the potency of close supportive networks in cohesive minority groups.

Work and depression

Work takes up a large proportion of most people's lives and is both a protective factor and a risk factor for depression. Working is good for mental health, providing income, resources, self-esteem, a source of social support and structure. On the other hand, unemployment has been linked with depression in factory-closure research and a range of other studies [128–130]. The effects of unemployment seem to be stronger in men than in women. Unemployment is associated with an increased suicide risk, which may be mediated through depression. Studies of unemployment suggest that it acts like a life event, with depression as the immediate reaction. With longer-term unemployment, mental health tends to improve as if some adaptation is taking place. The context of unemployment seems to be important: the risk of depression is less if the individual becomes unemployed in a setting where everyone else is unemployed. In this situation, the stigma of unemployment is less and the meaning less personally shameful. In a follow-up study of 49 men who became unemployed, higher depression scores at follow-up related to continuing unemployment and little social contact in the month before losing their jobs. It seems likely that the loss of social interaction at work combined with poor social support outside work may lead to increased vulnerability to developing depression [85].

Psychosocial work characteristics

Aspects of work that are risky for health can be divided into physical hazards (e.g. exposure to dust, heat, noise, long hours, shift work) and psychosocial risk factors. Karasek [131] described two key dimensions of the psychosocial work environment: psychological job demands and decision latitude, the latter comprising decision authority (control over work) and skill discretion (variety of work and opportunity for use of skills). According to Karasek's 'job strain model', the worst combination for health is to have high demands and low decision latitude. Work by Johnson and Theorell added an important further dimension of work social support to this model [132]. Siegrist has described an additional model of effort-reward imbalance [133]. In this model, the combination of putting in high effort at work (which may be both intrinsic effort, such as innate competitiveness and hostility, and high extrinsic work demands) and receiving by implication little reward in terms of salary, promotion or being valued is a powerful risk factor for ill-health.

Psychosocial work characteristics and mental health

There is consistent evidence from a number of cross-sectional [134–136] and longitudinal [137–142] studies that high levels of psychological demands, including high work pace and high conflicting demands, are predictive of poor mental health. Increasing job demands measured on two occasions have also been related to increased risk of psychological distress compared with people in whom job demands decreased or stayed the same over two occasions [142]. On the other hand, high levels of social support at work from colleagues and supervisors are protective of mental health in both cross-sectional [136,143] and longitudinal [137,138,140,142] studies.

Decision latitude has been associated with mental health outcomes either on its own or in combination with job demands. High levels of decision latitude have been found to be protective of mental health in both cross-sectional [144–146] and longitudinal [140,142] studies. Decision authority rather than skill discretion was found to be the strongest predictor of depression [146]. The effects of demands and decision latitude seem to be additive rather than multiplicative, not confirming

Karasek's original hypothesis of an interaction between high demands and low control. Nevertheless, high job strain, the combination of high demands and low decision latitude, has been associated with a higher prevalence of Clinical Interview Schedule-rated psychiatric morbidity in teachers [147] and higher rates of major depressive episode, depressive syndrome and dysphoria measured by the Diagnostic Interview Schedule in the Baltimore sample of the Epidemiologic Catchment Area Program [146]. The advantage of these two studies and that of Weinberg and Creed [143] is that they used structured interview measures of psychiatric morbidity that were likely to be more reliable and valid than the non-specific psychological distress scales. High job demands in women, and low social support and low skill discretion in both men and women, have also been associated with higher rates of psychiatric sickness absence for depression and anxiety [139]. There is some evidence that job demands, which may contain the threat of becoming overloaded, are related specifically to anxiety symptoms, while low decision latitude, which perhaps implies loss or insufficient control, are more related to depressive symptoms [134,145].

Effort–reward imbalance has a powerful impact on increasing the risk of psychological distress, which was largely independent of the effects of decision authority [142]. Associations between work and psychiatric morbidity might be confounded by the effects on depression of problems outside work. A well-constructed case–control study of healthcare staff found that although acute stressful situations and chronic difficulties outside work were important in depressive disorders, there were also independent effects of 'conflict of work role' and 'lack of management support at work' [143].

Psychosocial work characteristics, personality and depression

The sceptical reader may ask whether the associations between self-reported work characteristics and self-reported mental health outcomes are not entirely the result of confounding by a third factor such as personality. Negative affectivity accounts for some of the variance in the association between work characteristics and mental health [148]. Statistical adjustment by controlling for negative affectivity and hostility in the Whitehall II study had little effect on the risk of psychological distress associated with decision authority, increased the effects of job demands in women but not men, and reduced the effects of low skill discretion on the risk of psychological distress [142]. Personality measures such as hostility and attributes such as low self-esteem do not seem to explain the association between work characteristics and depressive symptoms in the French GAZEL study, a longitudinal occupational study of gas and electricity workers [149]. This is further evidence that the psychosocial environment at work is important and that these associations are not simply a form of response bias. One puzzle remains, however: most studies that have not relied on self-reports of work but have used assessments of the work environment, external to the person reporting psychological distress, have not found associations between work and mental health. Although this would tend to support the response bias argument, it is possible that the subjective perceptions of work are a necessary mediating step between the work environment and psychological distress.

Psychosocial risk factors and depression in the elderly

The majority of this chapter has dealt with psychosocial factors and depression in the adult population. Do the same findings apply to elderly populations? First, it is important to recognise that the incidence of depression is not invariant across old age. There is usually a decline in the incidence of depressive illness [150,151] in the fifth and sixth decades. Thereafter, the incidence increases with ageing in relation to the onset of physical illness. Additionally, although many older people with depression have their first onset of depression in young adulthood, there is also a group of elderly people who develop depression for the first time in old age. A syndrome of vascular depression has been described associated with cerebral arteriosclerosis and subcortical neurological dysfunction [152]. There is a concern about under-diagnosis of depressive illness in elderly people related to inappropriateness of adult depression criteria in the elderly, misattribution of physical symptoms, and sampling bias, with the most disabled individuals being excluded from community samples [153]. Thus, rates of depressive illness in old age may be underestimated. Depressive symptoms show a more curvilinear pattern across the life course, with, in general, an increase in symptoms in the mid seventies [153,154]. Unlike the case for depressive illness, there is a concern that these depressive symptom scales may overestimate the prevalence of depression because elderly people who are physically ill or frail, but not depressed, may positively endorse somatic symptoms on depressive symptom scales [154]. This is a complicated issue because depressive illness, especially in elderly people, often presents with prominent somatic symptoms [155,156].

The distribution and response to psychosocial stressors may differ in younger and older adulthood. As Bruce [157] points out 'widowhood, medical events, disability, and declining social support systems are not inevitable but increasingly likely as adults age'. Taking a developmental perspective, the risk of depressive onset seems more associated with psychological vulnerability, stressors and genetic factors in younger adults, and more associated with physical illness and disability in older adults [153]. Psychological vulnerability to depression appears to decline through adulthood [153]. There is also a suggestion of survivor effects – i.e. if an individual exposed to chronic stressors survives into old age without the onset of depression, then it is unlikely that new depressive onsets will occur for the first time in old age [157].

Having discussed the differences between younger and older adults, there is also a lot of continuity across the lifespan in the response to stressors [158,159], even though not all studies find increased risk of depression associated with life events [160]. Strong associations have been found between the onset of physical illness and the risk of depression, with an increased risk of up to three times [95]. This risk is maintained even after adjusting for confounding factors [161]. The onset of new physical illness in elderly people symbolises the advent of disability and intimations of mortality, which may increase the risk for depression. The onset of disability itself is a powerful risk factor for depression and is often accompanied by loss of independence, perception of loss of control over the environment, loss of productivity and a shaming inability to perform everyday role activities [95,157]. Methodologically, it is often difficult to separate out the direction of causation, because although disability is a risk factor for depression, depression may also increase levels of disability (see Chapter 6). Death of a spouse, which is more likely to occur in elderly people, is an evident risk factor for the onset of depression [157,162]; but there is variability of response to death of a spouse, depending on whether the death was expected and whether it was preceded by illness and disability and caregiving demands.

There have been several prospective studies of social support and depression in elderly people [91,95,151,161]. Lack of a relative or friend in whom to confide predicted late-life suicide in a North American community survey [163]. Lack of contact with friends predicted depression and modified the association between depression and disability, a powerful predictor of depression [95]. In a similar way, having a marital partner or, if unmarried, having social support significantly reduced the impact of functional disabilities on depression [161]. Hence, in a situation where provision of practical and emotional support may have profound effects on an elderly person's quality of life and functioning, a clear protective effect of social support was found. Lack of social support has not been associated with increased risk of depression in elderly people in all studies [161]. Some of this variation may relate to the changing pattern of social relationships in old age as friends and relatives die, and with increasing disability, the support from children and statutory services becomes more important.

Associations of psychosocial factors with depression and physical illness

There is good evidence that a range of stressors (early adverse experiences, life events, socioeconomic disadvantage, chronic difficulties, job demands, job insecurity, unemployment) are risk factors for the onset of depression. Many of these stressors are not specific to depression but are also implicated in the causation of physical illness. Job strain and social isolation have been identified as risk factors for coronary heart disease [164,165]. Some psychosocial risk factors seem more specific to physical illness, and others to mental illness, while some carry a common cause (e.g. work) [166]. Thus, psychosocial risk factors may play a direct role in the aetiology of physical illness or may exert their effects indirectly, mediated through the development of depression. As other chapters in this book suggest, depression may subsequently exert a direct influence on the development of physical illness.

REFERENCES

1. M. M. Weissman, G. L. Klerman, Sex differences and the epidemiology of depression. *Arch. Gen. Psychiatry* **34** (1977), 98–111.

2. T. B. Ustun, Cross-national epidemiology of depression and gender. *J. Gend. Specif. Med.* **3** (2000), 54–8.

3. M. Piccinelli, G. Wilkinson, Gender differences in depression: critical review. *Br. J. Psychiatry* **177** (2000), 486–92.

4. B. Rodgers, Pathways between parental divorce and adult depression. *J. Child Psychol. Psychiatry* **35** (1994), 1289–308.

5. K. S. Kendler, M. Neale, R. Kessler, A. Heath, L. Eaves, A twin study of recent life events and difficulties. *Arch. Gen. Psychiatry* **50** (1993), 789–96.

6. N. Breslau, L. Schultz, E. Peterson, Sex differences in depression: a role for preexisting anxiety. *Psychiatry Res.* **58** (1995), 1–12.

7. J. Y. Nazroo, A. C. Edwards, G. W. Brown, Gender differences in the onset of depression following a shared life event: a study of couples. *Psychol. Med.* **27** (1997), 9–19.

8. P. Moen, Social integration and longevity: an event history analysis of women's roles and resilience. *Am. Sociol. Rev.* **54** (1989), 635–47.

9. M. R. Frone, Work–family conflict and employee psychiatric disorders: the National Comorbidity Survey. *J. Appl. Psychol.* **85** (2000), 888–95.

10. S. Stansfeld, J. Head, V. Cattell, J. Wardle, R. Fuhrer, Work, partner's employment status and depressive symptoms in women. *Trends Evidence Based Neuropsychiatry* **6** (2004), 31–6.

11. E. M. Hall, Double exposure: the combined impact of the home and work environments on psychosomatic strain in Swedish women and men. *Int. J. Health Serv.* **22** (1992), 239–60.

12. C. Schooler, Work for the household: its nature and consequences for husbands and wives. *Am. J. Sociol.* **90** (1984), 97–124.

13. E. M. Hall, J. V. Johnson, Depression in unemployed Swedish women. *Soc. Sci. Med.* **27** (1988), 1349–55.

14. S. Weich, A. Sloggett, G. Lewis, Social roles and gender difference in the prevalence of common mental disorders. *Br. J. Psychiatry* **173** (1998), 489–93.

15. R. Jenkins, Sex differences in minor psychiatric morbidity. *Psychol. Med. Monogr. Suppl.* **7** (1985), 1–53.

16. S. Wyke, G. Ford, Competing explanations for associations between marital status and health. *Soc. Sci. Med.* **34** (1992), 523–32.

17. P. E. Bebbington, Sex and depression. *Psychol. Med.* **28** (1998), 1–8.

18. I. Waldron, M. E. Hughes, T. L. Brooks, Marriage protection and marriage selection: prospective evidence for reciprocal effects of marital status and health. *Soc. Sci. Med.* **43** (1996), 113–23.

19. C. A. Mathews, V. I. Reus, Assortative mating in the affective disorders: a systematic review and meta-analysis. *Compr. Psychiatry* **42** (2001), 257–62.

20. D. Melzer, T. Fryers, R. Jenkins, T. Brugha, B. McWilliams, Social position and the common mental disorders with disability: estimates from the National Psychiatric Survey of Great Britain. *Soc. Psychiatry Psychiatr. Epidemiol.* **38** (2003), 238–43.

21. D. Melzer, T. Fryers, R. Jenkins, *Social Inequalities and the Distribution of the Common Mental Disorders* (Hove: Psychology Press, 2004).

22. J. M. Murphy, D. C. Olivier, R. R. Monson, *et al.* Depression and anxiety in relation to social status: a prospective epidemiologic study. *Arch. Gen. Psychiatry* **48** (1991), 223–9.

23. V. Lorant, D. Deliege, W. Eaton, *et al.*, Socioeconomic inequalities in depression: a meta-analysis. *Am. J. Epidemiol.* **157** (2003), 98–112.

24. S. Aro, H. Aro, I. Keskimaki, Socio-economic mobility among patients with schizophrenia or major affective disorder: a 17-year retrospective follow-up. *Br. J. Psychiatry* **166** (1995), 759–67.

25. S. Weich, G. Lewis, Material standard of living, social class, and the prevalence of the common mental disorders in Great Britain. *J. Epidemiol. Community Health* **52** (1998), 8–14.

26. S. Weich, G. Lewis, Poverty, unemployment, and common mental disorders: population based cohort study. *Br. Med. J.* **317** (1998), 115–19.

27. T. Fryers, D. Melzer, R. Jenkins, Social inequalities and the common mental disorders: a systematic review of the evidence. *Soc. Psychiatry Psychiatr. Epidemiol.* **38** (2003), 229–37.

28. B. P. Dohrenwend, I. Levav, P. E. Shrout, *et al.*, Socioeconomic status and psychiatric disorders: the causation-selection issue. *Science* **255** (1992), 946–52.

29. J. K. Myers, J. J. Lindenthal, M. P. Pepper, D. R. Ostrander, Social class, life events and psychiatric symptoms: a longitudinal study. In *Stressful Life Events: Their Nature and Effects*, ed. B. S. Dohrenwend and B. P. Dohrenwend. (New York: John Wiley & Sons, 1974), pp. 91–206.

30. R. C. Kessler, K. A. McGonagle, S. Zhao, *et al.*, Lifetime and 12-month prevalence of DSM-III-R psychiatric disorders in the United States: results from the National Comorbidity Survey. *Arch. Gen. Psychiatry* **51** (1994), 8–19.

31. R. S. Kahn, P. H. Wise, B. P. Kennedy, I. Kawachi, State income inequality, household income, and maternal mental and physical health: cross sectional national survey. *Br. Med. J.* **321** (2000), 1311–15.

32. S. A. Everson, S. C. Maty, J. W. Lynch, G. A. Kaplan, Epidemiologic evidence for the relation between socioeconomic status and depression, obesity, and diabetes. *J. Psychosom. Res.* **53** (2002), 891–5.

33. M. Broese, I. van Groenou, [Unequal chances for reaching 'a good old age': socio-economic health differences among older adults from a life course perspective.] *Tijdschr. Gerontol. Geriatr.* **34** (2003), 196–207.

34. M. Benzeval, K. Judge, Income and health: the time dimension. *Soc. Sci. Med.* **52** (2001), 1371–90.

35. S. E. Gilman, I. Kawachi, G. M. Fitzmaurice, S. L. Buka, Socioeconomic status in childhood and the lifetime risk of major depression. *Int. J. Epidemiol.* **31** (2002), 359–67.

36. M. Marmot, M. Shipley, E. Brunner, H. Hemingway, Relative contribution of early life and adult socioeconomic factors to adult morbidity in the Whitehall II study. *J. Epidemiol. Community Health* **55** (2001), 301–7.

37. E. Goodman, The role of socioeconomic status gradients in explaining differences in US adolescents' health. *Am. J. Public Health* **89** (1999), 1522–8.

38. J. E. Ritsher, V. Warner, J. G. Johnson, B. P. Dohrenwend, Inter-generational longitudinal study of social class and depression: a test of social causation and social selection models. *Br. J. Psychiatry Suppl.* **40** (2001), 584–90.

39. R. J. Turner, F. Marino, Social support and social structure: a descriptive epidemiology. *J. Health Soc. Behav.* **35** (1994), 193–212.

40. B. H. Brummett, J. C. Barefoot, P. P. Vitaliano, I. C. Siegler, Associations among social support, income, and symptoms of depression in an educated sample: the UNC Alumni Heart Study. *Int. J. Behav. Med.* **10** (2003), 239–50.

41. R. J. Turner, D. A. Lloyd, P. Roszell, Personal resources and the social distribution of depression. *Am. J. Community Psychol.* **27** (1999), 643–72.

42. S. A. Stansfeld, J. Head, M. G. Marmot, Explaining social class differences in depression and well-being. *Soc. Psychiatry Psychiatr. Epidemiol.* **33** (1998), 1–9.

43. B. P. Dohrenwend, The role of adversity and stress in psychopathology: some evidence and its implications for theory and research. *J. Health Soc. Behav.* **41** (2000), 1–19.

44. R. Finlay-Jones, G. W. Brown, Types of stressful life event and the onset of anxiety and depressive disorders. *Psychol. Med.* **11** (1981), 803–15.

45. G. W. Brown, T. O. Harris, *Social Origins of Depression: A Study of Psychiatric Disorder in Women* (London: Tavistock, 1978).

46. E. S. Paykel, Contribution of life events to causation of psychiatric illness. *Psychol. Med.* **8** (1978), 245–53.

47. E. S. Paykel, Life events and affective disorder. *Acta Psychiatr. Scand. Suppl.* **418** (2003), 61–6.

48. E. Frank, B. Anderson, C. F. Reynolds, III, A. Ritenour, D. J. Kupfer, Life events and the research diagnostic criteria endogenous subtype: a confirmation of the distinction using the Bedford College methods. *Arch. Gen. Psychiatry* **51** (1994), 519–24.

49. G. W. Brown, T. O. Harris, C. Hepworth, Loss, humiliation and entrapment among women developing depression: a patient and non-patient comparison. *Psychol. Med.* **25** (1995), 7–21.

50. M. E. P. Seligman, *Helplesssness*. (San Francisco, CA: Freeman, 1975).

51. G. W. Brown, L. Lemyre, A. Bifulco, Social factors and recovery from anxiety and depressive disorders: a test of specificity. *Br. J. Psychiatry* **161** (1992), 44–54.

52. A. S. Leenstra, J. Ormel, R. Giel, Positive life change and recovery from depression and anxiety: a three-stage longitudinal study of primary care attenders. *Br. J. Psychiatry* **166** (1995), 333–43.

53. T. Harris, Recent developments in understanding the psychosocial aspects of depression. *Br. Med. Bull.* **57** (2001), 17–32.

54. M. L. Bruce, K. M. Kim, Differences in the effects of divorce on major depression in men and women. *Am. J. Psychiatry* **149** (1992), 914–17.

55. K. S. Kendler, L. M. Thornton, C. A. Prescott, Gender differences in the rates of exposure to stressful life events and sensitivity to their depressogenic effects. *Am. J. Psychiatry* **158** (2001), 587–93.

56. R. Fuhrer, S. A. Stansfeld, J. Chemali, M. J. Shipley, Gender, social relations and mental health: prospective findings from an occupational cohort (Whitehall II study). *Soc. Sci. Med.* **48** (1999), 77–87.

57. G. W. Brown, P. M. Moran, Single mothers, poverty and depression. *Psychol. Med.* **27** (1997), 21–33.

58. R. Plomin, P. Lichtenstein, N. L. Pedersen, G. E. McClearn, J. R. Nesselroade, Genetic influence on life events during the last half of the life span. *Psychol. Aging* **5** (1990), 25–30.

59. K. L. Harkness, S. M. Monroe, A. D. Simons, M. Thase, The generation of life events in recurrent and non-recurrent depression. *Psychol. Med.* **29** (1999), 135–44.

60. L. A. Champion, G. Goodall, M. Rutter, Behaviour problems in childhood and stressors in early adult life: I. A 20 year follow-up of London school children. *Psychol. Med.* **25** (1995), 231–46.

61. A. Caspi, K. Sugden, T. E. Moffitt, *et al.*, Influence of life stress on depression: moderation by a polymorphism in the *5-HTT* gene. *Science* **301** (2003), 386–9.

62. G. W. Brown, B. Andrews, T. Harris, Z. Adler, L. Bridge, Social support, self-esteem and depression. *Psychol. Med.* **16** (1986), 813–31.

63. B. Andrews, G. W. Brown, Self-esteem and vulnerability to depression: the concurrent validity of interview and questionnaire measures. *J. Abnorm. Psychol.* **102** (1993), 565–72.

64. B. Andrews, G. W. Brown, Stability and change in low self-esteem: the role of psychosocial factors. *Psychol. Med.* **25** (1995), 23–31.

65. G. Parker, Parental 'affectionless control' as an antecedent to adult depression: a risk factor delineated. *Arch. Gen. Psychiatry* **40** (1983), 956–60.

66. C. Tennant, P. Bebbington, J. Hurry, Parental death in childhood and risk of adult depressive disorders: a review. *Psychol. Med.* **10** (1980), 289–99.

67. G. W. Brown, T. O. Harris, M. J. Eales, Aetiology of anxiety and depressive disorders in an inner-city population: 2. Comorbidity and adversity. *Psychol. Med.* **23** (1993), 155–65.

68. A. Bifulco, G. W. Brown, T. O. Harris, Childhood Experience of Care and Abuse (CECA): a retrospective interview measure. *J. Child. Psychol. Psychiatry* **35** (1994), 1419–35.

69. J. Hill, R. Davis, M. Byatt, *et al.*, Childhood sexual abuse and affective symptoms in women: a general population study. *Psychol. Med.* **30** (2000), 1283–91.

70. A. Bifulco, G. W. Brown, P. Moran, C. Ball, C. Campbell, Predicting depression in women: the role of past and present vulnerability. *Psychol. Med.* **28** (1998), 39–50.

71. G. W. Brown, P. Moran, Clinical and psychosocial origins of chronic depressive episodes: I. A community survey. *Br. J. Psychiatry* **165** (1994), 447–56.

72. S. E. Gilman, I. Kawachi, G. M. Fitzmaurice, L. Buka, Socio-economic status, family disruption and residential stability in childhood: relation to onset, recurrence and remission of major depression. *Psychol. Med.* **33** (2003), 1341–55.

73. B. Andrews, G. W. Brown, L. Creasey, Intergenerational links between psychiatric disorder in mothers and daughters: the role of parenting experiences. *J. Child. Psychol. Psychiatry* **31** (1990), 1115–29.

74. G. Parker, K. Wilhelm, A. Asghari, Depressed mood states and their inter-relationship with clinical depression. *Soc. Psychiatry Psychiatr. Epidemiol.* **33** (1998) 10–15.

75. S. Cohen, S. L. Syme, *Social Support and Health* (London: Academic Press, 1985).

76. S. Cobb, Presidential address – 1976: social support as a moderator of life stress. *Psychosom. Med.* **38** (1976), 300–314.

77. S. Cohen, T. A. Wills, Stress, social support and the buffering hypothesis. *Psychol. Bull.* (1985), 310–57.

78. R. C. Kessler, J. D. McLeod, *Social Support and Mental Health in Community Samples* (New York: Academic Press, 1985).

79. B. A. Husaini, J. A. Neff, J. R. Newborough, M. C. Moore, The stress-buffering role of social support and personal competence among the rural married. *J. Commun. Psychol.* **10** (1982), 409–26.

80. R. C. Kessler, M. Essex, Marital status and depression: the role of coping resources. *Social Forces* **61** (1982), 484–507.

81. A. S. Henderson, Social relationships, adversity and neurosis: an analysis of prospective observations. *Br. J. Psychiatry* **138** (1981), 391–8.

82. L. I. Pearlin, M. A. Lieberman, E. G. Menaghan, J. T. Mullan, The stress process. *J. Health Soc. Behav.* **22** (1981), 337–56.

83. C. Tennant, P. Bebbington, The social causation of depression: a critique of the work of Brown and his colleagues. *Psychol. Med.* **8** (1978), 565–75.

84. R. C. Kessler, W. J. Magee, Childhood family violence and adult recurrent depression. *J. Health Soc. Behav.* **35** (1994), 13–27.

85. W. Bolton, K. Oatley, A longitudinal study of social support and depression in unemployed men. *Psychol. Med.* **17** (1987), 453–60.

86. T. S. Brugha, H. M. Sharp, S. A. Cooper, *et al.*, The Leicester 500 project: social support and the development of postnatal depressive symptoms – a prospective cohort survey. *Psychol. Med.* **28** (1998), 63–79.

87. S. A. Stansfeld, R. Fuhrer, M. J. Shipley, Types of social support as predictors of psychiatric morbidity in a cohort of British civil servants (Whitehall II Study). *Psychol. Med.* **28** (1998), 881–92.

88. T. L. Schuster, R. C. Kessler, R. H. Aseltine, Jr, Supportive interactions, negative interactions, and depressed mood. *Am. J. Community Psychol.* **18** (1990), 423–38.

89. K. S. Rook, The negative side of social interaction: impact on psychological well-being. *J. Pers. Soc. Psychol.* **46** (1984), 1097–108.

90. M. M. Burg, T. E. Seeman, Families and health: the negative side of social ties. *Ann. Behav. Med.* **16** (1994), 109–15.

91. T. E. Oxman, L. F. Berkman, S. Kasl, D. H. Freeman, Jr, J. Barrett, Social support and depressive symptoms in the elderly. *Am. J. Epidemiol.* **135** (1992), 356–68.

92. B. Andrews, G. W. Brown, Social support, onset of depression and personality: an exploratory analysis. *Soc. Psychiatry Psychiatr. Epidemiol.* **23** (1988), 99–108.

93. D. Quinton, M. Rutter, C. Liddle, Institutional rearing, parenting difficulties and marital support. *Psychol. Med.* **14** (1984), 107–24.

94. T. S. Brugha, P. E. Bebbington, B. MacCarthy, *et al.*, Gender, social support and recovery from depressive disorders: a prospective clinical study. *Psychol. Med.* **20** (1990), 147–56.

95. M. J. Prince, R. H. Harwood, A. Thomas, A. H. Mann, A prospective population-based cohort study of the effects of disablement and social milieu on the onset and maintenance of late-life depression: the Gospel Oak Project VII. *Psychol. Med.* **28** (1998), 337–50.

96. H. O. Veiel, C. Kuhner, Relatives and depressive relapse: the critical period after discharge from in-patient treatment. *Psychol. Med.* **20** (1990), 977–84.

97. G. Fadden, P. Bebbington, L. Kuipers, Caring and its burdens: a study of the spouses of depressed patients. *Br. J. Psychiatry* **151** (1987), 660–6.

98. J. Y. Nazroo, *Ethnicity and Mental Health* (London: Policy Studies Institute, 1997).

99. R. Cochrane, S. S. Bal, Ethnic density is unrelated to incidence of schizophrenia. *Br. J. Psychiatry* **153** (1988), 363–6.

100. D. Bhugra, Setting up psychiatric services: cross-cultural issues in planning and delivery. *Int. J. Soc. Psychiatry* **43** (1997), 16–28.

101. K. Sproston J. Y. Nazroo, *Ethnic Minority Psychiatric Illness Rates in the Community (EMPIRIC): Quantitative Report* (London, The Stationery Office, 2002).

102. D. R. Williams, Race, stress and mental health. In *Minority Health in America: Findings and Policy Implications from the Commonwealth Fund Minority Health Survey*, ed. C. J. R. Hogue, M. A. Hargreaves, K. S. Collins (Baltimore, MD: John Hopkins Press, 2000), pp. 194–208.

103. D. Halpern, Minorities and mental health. *Soc. Sci. Med.* **36** (1993), 597–607.

104. R. E. Faris, H. W. Dunham, *Mental Disorders in Urban Areas* (Chicago, IL: University of Chicago Press, 1939).

105. L. Levy, L. Rowitz, *The Ecology of Mental Disorder* (New York: Behavioral Publications, 1973).

106. J. G. Rabkin, Ethnic density and psychiatric hospitalisation: hazards of minority status. *Am. J. Psychiatry* **136** (1979), 1562–6.

107. G. L. Mulhin, Mental hospitalisation of the foreign born and the role of cultural isolation. *Int. J. Soc. Psychiatry* **25** (1979), 258–66.

108. D. Halpern, J. Y. Nazroo, The ethnic density effect: results from a national community survey of England and Wales. *Int. J. Soc. Psychiatry* **46** (1999), 34–46.

109. M. Stopes-Roe, R. Cochrane, Support networks of Asian and British families: comparisons between ethnicities and between generations. *Soc. Behav.* **5** (1990), 71–85.

110. S. K. Hoppe, R. L. Leon, J. P. Realini, Depression and anxiety among Mexican Americans in a family health center. *Soc. Psychiatry Psychiatr. Epidemiol.* **24** (1989), 63–8.

111. T. Joiner, J. C. Coyne, *The Interactive Nature of Depression: Advances in Interpersonal Approaches* (Washington, DC: American Psychological Association, 1999).

112. C. J. Holahan, R. H. Moos, C. K. Holahan, R. C. Cronkite, Resource loss, resource gain, and depressive symptoms: a 10-year model. *J. Pers. Soc. Psychol.* **77** (1999), 620–9.

113. C. J. Holahan, R. H. Moos, C. K. Holahan, R. C. Cronkite, Long-term posttreatment functioning among patients with unipolar depression: an integrative model. *J. Consult. Clin. Psychol.* **68** (2000), 226–32.

114. S. E. Hobfoll, R. J. Johnson, N. Ennis, A. P. Jackson, Resource loss, resource gain, and emotional outcomes among inner city women. *J. Pers. Soc. Psychol.* **84** (2003), 632–43.

115. H. R. Markus, S. Kitayama, Culture and the self: implications for cognition, emotion and motivation. *Psychol. Rev.* **98** (1991), 224–53.

116. G. Marin, H. C. Triandis, Allocentrism as an important characteristic of the behavior of Latin Americans and Hispanics. In ed. *Cross-cultural and National Studies in Social Psychology*, ed. R. Diaz-Guerrero (Amsterdam: North-Holland, 1985), pp. 85–104.

117. E. A. Plant, N. Sachs-Ericsson, Racial and ethnic differences in depression: the roles of social support and meeting basic needs. *J. Consult. Clin. Psychol.* **72** (2004), 41–52.

118. D. R. Williams, D. T. Takeuchi, R. K. Adair, Marital status and psychiatric disorders among blacks and whites. *J. Health Soc. Behav.* **33** (1992), 140–57.

119. R. J. Taylor, C. B. Hardison, L. M. Chatters, Kin and non-kin as sources of informal assistance. In *Mental Health in Black America*, ed. H. W. Neighbours, J. S. Jackson (Thousand Oaks, CA: Sage, 1996), pp. 130–45.

120. US Department of Health and Human Sciences. *Mental Health: Culture, Race and Ethnicity. A Supplement to Mental Health: A Report of the Surgeon General* (Rockville, MD: Substance Abuse and Mental Health Services Administration, Centre for Mental Health Services, 2001).

121. C. J. Holahan, R. H. Moos, Risk, resistance, and psychological distress: a longitudinal analysis with adults and children. *J. Abnorm. Psychol.* **96** (1987), 3–13.

122. N. E. Ennis, S. E. Hobfoll, K. E. Schroder, Money doesn't talk, it swears: how economic stress and resistance resources impact inner-city women's depressive mood. *Am. J. Community Psychol.* **28** (2000), 149–73.

123. J. D. Hovey, Religion and suicidal ideation in a sample of Latin American immigrants. *Psychol. Rep.* **85** (1999), 171–7.

124. W. J. Strawbridge, S. J. Shema, R. D. Cohen, G. A. Kaplan, Religious attendance increases survival by improving and maintaining good health behaviors, mental health, and social relationships. *Ann. Behav. Med.* **23** (2001), 68–74.

125. K. S. Kendler, X. Q. Liu, C. O. Gardner, M. E. McCullough, D. Larson, C. A. Prescott, Dimensions of religiosity and their relationship to lifetime psychiatric and substance use disorders. *Am. J. Psychiatry* **160** (2003), 496–503.

126. D. Bhugra, O. Ayonrinde, Depression in migrants and ethnic minorities. *Adv. Psychiatr. Treat.* **10** (2004), 13–17.

127. A. Kleinman, Anthropology and psychiatry: the role of culture in cross-cultural research on illness. *Br. J. Psychiatry* **151** (1987), 447–54.

128. N. Beale, S. Nethercott, The nature of unemployment morbidity. 2. Description. *J. R. Coll. Gen. Pract.* **38** (1988), 200–202.

129. S. Platt, N. Kreitman, Long term trends in parasuicide and unemployment in Edinburgh, 1968–87. *Soc. Psychiatry Psychiatr. Epidemiol.* **25** (1990), 56–61.

130. R. C. Kessler, J. S. House, J. B. Turner, Unemployment and health in a community sample. *J. Health Soc. Behav.* **28** (1987), 51–9.

131. R. A. Karasek, Job demands, job decision latitude and mental strain: implications for job redesign. *Admin. Sci. Q.* **24** (1979), 285–306.

132. R. Karasek, T. Theorell, *Healthy Work: Stress, Productivity and the Reconstruction of Working Life* (New York: Basic Books, 1990).

133. J. Siegrist, Adverse health effects of high-effort/low-reward conditions. *J. Occup. Health Psychol.* **1** (1996), 27–41.

134. D. E. Broadbent, The clinical impact of job design. *Br. J. Clin. Psychol.* **24** (1985), 33–44.

135. M. Estryn-Behar, M. Kaminski, E. Peigne, *et al.*, Stress at work and mental health status among female hospital workers. *Br. J. Ind. Med.* **47** (1990), 20–28.

136. E. J. Bromet, M. A. Dew, D. K. Parkinson, S. Cohen, J. E. Schwartz, Effects of occupational stress on the physical and psychological health of women in a microelectronics plant. *Soc. Sci. Med* **34** (1992), 1377–83.

137. N. Kawakami, T. Haratani, S. Araki, Effects of perceived job stress on depressive symptoms in blue-collar workers of an electrical factory in Japan. *Scand. J. Work Environ. Health* **18** (1992), 195–200.

138. K. R. Parkes, C. A. Mendham, C. Von Rabenau, Social support and the demand–discretion model of job stress: tests of additive and interactive effects in two samples. *J. Voc. Behav.* **44** (1994), 91–113.

139. S. A. Stansfeld, R. Fuhrer, J. Head, J. Ferrie, M. Shipley, Work and psychiatric disorder in the Whitehall II study. *J. Psychosom. Res.* **43** (1997), 73–81.

140. I. Niedhammer, M. Goldberg, A. Leclerc, I. Bugel, S. David, Psychosocial factors at work and subsequent depressive symptoms in the Gazel cohort. *Scand. J. Work Environ. Health* **24** (1998), 197–205.

141. Y. Mino, J. Shigemi, T. Tsuda, N. Yasuda, P. Bebbington, Perceived job stress and mental health in precision machine workers of Japan: a 2 year cohort study. *Occup. Environ. Med.* **56** (1999), 41–5.

142. S. A. Stansfeld, R. Fuhrer, M. J. Shipley, M. G. Marmot, Work characteristics predict psychiatric disorder: prospective results from the Whitehall II study. *Occup. Environ. Med.* **56** (1999), 302–7.

143. A. Weinberg, F. Creed, Stress and psychiatric disorder in healthcare professionals and hospital staff. *Lancet* **355** (2000), 533–7.

144. B. Hesketh, G. Shouksmith, Job and non-job activities, job satisfaction and mental health among veterinarians. *J. Occup. Behav.* **7** (1986), 325–9.

145. P. B. Warr, Decision latitude, job demands and employee well being. *Work Stress* **4** (1990), 285–94.

146. H. Mausner-Dorsch, W. W. Eaton, Psychosocial work environment and depression: epidemiologic assessment of the demand-control model. *Am. J. Public Health* **90** (2000), 1765–70.

147. M. Cropley, A. Steptoe, K. Joekes, Job strain and psychiatric morbidity. *Psychol. Med.* **29** (1999), 1411–16.

148. A. P. Brief, M. J. Burke, J. M. George, B. S. Robinson, J. Webster, Should negative affectivity remain an unmeasured variable in the study of job stress? *J. Appl. Psychol.* **73** (1988), 193–8.

149. S. Paterniti, I. Niedhammer, T. Lang, S. M. Consoli, Psychosocial factors at work, personality traits and depressive symptoms: longitudinal results from the GAZEL study. *Br. J. Psychiatry* **181** (2002), 111–17.

150. D. A. Regier, J. H. Boyd, J. D. Burke, Jr, *et al.*, One-month prevalence of mental disorders in the United States: based on five epidemiologic catchment area sites. *Arch. Gen. Psychiatry* **45** (1988), 977–86.

151. A. S. Henderson, A. E. Korten, P. A. Jacomb, *et al.*, The course of depression in the elderly: a longitudinal community-based study in Australia. *Psychol. Med.* **27** (1997), 119–29.

152. R. C. Baldwin, J. O'Brien, Vascular basis of late-onset depressive disorder. *Br. J. Psychiatry* **180** (2002), 157–60.

153. M. J. Karel, Aging and depression: vulnerability and stress across adulthood. *Clin. Psychol. Rev.* **17** (1997), 847–79.

154. R. C. Kessler, C. Foster, P. S. Webster, J. S. House, The relationship between age and depressive symptoms in two national surveys. *Psychol. Aging* **7** (1992), 119–26.

155. M. D. Blumenthal, Depressive illness in old age: getting behind the mask. *Geriatrics* **35** (1980), 34–43.

156. B. H. Mulsant, M. Ganguli, Epidemiology and diagnosis of depression in late life. *J. Clin. Psychiatry* **60**: Suppl 20 (1999), 9–15.

157. M. L. Bruce, Psychosocial risk factors for depressive disorders in late life. *Biol. Psychiatry* **52** (2002), 175–84.

158. E. Murphy, Social origins of depression in old age. *Br. J. Psychiatry* **141** (1982), 135–42.

159. E. I. Brilman, J. Ormel, Life events, difficulties and onset of depressive episodes in later life. *Psychol. Med.* **31** (2001), 859–69.

160. C. M. Mazure, P. K. Maciejewski, S. C. Jacobs, M. L. Bruce, Stressful life events interacting with cognitive/personality styles to predict late-onset major depression. *Am. J. Geriatr. Psychiatry* **10** (2002), 297–304.

161. R. A. Schoevers, A. T. Beekman, D. J. Deeg, *et al.*, Risk factors for depression in later life: results of a prospective community based study (AMSTEL). *J. Affect. Disord.* **59** (2000), 127–37.

162. B. Pitt, Loss in late life. *Br. Med. J.* **316** (1998), 1452–4.

163. C. L. Turvey, Y. Conwell, M. P. Jones, *et al.*, Risk factors for late-life suicide: a prospective, community-based study. *Am. J. Geriatr. Psychiatry* **10** (2002), 398–406.

164. M. Marmot, T. Theorell, J. Siegrist, Work and coronary heart disease. In *Stress and the Heart: Psychosocial Pathways to Coronary Heart Disease*, ed. S. A. Stansfeld, M. G. Marmot (London: BMJ Books, 2002), pp. 50–71.

165. S. A. Stansfeld, R. Fuhrer, Depression and coronary heart disease. In *Stress and the Heart: Psychosocial Pathways to Coronary Heart Disease*, ed. S. A. Stansfeld, M. G. Marmot (London: BMJ Books, 2002), pp. 101–23.

166. S. A. Stansfeld, J. Head, R. Fuhrer, J. Wardle, V. Cattell, Social inequalities in depressive symptoms and physical functioning in the Whitehall II study: exploring a common cause explanation. *J. Epidemiol. Community Health* **57** (2003), 361–7.

Part 2

Depression and specific health problems

3

Depression and the development of coronary heart disease

Andrew Steptoe

Introduction

This chapter is concerned with the role of depression in the development of coronary atherosclerosis and in the aetiology of coronary heart disease (CHD). Chapter 4 discusses the association between depression and prognosis in patients with existing CHD. The relationship of depression with cardiovascular disease has been a topic of intense research interest over the past 15 years and has driven much contemporary thinking about how physical illness and depression are linked. It has stimulated work on a variety of biological processes that potentially mediate the relationship, including platelet activation [1], vascular inflammation [2], endothelial dysfunction [3], reduced baroreceptor reflex sensitivity [4], sympathovagal imbalance [5] and neuroendocrine dysfunction [6].

The purpose of this chapter is to evaluate the strength and consistency of the association between depression and future CHD, to evaluate the specificity of the relationship, and to describe the biological processes that are probably involved. The chapter is divided into five sections. The first section provides a critical review of existing evidence from longitudinal observational studies that depression and depressive symptoms are associated prospectively with CHD in initially healthy adults. Studies of this topic have generated rather variable results, and so it is worth considering what accounts for the discrepancies. The chapter then questions whether there is a specific link between depression and CHD, or whether comparable associations are present for anxiety and more general psychological distress. It could be that depression promotes the clinical manifestation of CHD, rather than the long-term development of atherosclerosis, and so the relationship of depression with subclinical atherosclerosis is the topic of the third section. Next, the chapter discusses the time course of relationships between depressive symptoms and CHD, and whether depression in the days or even hours preceding acute

Depression and Physical Illness, ed. A. Steptoe.
Published by Cambridge University Press. © Cambridge University Press 2006.

cardiac events is relevant. The final section of the chapter outlines the different pathways that may translate depressive emotional experience into CHD. It touches on several of the biological and behavioural processes discussed in detail in later chapters, but it addresses them specifically in relation to coronary atherosclerosis and CHD. Throughout the chapter, methodological problems in this literature are highlighted, some of which arise from the difficulty of establishing associations between a subjective experience such as depression and a physical illness such as CHD, while others concern issues such as confounding and biological plausibility that apply to studies of many risk factors.

Longitudinal studies of depression and CHD

The first issue to resolve when studying depression and CHD is whether there is consistent and reliable evidence that people who are depressed or have elevated levels of depressive symptoms are at increased risk for future CHD. Cross-sectional studies can establish whether depression is more common in CHD patients than in comparable healthy populations, and there have been numerous studies of this kind. For example, INTERHEART is a multicentre case–control study involving more than 11 000 first myocardial infarction patients and matched controls from 52 countries. Depressive symptoms over the 12 months before admission were consistently more common in cases than controls, and the population attributable risk was estimated to be 9% [7]. However, cross-sectional studies cannot establish accurately the temporal relationship between depressive episodes and CHD, and so longitudinal observational studies of initially healthy populations are required.

Three particular difficulties arise in investigating this topic. The first is case ascertainment and how CHD outcomes are defined. The clinical manifestations of CHD include cardiac death, acute coronary syndromes (ST-elevation myocardial infarction, non ST-elevation myocardial infarction, and unstable angina) and angina pectoris. Angina pectoris is a subjective experience of chest pain or discomfort under defined physical activity conditions. Subjective reports of chest pain may be subject to bias, with more depressed or stressed individuals perhaps being more likely to rate their chest discomfort above the thresholds for definition of angina pectoris. Some prospective studies have relied on self-reports of angina, either alone or in combination with objective clinical events, as CHD outcomes, and thereby run the risk of reporting bias. This review is therefore limited to outcomes such as myocardial infarction, fatal CHD and electrocardiographic (ECG) changes indicative of ischaemia.

The second issue is the confounding of depression with other determinants of CHD. Conventionally, multivariate analysis is employed to assess whether exposure to a putative risk factor is associated independently with disease incidence or whether it overlaps with other known risk factors. In the studies described here, the association between depression and CHD was typically evaluated after taking into account a variety of factors, such as age, sex, blood pressure, smoking, cholesterol level, body mass, diabetes and socioeconomic status. However, a difficulty that arises is that some confounding factors may actually be mediators of the association between depression and CHD. Later chapters in this book document relationships between depression, smoking and physical activity. Depression may also be linked positively with risk factors such as high blood pressure [8]. If these factors are statistically co-varied, then there is a danger that associations between depression and CHD could be attenuated.

The third difficulty arises from the nature of CHD. Clinical cardiac events are the end product of the progressive development of coronary atherosclerosis. Post-mortem studies of victims of accidental or violent death have shown significant coronary atherosclerosis in adolescents and young adults, related to risk factors such as smoking and high serum cholesterol [9]. No longitudinal studies of depression that began even in early adult life have yet been able to rule out the possibility that subclinical atherosclerosis was already more advanced in depressed individuals. The impact of depression at different stages of CHD aetiology is discussed more fully later in this chapter.

Table 3.1 summarises results from 27 longitudinal observational studies published between 1964 and 2005. Studies were identified through systematic searches on PubMed and PsychInfo and scrutiny of existing reviews [10–12]. Studies were excluded if fatal CHD and myocardial infarction were not used as outcome measures. Many of these studies had several outcomes adjusted for different covariates. The relative risks shown in Table 3.1 are those that were calculated for analyses adjusting for the standard demographic, clinical and behavioural risk factors that were available. Some studies included individuals with suspected or definite cardiac disease at baseline, but the present results exclude such cases. Outcomes are presented as relative risks with 95% confidence intervals (CI).

In purely numerical terms, the findings are weighted towards positive associations being present. Out of the 27 studies reviewed, 16 showed at least 1 significant association between depression and future CHD, while 11 did not. It should also be noted that some of the effect sizes in the null studies were quite substantial, even though the confidence intervals crossed 1 [13–15]. None of these prospective studies has shown that depressive symptoms were protective against CHD.

One representative study to find a positive effect was the analysis of the National Health Examination Follow-up study described by Anda *et al.* [16]: 11.1% of the cohort of 2832 men and women aged 45–77 years had depressed affect at baseline, as assessed with the General Wellbeing Schedule. Depressed affect was associated with female gender, African American ethnicity, low education, unmarried status,

Table 3.1 Depression as a predictor of future coronary heart disease (CHD)

Ref.	Country, study	n	Age range (years)	Follow-up (years)	Depression measure	Outcome	Adjustments, covariates	Relative risk (95% CI)	Effect?	Issues
Ostfeld et al. [149]	USA	1885	40–55	4.5	MMPI-derived	MI, angina	None	0	0	Angina included in outcome, only men studied, no co-variates
Hallstrom et al. [150]	Sweden	795	38–54	12 (max.)	DIS and Hamilton scale	MI, ECG changes	Age, SES, marital, standard risk factors	NS	0	Only women studied
Haines et al. [13]	Northwick Park Heart Study, UK	1457	40–64	10	Crown-Crisp Experiential Index	Fatal CHD, NF MI	None	Fatal CHD: 3.3 (0.9–5.6) NF MI: 2.2 (0.8–5.6)	0 0	No co-variates, only men studied
Anda et al. [16]	NHANES, USA	2832	45–77	12.4	General wellbeing schedule	Fatal CHD	Age, sex, education, BMI, standard risk factors, alcohol, PA, race, marital status	Fatal: 1.5 (1.0–2.3)	+	
Aromaa et al. [27]	Finland	3811	40–64	6.6	Present State Examination	Fatal CHD	Age	3.36 (significant)	+	Limited co-variates
Barefoot and Schroll [151]	Denmark	730	50 or 60	17 or 27	MMPI scale	Fatal and NF MI	Age, sex, standard risk factors, PA	1.72 (1.18–2.51)	+	
Pratt et al. [29]	ECA study, USA	1551	18–64	13	Major depression Dysphoria	NF MI	Age, sex, education, smoking, BP, marital status, diabetes	Major: 4.14 (1.48–11.6) Dysphoria: 2.06 (1.15–3.72)	+ +	
Wassertheil-Smoller et al. [23]	USA	4367	> 60	4.5	CES-D	Fatal and NF MI	Age, sex, education, smoking, history of MI, stroke, diabetes, race.	Per 5-point increase in CES-D score: 1.14 (0.97–1.34)	+	

Study	Cohort/Location	N	Age	Follow-up	Depression measure	Outcome	Covariates	Risk estimate	Effect	Comments
Mendes de Leon et al. [14]	EPESE, USA	2391	65–99	9	CES-D	Fatal CHD, NF MI	Age, education, smoking, BP, diabetes	Women: 1.67 (0.96–2.9) Men: 0.7 (0.34–1.42)	0 0	
Ford et al. [28]	USA	1190	26 (mean)	37	Self-reported clinical depression	MI and sudden death	Age, standard risk factors, PA, diabetes, family history	2.1 (1.1–4.1)	+	Only men studied, all former Johns–Hopkins medical students
Penninx et al. [21]	EPESE, USA	3701	70–103	4	CES-D	CHD events	Age, sex, standard risk factors, BMI, alcohol, medical history	Chronic depression: Men: 1.19 (0.58–2.46) Women: 1.12 (0.76–1.65) Newly depressed: Men: 2.03 (1.28–3.24) Women: 1.22 (0.83–1.8)	0 0 + 0	Effects only in men
Schwartz et al. [152]	USA	2960	65–101	3	CES-D	Fatal and NF MI	Age, sex	2.23 (1.34–3.71)	+	Short follow-up, limited co-variates
Sesso et al. [15]	Normative Aging Study, USA	1305	21–80	7	MMPI scale	Fatal CHD and NF MI	Age, standard risk factors, BMI, alcohol, family history	1.88 (0.77–4.59)	0	Only men studied
Whooley and Browner [153]	USA	7518	67+	6	Geriatric Depression Scale	CHD death	Age, smoking, BP, diabetes, CVD history	1.7 (1.0–3.0)	+	Only women studied
Cole et al. [154]	College Alumni Health Study, USA	5053	65 (mean)	12 (max.)	Self-reported physician-diagnosed depression	Fatal CHD	Age, smoking, BP, BMI, PA, alcohol, diabetes	1.20 (0.53–2.71)	0	Only men studied

(cont.)

Table 3.1 (*cont.*)

Ref.	Country, study	n	Age range (years)	Follow-up (years)	Depression measure	Outcome	Adjustments, covariates	Relative risk (95% CI)	Effect?	Issues
Ariyo et al. [20]	USA	4493	65–98	6	CES-D	MI	Age, sex, education, standard risk factors, PA, BMI, alcohol, diabetes, angina, heart failure, race, marital status	Per 5-point increase in CES-D score MI: 1.12 (0.97–1.29)	0	
Cohen et al. [41]	USA	54 997	43 (mean)	3.6	Antidepressant use	Fatal or NF MI	Age, sex, hypertension, hyperlipidaemia, diabetes, heart disease, anxiety, cancer	1.8 (1.1–3.1)	+	
Ferketich et al. [76]	NHANES 1, USA	7893	55 (mean)	8.3	CES-D	Fatal CHD	Age, race, smoking, hypertension, BMI, diabetes, poverty	Men: 2.34 (1.54–3.56) Women: 0.74 (0.4–1.48)	+ 0	Effects seen only in men
Chang et al. [155]	NHANES, USA	10 766	35–74	21 (max.)	General Wellbeing Schedule	Fatal CHD	Age, sex, education, standard risk factors, BMI, PA, diabetes	NS	0	
Cohen et al. [117]	USA	5564	53 (mean)	4.9	History of treatment	MI	Age, sex, education, standard risk factors, BMI, alcohol, diabetes, CVD history, left ventricular hypertrophy, race, marital status	2.10 (1.04–4.23)	+	
Haines et al. [26]	Northwick Park Heart Study, UK	1408	40–64	20.9	Crown–Crisp Experiential Index	Fatal CHD	Age, standard risk factors, BMI, fibrinogen, factor V11c, social class	1-point increase: 1.07 (0.99–1.2)	0	Only men studied
Penninx et al. [22]	NL	2397	55–85	4.2	DIS for major depression, CES-D for symptoms	Cardiac mortality	Age, sex, education, smoking, BP, BMI, alcohol, diabetes, stroke, lung disease, cancer	DIS: 3.9 (1.4–10.9) Minor depression: NS	+	Effect for major depression only

Study	Country	N	Age		Depression measure	Outcome	Adjustments	Result	Effect	Notes
Yasuda et al. [156]	Japan	817	65–84	7.5	GHQ depression scale	Cardiac mortality	Age, chronic disease, PA, social networks	Men: 0.65 (0.37–1.14) Women: 2.03 (1.17–3.50)	0 +	Participants with disability excluded
Everson-Rose et al. [157]	USA	3617	25+	7.5	CES-D	Fatal CVD	Age, sex, race, education, income, BMI, smoking, alcohol, hypertension, functional impairment, serious illness	NS	0	
Wassertheil-Smoller et al. [24]	USA	93 676	50–79	4.1	CES-D	CHD, fatal CVD	Age, race, education, income, standard risk factors, BMI, diabetes, hormone therapy, PA	CHD: 1.12 (0.89–1.41) Fatal CVD: 1.59 (1.12–2.10)	0 +	Only women studied
Gump et al. [158]	MRFIT	12 866	41–63	18	CES-D	Fatal	Age, race, education, standard risk factors, alcohol	1.10 (0.91–1.32)	0	Only men studied; all at above average CHD risk
Rowan et al. [25]	Canada	1302	45+	4	CES-D	Fatal CHD, NF MI	Age, gender, education, standard risk factors, diabetes, family history, alcohol, BMI, PA	1-point increase: 1.32 (1.07–1.71)	+	

BP, blood pressure; CI, confidence interval; CVD, cardiovascular disease; ECG, electrocardiogram; ECA, Ecological Catchment Area; EPESE, Established Populations for the Epidemiologic Studies of the Elderly; MRFIT, Multiple Risk Factor Intervention Trial; NHANES, National Health and Nutrition Examination Survey; MMPI, Minnesota Multiphasic Personality Inventory; DIS, Diagnositc Interview Schedule; CES-D, Center for Epidemiological Studies depression scale; GHQ, General Health Questionnaire; NF CHD, non-fatal coronary heart disease; NF MI, non-fatal myocardial infarction; Standard risk factors, blood pressure, smoking, cholesterol; marital, marital status; SES, socioeconomic status; BMI, body mass index; PA, physical activity; NS, not significant; *Effect*: + = positive association with 95% CI not crossing 1 after adjustement; 0 = association either not significant or with CI crossing 1 after adjustment.

smoking and physical inactivity. Over the follow-up period of more than 12 years, 6.7% died from CHD. The rate of fatal CHD was 7.1 per 1000 person-years in depressed people, compared with 5.2 in the non-depressed participants, with a relative risk (RR) adjusted for other factors of 1.5 (95% CI 1.0 to 2.3).

One prospective study that has not been included in Table 3.1 because some participants had CHD at baseline is the eight-year follow-up of a representative sample of people aged 70 years or older in north Finland [17]. Elevated scores on the Zung depression rating scale predicted sudden cardiac death, but not cardiac mortality in general, or non-fatal myocardial infarction. Although a proportion of participants had a history of myocardial infarction, chest pain and heart failure at baseline, the multivariate hazard ratio was significant for those with high depression scores (1.70, 95% CI 1.37 to 2.10) after these factors had been taken into account along with gender, age, diabetes and body mass index (BMI). Similarly, in the Italian Longitudinal Study on Aging, depressive symptoms were associated independently with future cardiovascular mortality in men after adjusting for risk factors and pre-existing clinical conditions [18].

Another study not included in Table 3.1 because it presented results as a case–control analysis instead of a prospective cohort analysis is the Prospective Epidemiological Study of Myocardial Infarction (PRIME) carried out in France and Northern Ireland [19]. Depressive mood, assessed with a subscale from the Minnesota Multiphasic Personality Inventory (MMPI), was assessed in some 8600 initially healthy men aged 50–59 years who were followed up for five to six years. A total of 335 men with a first CHD event (angina, non-fatal myocardial infarction or cardiac death) were compared with 670 controls matched by age and date of baseline assessment. The odds ratio for the association of CHD with depressive mood was 1.50 (95% CI 1.04 to 2.15) after adjusting for smoking, cholesterol, BMI, education and marital status.

There are no clear distinctions between the studies that showed positive and null effects in terms of age of the samples, gender or length of follow-up. The same measures of depression, such as the Center for Epidemiological Studies Depression (CES-D) scale generated both positive and null findings [14,20–25]. However, two analyses from the same British sample involving the less established measure of depression from the Crown–Crisp Experiential Index generated null findings [13,26]. One factor that might be important is the intensity of depression. It is interesting that most studies that involved clinical diagnoses or treatment-based criteria as opposed to measures on questionnaires reported positive associations [27–29]. Pratt et al. [29] showed a larger relative risk for major depression than dysphoria, and an intensity effect was also found in the Amsterdam Longitudinal Aging Study [22]. Similarly, Everson et al. [30] analysed the related construct of hopelessness in the Kuopio study from Finland and observed a higher risk of cardiac death over six years in participants with severe compared with moderate hopelessness (relative risk 3.66 and 2.52, respectively).

A related construct to depression is vital exhaustion, a syndrome of fatigue, tiredness and hopelessness. Vital exhaustion has been associated with CHD in cross-sectional and longitudinal studies [31]. For example, Prescott *et al.* [32] tracked 9563 Danish adults for up to six years. The risk of a first myocardial infarction requiring hospitalisation in apparently healthy individuals at baseline was 2.20 (95% CI 1.53 to 3.17) for those with high vital exhaustion ratings, after adjustment for age, blood pressure, cholesterol, smoking, BMI, waist/hip ratio, diabetes, family history of CHD, physical activity, alcohol consumption, education and household income.

A positive though rather mixed picture for the relationship between depression and future CHD emerges from this survey. Other reviews that have been more select-ive in their inclusion criteria have perhaps come to even more positive conclusions [10–12]. Nonetheless, the inconsistencies in this literature are substantial.

CHD in patients with clinical depression

The survey in Table 3.1 suggests that more consistent associations with CHD may be present among individuals with severe depression as opposed to only moderate symptoms of depression. One way of addressing this issue is to investigate CHD incidence in clinically depressed populations. Several of the studies summarised in Table 3.1 included participants with clinically diagnosed depression, but these were individuals who happened to be in the larger population cohorts. Other researchers have specifically tracked patients with psychiatric histories in order to assess their CHD rates.

These studies have mostly found associations between clinical depression and future CHD, but results are not conclusive. Some early work on pharmacologically treated psychiatric patients reported elevations in cardiovascular mortality in com-parison with population norms [33], but no differences were found by other inves-tigators [34]. A record-linkage study in Iowa, USA, showed a higher than expected death rate from CHD only in women [35], while in the Stirling County study in Canada death rates from circulatory disorders were elevated in men with affective disorders [36]. Allgulander [37] analysed the national psychiatric case register in Sweden, identifying individuals diagnosed with depressive neuroses over a ten-year period. There was an elevation in CHD death rates among patients diagnosed with either anxiety neurosis or depression in comparison with national statistics. More recently, Coryell *et al.* [38] assessed patients seeking treatment for major depressive disorder, mania or schizoaffective disorder in five academic treatments centres over an 11-year period. There was no association between the persistence of depressive morbidity and cardiovascular death, but comparisons were not made with death rates in non-psychiatric populations.

Many of the samples investigated in these studies have not been well suited to analysing CHD. Comparisons have been made with national mortality rates rather than appropriate controls. Few have included measures of standard cardiovascular risk factors, thereby complicating the interpretation of results. Lifestyle factors such as cigarette smoking and heavy alcohol consumption are common in depressed populations, and it is not known whether risk factors such as high blood pressure are treated as vigorously in psychiatrically ill patients compared with non-depressed individuals. Some studies of psychiatric patients have assessed relatively young samples in which cardiovascular mortality is rare and so have limited power for identifying associations, and many early studies focused on institutionalised patients.

Even if a relationship was found between clinical depression and CHD mortality, interpretation is difficult. There is evidence that procedures such as coronary revascularisation are used less frequently in patients with mental disorders compared with cardiac patients who do not have psychiatric problems, and so prognosis may be adversely affected [39]. Some CHD may be iatrogenic in patients treated with antidepressants. Hippisley-Cox et al. [40] reported a case–control study of CHD patients recruited from general practice. The odds of CHD were significantly elevated among individuals prescribed tricyclic antidepressants, adjusting for cardiovascular risk factors. Similarly, in Cohen and colleagues' [41] community-based study listed in Table 3.1, the excess risk of myocardial infarction was limited to patients who had been prescribed tricyclic medications. Consequently, the inferences that can be drawn about the role of depression in CHD aetiology from studies of psychiatric populations are, unfortunately, limited.

Anxiety and psychological distress in relation to CHD

Although the primary focus of research over recent years has been on depression, it is possible that other negative emotional states are also relevant to CHD. The incidence of CHD has been associated prospectively with various forms of stress and adversity, notably work stress and social isolation [12,42]. These experiences frequently engender feelings of distress, and so relationships with other psychological states are plausible.

There have been rather fewer prospective observational studies of psychological distress and anxiety than of depression, although cross-sectional associations between CHD and elevated distress are marked [43]. A review of this literature comparable with that detailed in the previous section was conducted, and the studies that measured objective cardiovascular endpoints in initially apparently healthy populations are summarised in Table 3.2. A range of standardised measures of distress have been used, including the General Health Questionnaire (GHQ) and subscales from the Crown–Crisp Experiential Index [13,44–49]. Results have generally been positive, particularly in men, with significant associations between psychological distress and future CHD that simply were independent of standard cardiovascular risk factors and demographic indices as well. However, this conclusion must be treated with caution, since the number of studies is small and it is possible that analyses of other cohorts that failed to show significant associations simply were not published.

The issue of confounding is particularly vexed for anxiety and distress, since risky behaviours such as smoking and excessive alcohol consumption are linked strongly with these psychological states. For example, Kawachi *et al.* [50] conducted a nested case–control analysis relating anxiety with fatal CHD and non-fatal myocardial infarction in a 32-year follow-up of the Normative Aging Study. An age-adjusted odds ratio of 3.20 (95% CI 1.27 to 8.09) emerged for fatal CHD, and this was even higher when analysis was limited to cases of sudden death (OR 5.73, 95% CI 1.26 to 26.1). But when smoking, alcohol consumption and standard risk factors were taken into account, the multivariate odds ratios became non-significant (OR 1.94, 95% CI 0.70 to 5.41 for fatal CHD; OR 4.46, 95% CI 0.93 to 8.25 for sudden death). It is arguable whether the non-significance of such adjusted effects should be regarded as disproving the impact of anxiety.

A number of researchers have also investigated perceived stress in relation to CHD in prospective observational studies. Perceived stress occupies an intermediate position between measures of specific exposures such as excessive job demands and burdensome caregiving on the one hand, and measures of emotional state such as anxiety and depression on the other hand. Results have been rather variable, due in part to differences in measures and their application in diverse populations. A study of more than 73 000 Japanese men and women used a single question about the level of stress in everyday life [51]. Over a 7.9-year follow-up period, the risk of myocardial infarction was elevated significantly in women reporting high stress after adjustment for age, BMI, smoking, alcohol intake, diabetes, hypertension and physical exercise. In Sweden, a 21-year follow-up has been reported of 13 609 men and women who answered two simple questions about stress [52]. Risk of incident CHD and stroke was raised in individuals reporting higher stress, with the most consistent effects being observed for death from stroke in men. By contrast, a smaller study of middle-aged men from Scotland who completed a four-item perceived stress inventory showed no significant association with CHD mortality over 21 years after adjustment for risk factors [53]. The measures of perceived stress in these studies have differed in the extent to which they tapped transient

Table 3.2 Psychological distress and anxiety as predictors of future coronary heart disease (CHD)

Ref.	Country/study	n	Age range (years)	Follow-up (years)	Distress measure	Outcome	Adjustments, co-variates	Relative risk (95% CI)	Effect	Issues
Haines et al. [13]	Northwick Park Heart Study, UK	1457	40–64	10	Phobic anxiety	Fatal CHD, NF MI	Age, sex, BMI, standard risk factors, fibrinogen, SES	Fatal CHD: 3.77 (1.64–8.64) NF MI: 1.26 (0.62–2.54)	+ 0	
Eaker et al. [159]	Framingham, USA	749	45–64	20 (max.)	Anxiety	Fatal CHD, NF MI	Age, standard risk factors, BMI, diabetes	7.8 (1.9–32.3)	+	Only women studied; effect in homemakers but not employed women
Kawachi et al. [46]	Health Professionals, USA	33 999	42–77	2	Phobic anxiety	Fatal CHD, NF MI	Age, smoking, BMI, diabetes, hypertension, alcohol, hypercholesterolaemia, exercise, family history	Fatal CHD: 2.45 (1.0–5.96) NF MI: 0.89 (0.45–1.79)	+ 0	Short follow-up
Kubzansky et al. [160]	Normative Aging Study, USA	1759	21–80	20 (max.)	Worry about social conditions	Fatal CHD, NF MI	Age, standard risk factors, BMI, alcohol, family history	Fatal CHD: 0.81 (0.45–1.44) NF MI: 2.41 (1.40–4.13)	0 +	Only men studied

Study	Cohort	N	Age	Years	Exposure	Outcome	Adjustments	Effect size (95% CI)	Effect	Comments
Haines et al. [26]	Northwick Park Heart Study, UK	1408	40–64	20.9	Phobic anxiety	Fatal CHD	Age, standard risk factors, BMI, alcohol, fibrinogen, SES	1-point increase on scale: 1.07 (0.99–1.15)	0	Only men studied
Stansfeld et al. [44]	Whitehall II study, UK	7081	35–55	5	Distress	ECG ischaemia	Age, smoking, BMI, diet, alcohol, physical activity, SES	Men: 1.47 (1.0–2.1); Women: 0.68 (0.4–1.3)	+; 0	Effects seen only in men
Robinson et al. [45]	UK	4501	18–75	8 (max.)	Distress	Fatal CHD	Age, gender, smoking, deprivation, pain	1.90 (1.08–3.35)	+	
Rasul et al. [47]	Midspan study, UK	4941	45–64	5	Distress	Fatal CHD	Age, standard risk factors, marital status, SES, BMI, glucose	Men:1.29 (0.6–2.98); Women: 0.62 (0.4–2.36)	0; 0	Small number of deaths
Albert et al. [48]	Nurses Health study, USA	72 359	30–55	12	Phobic anxiety	Fatal CHD, NF MI	Age, smoking, BMI, PA, hypertension, family history, hypercholesterolaemia, alcohol, menopausal status, aspirin	Fatal CHD: 1.30 (1.02–1.67) NF; MI: 0.88 (0.76–1.01)	+; 0	Only women studied
Rasul et al. [49]	Midspan study, UK	6575	45–64	5	Distress	Hospital admission for CHD	Age, standard risk factors, marital status, SES, BMI, glucose, physical illness	Men: 1.61 (1.02–2.55); Women: 1.37 (0.59–3.19)	+; 0	

BP, blood pressure; CI, confidence interval; CVD, cardiovascular disease; ECG, electrocardiogram; ECA, Ecological Catchment Area; EPESE, Established Populations for the Epidemiologic Studies of the Elderly; MRFIT, Multiple Risk Factor Intervention Trial; NHANES, National Health and Nutrition Examination Survey; MMPI, Minnesota Multiphasic Personality Inventory; DIS, Diagnositc Interview Schedule; CES-D, Center for Epidemiological Studies depression scale; GHQ, General Health Questionnaire; NF CHD, non-fatal coronary heart disease; NF MI, non-fatal myocardial infarction; Standard risk factors, blood pressure, smoking, cholesterol; marital, marital status; SES, socioeconomic status; BMI, body mass index; PA, physical activity; NS, not significant; Effect: + = positive association with 95% CI not crossing 1 after adjustement; 0 = association either not significant or with CI crossing 1 after adjustment; Phobic anxiety, Crown–Crisp Experiential Index; anxiety, Framingham measure; worry about social conditions, Normative Aging Study measure; distress, General Health Questionnaire.

moods, genuine experience of adversity, and dysphoric dispositions. There may also be important variations in the extent that individuals from diverse cultures are prepared to acknowledge relatively non-specific negative feelings. Nonetheless, studies of psychological distress and anxiety suggest that associations with CHD may not be exclusive to depression.

Depression and subclinical atherosclerosis

The question of whether depression contributes to the long-term evolution of atherosclerosis, or to the clinical manifestations of the disease, has begun to be investigated over recent years as a result of the introduction of non-invasive indices of atherosclerosis. The thickness of the intima-medial layer (IMT) and the presence of plaque in the carotid arteries can be imaged with ultrasonography and appear to mirror the disease present in the coronary arteries, since carotid measures predict clinical CHD prospectively [54,55]. Carotid IMT and the presence of plaque have been associated longitudinally with work stress [56], with low socioeconomic status [57] and with acute cardiovascular stress reactivity [58]. More recent studies have assessed associations with depression as well.

Jones *et al.* [59] assessed 336 healthy women in whom lifetime history of major depression was associated positively with carotid plaque independently of blood pressure, age, smoking and race. In the Work Site Blood Pressure Study, depressed mood at baseline predicted carotid plaque ten years later after adjustment for cardiovascular risk factors, including age, gender, ethnicity, education, cholesterol, BMI, diabetes, smoking, blood pressure and family history [60].

Three studies have used computed tomography (CT) to assess coronary artery calcification, a more direct measure than carotid IMT of coronary disease [61]. No relationship with depression was reported by O'Malley *et al.* [62]; however, this study was carried out with US military personnel aged 39–45 years on active duty, and selection factors in terms of both physical and mental health may have reduced the chances of observing consistent associations. A larger investigation of more than 4000 men and women aged 60 years and older in Rotterdam showed positive associations between depressive disorders and coronary artery and aortic calcification [63]. Agatisa *et al.* [64] measured coronary artery calcification in 206 middle-aged women with no heart disease history. The 53 women who had a history of major depression according to a structured diagnostic interview had an increased likelihood of coronary artery calcification that was independent of demographic and cardiovascular risk factors. However, the association was attenuated by the inclusion of the waist/hip ratio in the model, suggesting that abdominal adiposity might partly mediate the effect.

Evidence for relationships between subclinical atherosclerosis and indices of distress such as anxiety and psychological strain has also emerged. Rather convincing findings were reported from a study of 726 French men and women aged 59–71 years [65]. Participants had no history of CHD, either at baseline or two years later. But men with high anxiety scores at both time points showed greater progression in carotid IMT over a four-year period than did less anxious individuals, with a similar but weaker effect among women. Cross-sectionally, psychological strain was associated with carotid plaque in a large German sample independently of standard risk factors, body mass, alcohol consumption and family history [66]. By contrast, hostile attitudes but not anxiety were associated with carotid IMT in a smaller study of postmenopausal women [67]. Thus, although the evidence is not yet comprehensive, there is reason to suppose that depression and allied negative mood states are associated not only with manifest CHD but also with subclinical disease.

Timing of associations with depression

Another method that has been used in longitudinal observational studies to determine whether depression is associated with underlying disease rather than its acute clinical manifestation is to exclude cardiac events that took place soon after the assessment of depression. For example, in the study based on the National Health and Nutrition Examination Survey (NHANES) sample described in Table 3.1, Anda et al. [16] excluded cardiac events that took place within two years of psychological assessment. Similarly, Robinson et al. [45] reported that a positive association between psychological distress assessed with the GHQ and fatal CHD was maintained after excluding deaths that occurred with 24 months of questionnaire administration.

The rationale behind this approach is that if depression or distress was a catalyst for acute cardiac events only in people with advanced disease, then such effects would be expected to take place within a relatively short time. However, this raises the question of how important depression or distress is at different stages of the life course for risk of future CHD. Since most studies have assessed psychological state at a single point, it is difficult to know whether one episode of major depression in early life would be associated with the same risk as one in middle age, or whether chronic low-level dysphoria would be more relevant than transient severe depression. One relevant finding comes from the analysis reported by Penninx et al. [21] of CHD events in a sample of 3701 men and women aged 70–103 years. Participants completed the CES-D three times over a six-year period and were divided into chronically depressed (those with high CES-D scores both at the latest and one of the two earlier assessments) and newly depressed (people with high scores only on the latest assessment) groups. Over a median four-year follow-up, an association with CHD was observed only for newly depressed men, and not for chronically depressed participants. This suggests that recent depression might be particularly relevant. Such a conclusion is consistent with case–control studies that have measured depression for the 6 or 12 months before cardiac admission. In the INTERHEART study, for example, the relative risk for depression over the previous 12 months was 1.55 (95% CI 1.49 to 1.6) [7].

The rates of severe depressive symptoms in the months preceding acute myocardial infarction are not well characterised and vary substantially across studies. Lesperance *et al.* [68] reported that 5.4% of patients admitted for first-time myocardial infarction fulfilled Diagnostic and Statistical Manual of Mental Disorders, 3rd edn (DSM-III) criteria for major depression in the six months before myocardial infarction. By contrast, in a larger study in Manchester, 23.8% of myocardial infarction patients were depressed in the weeks before admission, on the basis of questionnaire scores that had been validated against clinical interview [69]. These rates may differ because of both the methods of assessment and the precise criteria for inclusion or exclusion from the studies. It should also be noted that assessments were made retrospectively, and it is conceivable that patients' evaluations of their previous mental states are coloured by their subsequent cardiac history.

An additional possibility is that depressive episodes might be acute triggers of cardiac events. Triggers are external stimuli, emotional states or activities that provoke acute pathophysiological change leading directly to the onset of coronary syndromes [70]. Triggering typically takes place against a background of long-term coronary artery disease and may operate over periods as short as one to two hours. It is thought that triggers act by disrupting coronary plaque through plaque rupture or erosion, leading to the development of thrombus [71]. Acute emotional triggers are difficult to study, since they generally involve retrospective assessments and reporting biases may operate. The case-crossover method was developed to analyse acute triggers and involves comparing the incidence of potential triggers during hazard and control periods on a within-subject basis [72]. This technique has been used to document an association between the experience of anger and increased risk of myocardial infarction in the subsequent two hours [73] and the impact of vigorous physical exertion on cardiac events in unfit individuals [74].

The author and his colleagues have studied whether depressed mood might act as an acute trigger in a manner analogous to anger. Data were collected from 295 men and women admitted to hospital with acute coronary syndromes and who were interviewed an average of 2.54 days after the cardiac event. They were questioned in detail about their emotional states in the two hours preceding symptom onset (hazard period) and for various control periods including the previous 24 hours and past 6 months. We found that 18.9% experienced depression in the two-hour hazard period. The relative risk of onset of an acute cardiac event following an episode of depression during the 2-hour hazard period compared with the previous 24 hours was 2.99 (95% CI 2.07 to 4.32), while the risk in comparison with the previous 6 months was 4.33 (95% CI 3.39 to 6.11). These findings suggest that depression might act as an acute precipitant of cardiac pathology in vulnerable individuals.

Pathways relating depression to CHD development

Longitudinal observational studies cannot by themselves demonstrate causation, and it is conceivable that the association between depression and future CHD is due to processes underlying both conditions or to residual confounding with other factors. In patients with more advanced coronary atherosclerosis, it is possible that vascular inflammatory processes result in both depressed mood and accelerated disease progression [75]. However, the argument that depression might contribute to the development of CHD can be strengthened if plausible pathways linking the two can be identified.

Psychosocial factors are thought to influence physical disease states through two broad sets of pathways: behavioural or lifestyle processes, and more direct biological processes. A number of behavioural factors contribute to CHD, including cigarette smoking, certain patterns of alcohol consumption, eating behaviour (both total caloric intake and consumption of particular nutrients) and physical activity. If depression was systematically related to behaviours that increased CHD risk, then associations could be mediated through these factors without invoking direct biological pathways.

It is notable that in many of the prospective studies summarised in Tables 3.1 and 3.2, depressive symptoms were associated with an increased likelihood of smoking, physical inactivity, higher levels of alcohol consumption, and greater BMI and abdominal obesity, e.g.[24,34,76]. The fact that associations between depression and CHD remain significant after taking account of these factors indicates that health behaviours are responsible only in part for mediation. However, this mediating role has yet to be investigated in great detail in prospective aetiological studies. Measures of health behaviour are often taken on only a single occasion, with relatively insensitive markers of dietary intake, physical activity and tobacco exposure, and so the impact of these factors may be underplayed.

The biological processes that could mediate the impact of depression on the development of CHD have been studied in rather more detail. Several of these processes may be relevant to explaining associations between depression and prognosis in patients following acute cardiac events, as outlined in Chapter 4. Here, the emphasis is on mechanisms that are involved in primary aetiology. It should be emphasised that depression does not appear to be related strongly to standard cardiovascular risk factors such as high blood pressure and elevated cholesterol, although, as noted earlier, some associations with hypertension have been described [8,77]. Other biological processes involved in atherogenesis have been implicated.

Endothelial function and vascular inflammation

The gradual accumulation of lipid in the walls of arteries used to be regarded as a largely passive process, depending on the concentration of cholesterol in the blood. More recent research has demonstrated that atherosclerotic lesions contain a variety of cells with highly specific inflammatory responses to lipid storage and vascular injury [78]. The early stages of atherosclerosis are characterised by functional alterations in the endothelial cell layer that lines the blood vessels. Endothelial injury arises from a variety of sources and may lead to endothelial dysfunction in which this protective layer develops pro-inflammatory and pro-thrombotic properties and becomes more permeable to low-density lipoprotein (LDL) cholesterol. Endothelial dysfunction is associated positively with cardiovascular risk factors and inflammation, even in childhood [79], and is an independent predictor of future carotid IMT [80] and CHD [54]. Nitric oxide (NO) production is an important feature of healthy endothelial function, and reduced levels of plasma metabolites and endothelial NO synthase activity have been described in patients with major depression [81]. Functional assessments have also demonstrated endothelial dysfunction in depressed adults without CHD [3], even when patients were in remission [82]. Psychological stress stimulates acute reversible impairment of endothelial function, which persists long after the stressor is terminated [83]. Such episodes might occur frequently during periods of depression, contributing to more sustained dysfunction.

Endothelial dysfunction results in the recruitment and adhesion of monocytes and T-lymphocytes to vulnerable sites on the vessel wall, a process that is mediated by up-regulation of cell adhesion modules. These are stimulated by pro-inflammatory cytokines such as interleukin (IL)-1, IL-6, tumour necrosis factor alpha (TNF-α) and interferon gamma (IFN-γ). These cytokines are also implicated in the activity of macrophages in lesions, the oxidation of LDL cholesterol and the migration of smooth muscle cell into lesions. The acute-phase protein C-reactive protein (CRP) stimulates the expression of tissue factor on macrophages and smooth muscle cells and pro-inflammatory cytokine production by macrophages, and facilitates the uptake of LDL cholesterol and the expression of adhesion molecules. Population studies indicate that elevated plasma CRP, IL-6, IFN-γ and circulating soluble cell-adhesion modules predict future CHD [84–86].

The literature relating inflammatory cytokines and other inflammatory molecules with depression is discussed by Irwin in Chapter 14. As noted by Irwin, many comparisons of depressed and non-depressed groups have been confounded by factors such as smoking, body weight, alcohol consumption and socioeconomic position, which can also influence inflammatory markers. Small studies of selected groups of healthy adults have shown associations between depressive symptoms and pro-inflammatory cytokines, including IL-6, IL-1β and TNF-α [87,88]. Population studies have been much less consistent, with positive associations being observed in some studies [89–91] but not others [92–94]. There are some indications that associations may be more pronounced in older cohorts [89,90,92]. However, if this is the case, then it may cast doubt on inflammatory processes being mediators of the relationship between depression and early atherosclerosis. An analysis from the PRIME study also suggests that inflammation is only part of the story. This study found an association between baseline CRP, IL-6 and soluble intercellular adhesion molecule 1 (ICAM-1) and future CHD, and between these inflammatory markers and depressive mood [19]. After adjustment for sociodemographic and cardiovascular risk factors, the 50% increase in odds ratio for depression being associated with CHD was reduced to 39% by including CRP, IL-6 and ICAM-1 in the model. This suggests that much of the association between CHD and depressive mood remained unaccounted for.

Haemostatic processes and platelet function

A second set of processes that might be implicated in the association between CHD and depression concern haemostasis and platelet function. Haemostatic processes are mechanisms that govern blood coagulation and the development of thrombi within the circulation. Coronary atherosclerosis is thought to progress through the disruption of coronary plaque and the subsequent formation of thrombus [95]. Plaque rupture is the commonest type of disruption, accounting for some 70% of fatal myocardial infarctions and sudden cardiac deaths, and occurs when the fibrous cap of the plaque is mechanically disturbed or disrupted by the action of matrix metalloproteinases [71]. In other cases, thrombus is superimposed on a plaque that is intact except for the loss of the endothelial cell layer, and injury is due to plaque erosion. It is evident from histological studies that episodic rupture is a frequent event that results only occasionally in acute coronary events, and the most angiographically severe lesions are not necessarily those at highest risk of disruption [96]. The local balance between pro-thrombotic and thrombolytic factors will determine whether a thrombus forms, whether vessel occlusion takes place or whether blood flow continues without impediment. Thus, the cascade of circulating and local coagulatory factors is crucial, including fibrinogen, von Willebrand factor, factors VII and VIII, fibrin D-dimer and plasminogen activator inhibitor (PAI). Meta-analyses of population-based prospective studies have shown that von Willebrand factor, factor VIII, plasma viscosity, fibrinogen and fibrin D-dimer all appear to be independent predictors of future CHD [97–99]. Platelets also play a key role, since they rapidly accumulate at the site of vascular injury, and the extent to which platelets are prone to activation may be critical [100].

It is known that psychological stress provokes acute haemostatic responses in healthy individuals and in patients with CHD [101]. Our group, for example, has shown that men and women without any history of CHD show increases in fibrinogen, von Willebrand factor, factor VIII, plasma viscosity and platelet activation following challenging behavioural tasks [102,103]. One study has explored the impact of depression and anxiety on haemostatic stress responses [104]. In a small sample of men and women with an average age of 71 years, it was found that anxiety and depression were associated positively with D-dimer responses but not with von Willebrand factor, PAI or tissue plasminogen activator responses. A substantial proportion of participants in this study had a history of cardiovascular disease, but the extent of coronary atherosclerosis is not known. A population study in Greece has documented a positive relationship between depressive symptoms and fibrinogen concentration that was independent of age, blood pressure, cholesterol, smoking, BMI, physical activity, medication and dietary habit [91].

There is a much larger literature relating platelet function with depression. Many of these studies were not carried out in order to assess whether depression is associated with platelet activation but were stimulated by the use of the serotonergic receptor on platelets as a model of brain-receptor functioning. Nevertheless, some researchers have tested whether platelet hyperactivity is characteristic of depression. This work has been reviewed systematically by von Kanel *et al.* [105]. Their conclusion is that the evidence is inconsistent: while 16 studies have demonstrated platelet hyperactivity in at least one measure, 18 have not. This may be due in part to the wide range of measures of platelet activity used. Modern techniques based on flow cytometry may elicit more consistent results than in vitro aggregation methods. There is certainly evidence that antidepressants affect platelet behaviour, but the implications of such studies for the involvement of platelets in mediating links with CHD is not yet clear.

Neuroendocrine and autonomic function

There is considerable evidence for depression being associated with disturbances of hypothalamic–pituitary–adrenocortical (HPA) axis function and the metabolism of cortisol. Corticotropin-releasing factor (CRF) and arginine vasopressin (AVP) are synthesised in the paraventricular nucleus of the hypothalamus and released via hypophyseal portal vessels to stimulate the production of adrenocorticotropin (ACTH) in the pituitary gland, which in turn elicits cortisol secretion from the adrenal glands. As noted by Goodyer in Chapter 13, HPA dysregulation is observed in some 50% of patients with unipolar depression and may contribute to associations between depressive symptoms and many types of physical disorder [6]. The effects of cortisol on obesity and diabetes may be particularly relevant in relation to CHD. The disturbances of HPA function present in obesity, and in particular abdominal adiposity, include heightened cortisol secretion, impaired feedback control, and changes in the peripheral metabolism and clearance of cortisol. Thus, impaired dexamethasone suppression of cortisol is associated with waist/hip ratio [106,107], as is the cortisol response to administration of CRF/AVP [108], and alterations in the metabolism of cortisol in the liver and adipose tissue have been described [109]. Cortisol responses to stress are correlated positively with waist/hip ratio, particularly in women [106,110], while the magnitude of cortisol responses following waking in the morning is associated positively with waist/hip ratio in men [111]. Abnormalities of cortisol metabolism have also been observed in patients with metabolic syndrome [112]. In type I diabetes, the rate of cortisol non-suppression following dexamethasone administration is elevated [113], and raised plasma cortisol levels in the morning have been described [114]. Rosmond *et al.* [115] reported a 5-year follow-up of 141 Swedish men and suggested that a flattened slope of cortisol decline over the day, coupled with low mean levels of cortisol and testosterone, was predictive of future type II diabetes. Phillips *et al.* [116] demonstrated a positive correlation between morning plasma cortisol concentration, systolic blood pressure, and other features of the metabolic syndrome in a cohort of British men.

However, many of the population studies shown in Table 3.1 have controlled statistically for blood pressure, diabetes and BMI and have nevertheless observed that relationships between depression and future CHD are still present [22,76,117]. There is little evidence for a more direct association between HPA dysfunction and CHD that does not involve adiposity or diabetes [6]. The evidence from population studies relating depression to insulin resistance is inconsistent, with insulin resistance being related to lower levels of depression in some studies [118,119] and to higher levels in others [120,121]. Thus, at present, there is limited support for the theory that HPA function and cortisol mediate the associations between CHD and depression that are not accounted for by these risk factors.

The paraventricular nucleus of the hypothalamus is involved in autonomic nervous system regulation as well as in HPA function, influencing brainstem autonomic control nuclei [122]. The hypothalamus in turn receives inputs from the limbic system, notably the central nucleus of the amygdala, which operates in close coordination with the prefrontal neocortex to integrate emotional and motivational behaviours [123]. A role for autonomic dysregulation in mediating associations between depression and CHD risk can, therefore, be postulated.

Three aspects of autonomic activity have been investigated: sympathoadrenal function, heart-rate levels and autonomic control processes governing cardiac

sympathovagal balance and baroreceptor reflex sensitivity. All have been implicated in CHD. Sympathoadrenal activation causes peripheral vasoconstriction
and increased haemodynamic load, which may promote disturbed blood flow
and endothelial sheer stress [124], which in turn increase local inflammation and
endothelial gene expression [125]. Elevated heart rate has been shown to predict
future CHD independently of standard cardiovascular risk factors in a number
of studies [126,127]. Autonomic cardiac control can be assessed both with simple
temporal measures, such as heart-rate variability, and with more elaborate power
spectrum analysis. Using the latter, high-frequency power is thought to indicate
parasympathetic or vagal tone, while low-frequency power probably reflects sympathovagal balance and baroreceptor reflex modulation of heart rate [128]. Low
levels of heart-rate variability and low parasympathetic tone predict future CHD in
apparently healthy individuals [129] and are strongly predictive of future morbidity
in patients following acute myocardial infarction [130].

The relationship between depression and sympathetic nervous system activity
indexed by measures such as plasma or urinary catecholamines has been studied
extensively in clinical cohorts but less extensively in population studies. Comparisons between clinically depressed patients and healthy individuals have shown elevated sympathetic nervous system activity [131,132], but such investigations have
difficulty controlling for factors such as smoking, body mass and physical activity,
which influence neuroendocrine function. Nevertheless, a recent investigation of
a population cohort of non-smoking healthy middle-aged women demonstrated
positive correlations between 24-hour urinary excretion of noradrenaline and both
depression and anxiety symptoms, after controlling for age, race and body mass
[133]. Sympathetic activation and reduced vagal tone are also known to reduce the
threshold for cardiac ventricular fibrillation and to stimulate ventricular arrhythmias [134]. However, such effects are unlikely to be involved in the association
between depression and the early aetiology and CHD, since they typically occur
among individuals who already have advanced coronary artery disease.

There is strong evidence from clinical studies that resting heart rate is higher in
depressed than non-depressed individuals without CHD [135–137]. Data concerning heart-rate variability and sympathovagal balance are more mixed. No association between heart-rate variability and depression has been observed in several
studies of depressed patients [137,138], while marginal differences have been shown
in others [135,136]. One group has found reduced cardiac baroreceptor reflex sensitivity in patients with treated depression [139], while another group showed that
cardiac baroreflex sensitivity was reduced only in depressed patients who were also
anxious [140]. Horsten *et al.* [141] described a population study of 300 healthy
women in whom the ratio of low- to high-frequency power in the 24-hour ECG
power spectrum was related negatively to depressive symptoms, but no differences

were found in four other spectral analytic measures. By contrast, a larger population study of 2627 postmenopausal women showed that on several different measures, heart-rate variability was reduced in those with depressive symptoms [142]. In CHD patients, depression has been associated with reduced heart-rate variability and baroreceptor reflex sensitivity in some studies [4,5] but not others [143]. The evidence relating sympathovagal balance, depression and CHD is, therefore, quite mixed. This mechanism has become increasingly difficult to study in clinical samples because of the widespread use of beta-blockade, and so the inconsistencies in the literature may be difficult to reconcile in the future.

Limitations to studies of mechanisms

The literature described in this section indicates that there is some evidence for inflammatory, haemostatic, neuroendocrine and autonomic mediators of the association between depression and CHD. However, the results at present have many limitations. Most studies have been cross-sectional, and it is not known whether these physiological mechanisms are pathways or correlates. Much of the work has been carried out with severely depressed patients and not representative samples from the population or the people with milder depressive symptoms shown to be at risk in observational studies. The extent to which mechanisms are related specifically to depression or are also implicated in the influence of anxiety and other psychosocial factors on CHD is not known. Nevertheless, there have been important findings that point to psychobiological mediators of at least part of the link of depression with CHD.

Conclusions

The consensus of longitudinal observational studies discussed in this chapter indicates that depression predicts future CHD in apparently healthy individuals, with some evidence of a relationship with symptom severity. It must be acknowledged that the results from different studies are quite variable. Considering that depression is often assessed on only a single occasion and that CHD is influenced by so many other factors, it is remarkable that positive associations have been recorded with any consistency at all. There is also reasonable evidence that other indicators of psychological distress are predictive of future disease, although again findings have been mixed. Given the present state of the evidence, it is prudent to conclude that depression does not have an exclusive association with CHD and that other manifestations of psychological distress may also be significant. It should be borne in mind that several other aspects of psychosocial adversity, including chronic work stress and social isolation, have been related prospectively with CHD [42,144].

The extent to which such effects are mediated through symptoms of psychological distress or are independent of affective state has not been clarified fully.

The time course of associations between depression or psychological distress and future CHD is understood poorly, due primarily to the use of single snapshots of psychological state. It could be that depression operates at several levels on aetiology, from the long-term development of atherosclerosis, through acceleration of disease development in more advanced cases, to acute triggering of plaque rupture and the development of acute coronary syndromes.

Depression and psychological distress appear to be associated with subclinical atherosclerosis, and not only with the clinical manifestations of disease. This is important, since it has implications for where the search for mediating mechanisms might be focused. However, the evidence to date is largely cross-sectional, and longitudinal studies of subclinical atherosclerosis are urgently required.

There is no dearth of candidate mechanisms that might translate depression into CHD risk, but convincing evidence is sparse. Studies are needed that decompose the depression–CHD link and compute the proportion of variance accounted for by different factors. A similar exercise has been conducted fruitfully in trying to understand the factors that contribute to the socioeconomic gradient in CHD. In a number of studies, between 45% and 60% of the social gradient in CHD has been accounted for by smoking, alcohol consumption, physical activity and body mass [145–147]. It is likely that both behavioural and psychobiological pathways are involved in the link with depression. But a striking feature of the studies of potential biological mediators that have been carried out to date is that evidence is stronger for their involvement in advanced CHD than in the early development of coronary atherosclerosis. Findings linking autonomic dysregulation or heightened vascular inflammatory markers with depression in younger individuals without apparent CHD are sparse. Impaired endothelial function may be a stronger candidate for involvement in the long-term influence of depression on disease risk, since it is an early event in atherosclerosis and can modify the association between risk factors and disease development [148]. Heightened sympathoadrenal activity may also be relevant from an early stage. However, perhaps we should not expect the association with any single potentially mediating mechanism to be very strong, since a combination of factors is most likely to be involved.

Acknowledgements

I am grateful to Emily Williams for helping to assemble the literature reviewed in this chapter, and to Amanda Nicholson for her helpful comments on the manuscript. This research was supported by the British Heart Foundation.

REFERENCES

1. C. B. Nemeroff, D. L. Musselman, Are platelets the link between depression and ischemic heart disease? *Am. Heart J.* **140** (2000), 57–62.

2. P.H. Black, L. D. Garbutt, Stress, inflammation and cardiovascular disease. *J. Psychosom. Res.* **52** (2002), 1–23.

3. S. Rajagopalan, R. Brook, M. Rubenfire, *et al.*, Abnormal brachial artery flow-mediated vasodilation in young adults with major depression. *Am. J. Cardiol.* **88** (2001), 196–8, A7.

4. L. L. Watkins, P. Grossman, Association of depressive symptoms with reduced baroreflex cardiac control in coronary artery disease. *Am. Heart J.* **137** (1999), 453–7.

5. R. M. Carney, J. A. Blumenthal, P. K. Stein, *et al.*, Depression, heart rate variability, and acute myocardial infarction. *Circulation* **104** (2001), 2024–8.

6. E. S. Brown, F. P. Varghese, B. S. McEwen, Association of depression with medical illness: does cortisol play a role? *Biol. Psychiatry* **55** (2004), 1–9.

7. A. Rosengren, S. Hawken, S. Ounpuu, *et al.*, Association of psychosocial risk factors with risk of acute myocardial infarction in 11119 cases and 13648 controls from 52 countries (the INTERHEART study): case–control study. *Lancet* **364** (2004), 953–62.

8. K. Davidson, B. S. Jonas, K. E. Dixon, J. H. Markovitz, Do depression symptoms predict early hypertension incidence in young adults in the CARDIA study? Coronary Artery Risk Development in Young Adults. *Arch. Intern. Med.* **160** (2000), 1495–500.

9. A. W. Zieske, G. T. Malcom, J. P. Strong, Natural history and risk factors of atherosclerosis in children and youth: the PDAY study. *Pediatr. Pathol. Mol. Med.* **21** (2002), 213–37.

10. R. Rugulies, Depression as a predictor for coronary heart disease: a review and meta-analysis. *Am. J. Prev. Med.* **23** (2002), 51–61.

11. H. S. Lett, J. A. Blumenthal, M. A. Babyak, *et al.*, Depression as a risk factor for coronary artery disease: evidence, mechanisms, and treatment. *Psychosom. Med.* **66** (2004), 305–15.

12. H. Hemingway, H. Kuper, M. Marmot, Psychosocial factors in the primary and secondary prevention of coronary heart disease: an updated systematic review of prospective cohort studies. In *Evidence-Based Cardiology*, 2nd edn, ed. S. Yusuf, J. A. Cairns, A. J. Camm, E. L. Fallen, B. J. Gersh (London: BMJ Books, 2003), pp. 181–218.

13. A. P. Haines, J. D. Imeson, T. W. Meade, Phobic anxiety and ischaemic heart disease. *Br. Med. J.* **295** (1987), 297–9.

14. C. F. Mendes de Leon, H. M. Krumholz, T. S. Seeman, *et al.*, Depression and risk of coronary heart disease in elderly men and women: New Haven EPESE, 1982–1991. Established Populations for the Epidemiologic Studies of the Elderly. *Arch. Intern. Med.* **158** (1998), 2341–8.

15. H. D. Sesso, I. Kawachi, P. S. Vokonas, D. Sparrow, Depression and the risk of coronary heart disease in the Normative Aging Study. *Am. J. Cardiol.* **82** (1998), 851–6.

16. R. Anda, D. Williamson, D. Jones, *et al.*, Depressed affect, hopelessness, and the risk of ischemic heart disease in a cohort of U.S. adults. *Epidemiology* **4** (1993), 285–94.

17. H. Luukinen, P. Laippala, H. V. Huikuri, Depressive symptoms and the risk of sudden cardiac death among the elderly. *Eur. Heart J.* **24** (2003), 2021–6.

18. C. Marzari, S. Maggi, E. Manzato, *et al.*, Depressive symptoms and development of coronary heart disease events: the Italian longitudinal study on aging. *J. Gerontol. A Biol. Sci. Med. Sci.* **60** (2005), 85–92.

19. J. P. Empana, D. H. Sykes, G. Luc, *et al.*, Contributions of depressive mood and circulating inflammatory markers to coronary heart disease in healthy European men: the Prospective Epidemiological Study of Myocardial Infarction (PRIME). *Circulation* **111** (2005), 2299–305.

20. A. A. Ariyo, M. Haan, C. M. Tangen, *et al.*, Depressive symptoms and risks of coronary heart disease and mortality in elderly Americans: Cardiovascular Health Study Collaborative Research Group. *Circulation* **102** (2000), 1773–9.

21. B. W. Penninx, J. M. Guralnik, C. F. Mendes, de Leon, *et al.*, Cardiovascular events and mortality in newly and chronically depressed persons > 70 years of age. *Am. J. Cardiol.* **81** (1998), 988–94.

22. B. W. Penninx, A. T. Beekman, A. Honig, *et al.*, Depression and cardiac mortality: results from a community-based longitudinal study. *Arch. Gen. Psychiatry* **58** (2001), 221–7.

23. S. Wassertheil-Smoller, W. B. Applegate, K. Berge, *et al.*, Change in depression as a precursor of cardiovascular events. SHEP Cooperative Research Group (Systolic Hypertension in the Elderly). *Arch. Intern. Med.* **156** (1996), 553–61.

24. S. Wassertheil-Smoller, S. Shumaker, J. Ockene, *et al.*, Depression and cardiovascular sequelae in postmenopausal women: the Women's Health Initiative (WHI). *Arch. Intern. Med.* **164** (2004), 289–98.

25. P. J. Rowan, D. Haas, J. A. Campbell, D. R. Maclean, K. W. Davidson, Depressive symptoms have an independent, gradient risk for coronary heart disease incidence in a random, population-based sample. *Ann. Epidemiol.* **15** (2005), 316–20.

26. A. Haines, J. Cooper, T. W. Meade, Psychological characteristics and fatal ischaemic heart disease. *Heart* **85** (2001), 385–9.

27. A. Aromaa, R. Raitasalo, A. Reunanen, *et al.*, Depression and cardiovascular diseases. *Acta Psychiatr. Scand. Suppl.* **377** (1994), 77–82.

28. D. E. Ford, L. A. Mead, P. P. Chang, *et al.*, Depression is a risk factor for coronary artery disease in men: the precursors study. *Arch Intern. Med.* **158** (1998), 1422–6.

29. L. A. Pratt, D. E. Ford, R. M. Crum, H. K. Armenian, J. J. Gallo, W. W. Eaton, Depression, psychotropic medication, and risk of myocardial infarction: prospective data from the Baltimore ECA follow-up. *Circulation* **94** (1996), 3123–9.

30. S. A. Everson, D. E. Goldberg, G. A. Kaplan, *et al.*, Hopelessness and risk of mortality and incidence of myocardial infarction and cancer. *Psychosom. Med.* **58** (1996), 113–21.

31. A. Appels, P. Mulder, Excess fatigue as a precursor of myocardial infarction. *Eur. Heart J.* **9** (1988), 758–64.

32. E. Prescott, C. Holst, M. Gronbaek, *et al.*, Vital exhaustion as a risk factor for ischaemic heart disease and all-cause mortality in a community sample: a prospective study of 4084 men and 5479 women in the Copenhagen City Heart Study. *Int. J. Epidemiol.* **32** (2003), 990–97.

33. B. Norton, L. J. Whalley, Mortality of a lithium-treated population. *Br. J. Psychiatry* **145** (1984), 277–82.

34. B. Ahrens, B. Muller-Oerlinghausen, M. Schou, *et al.*, Excess cardiovascular and suicide mortality of affective disorders may be reduced by lithium prophylaxis. *J. Affect. Disord.* **33** (1995), 67–75.

35. D. W. Black, G. Warrack, G. Winokur, Excess mortality among psychiatric patients: the Iowa Record-Linkage Study. *J. Am. Med. Assoc.* **253** (1985), 58–61.

36. J. M. Murphy, R. R. Monson, D. C. Olivier, A. M. Sobol, A. H. Leighton, Affective disorders and mortality: a general population study. *Arch. Gen. Psychiatry* **44** (1987), 473–80.

37. C. Allgulander, Suicide and mortality patterns in anxiety neurosis and depressive neurosis. *Arch. Gen. Psychiatry* **51** (1994), 708–12.

38. W. Coryell, C. Turvey, A. Leon, *et al.*, Persistence of depressive symptoms and cardiovascular death among patients with affective disorder. *Psychosom. Med.* **61** (1999), 755–61.

39. B. G. Druss, D. W. Bradford, R. A. Rosenheck, M. J. Radford, H. M. Krumholz, Mental disorders and use of cardiovascular procedures after myocardial infarction. *J. Am. Med. Assoc.* **283** (2000), 506–11.

40. J. Hippisley-Cox, M. Pringle, V. Hammersley, *et al.*, Antidepressants as risk factor for ischaemic heart disease: case–control study in primary care. *Br. Med. J.* **323** (2001), 666–9.

41. H. W. Cohen, G. Gibson, M. H. Alderman, Excess risk of myocardial infarction in patients treated with antidepressant medications: association with use of tricyclic agents. *Am. J. Med.* **108** (2000), 2–8.

42. S. A. Everson-Rose, T. T. Lewis, Psychological factors and cardiovascular diseases. *Annu. Rev. Public Health* **26** (2005), 469–500.

43. A. K. Ferketich, P. F. Binkley, Psychological distress and cardiovascular disease: results from the 2002 National Health Interview Survey. *Eur. Heart J.* **26** (2005), 1923–9.

44. S. A. Stansfeld, R. Fuhrer, M. J. Shipley, M. G. Marmot, Psychological distress as a risk factor for coronary heart disease in the Whitehall II study. *Int. J. Epidemiol.* **31** (2002), 248–55.

45. K. L. Robinson, J. McBeth, G. J. Macfarlane, Psychological distress and premature mortality in the general population: a prospective study. *Ann. Epidemiol.* **14** (2004), 467–72.

46. I. Kawachi, G. A. Colditz, A. Ascherio, *et al.*, Prospective study of phobic anxiety and risk of coronary heart disease in men. *Circulation* **89** (1994), 1992–7.

47. F. Rasul, S. A. Stansfeld, C. L. Hart, C. R. Gillis, G. D. Smith, Psychological distress, physical illness and mortality risk. *J. Psychosom. Res.* **57** (2004), 231–6.

48. C. M. Albert, C. U. Chae, K. M. Rexrode, J. E. Manson, I. Kawachi, Phobic anxiety and risk of coronary heart disease and sudden cardiac death among women. *Circulation* **111** (2005), 480–87.

49. F. Rasul, S. A. Stansfeld, C. L. Hart, G. Davey Smith, Psychological distress, physical illness, and risk of coronary heart disease. *J. Epidemiol. Community Health* **59** (2005), 140–45.

50. I. Kawachi, D. Sparrow, P. S. Vokonas, S. T. Weiss, Symptoms of anxiety and risk of coronary heart disease: the Normative Aging Study. *Circulation* **90** (1994), 2225–9.

51. H. Iso, C. Date, A. Yamamoto, *et al.*, Perceived mental stress and mortality from cardiovascular disease among Japanese men and women: the Japan Collaborative Cohort Study for Evaluation of Cancer Risk Sponsored by Monbusho (JACC Study). *Circulation* **106** (2002), 1229–36.

52. B. Ohlin, P. M. Nilsson, J. A. Nilsson, G. Berglund, Chronic psychosocial stress predicts long-term cardiovascular morbidity and mortality in middle-aged men. *Eur. Heart J.* **25** (2004), 867–73.

53. J. Macleod, Davey G. Smith, P. Heslop, *et al.*, Psychological stress and cardiovascular disease: empirical demonstration of bias in a prospective observational study of Scottish men. *Br. Med. J.* **324** (2002), 1247–51.

54. D. H. O'Leary, J. F. Polak, R. A. Kronmal, *et al.*, Carotid-artery intima and media thickness as a risk factor for myocardial infarction and stroke in older adults: Cardiovascular Health Study Collaborative Research Group. *N. Engl. J. Med.* **340** (1999), 14–22.

55. M. L. Bots, J. M. Dijk, A. Oren, D. E. Grobbee, Carotid intima-media thickness, arterial stiffness and risk of cardiovascular disease: current evidence. *J. Hypertens.* **20** (2002), 2317–25.

56. S. A. Everson, J. W. Lynch, M. A. Chesney, *et al.*, Interaction of workplace demands and cardiovascular reactivity in progression of carotid atherosclerosis: population based study. *Br. Med. J.* **314** (1997), 553–8.

57. M. Rosvall, P. O. Ostergren, B. Hedblad, *et al.*, Occupational status, educational level, and the prevalence of carotid atherosclerosis in a general population sample of middle-aged Swedish men and women: results from the Malmo Diet and Cancer Study. *Am. J. Epidemiol.* **152** (2000), 334–46.

58. J. R. Jennings, T. W. Kamarck, S. A. Everson-Rose, *et al.*, Exaggerated blood pressure responses during mental stress are prospectively related to enhanced carotid atherosclerosis in middle-aged Finnish men. *Circulation* **110** (2004), 2198–203.

59. D. J. Jones, J. T. Bromberger, K. Sutton-Tyrrell, K. A. Matthews, Lifetime history of depression and carotid atherosclerosis in middle-aged women. *Arch. Gen. Psychiatry* **60** (2003), 153–60.

60. D. C. Haas, K. W. Davidson, D. J. Schwartz, *et al.*, Depressive symptoms are independently predictive of carotid atherosclerosis. *Am. J. Cardiol.* **95** (2005), 547–50.

61. M. J. Pletcher, J. A. Tice, M. Pignone, W. S. Browner, Using the coronary artery calcium score to predict coronary heart disease events: a systematic review and meta-analysis. *Arch. Intern. Med.* **164** (2004), 1285–92.

62. O'Malley PG, D. L. Jones, I. M. Feuerstein, A. J. Taylor, Lack of correlation between psychological factors and subclinical coronary artery disease. *N. Engl. J. Med.* **343** (2000), 1298–304.

63. H. Tiemeier, W. van Dijck, A. Hofman, *et al.*, Relationship between atherosclerosis and late-life depression: the Rotterdam Study. *Arch. Gen. Psychiatry* **61** (2004), 369–76.

64. P. K. Agatisa, K. A. Matthews, J. T. Bromberger, *et al.*, Coronary and aortic calcification in women with a history of major depression. *Arch. Intern. Med.* **165** (2005), 1229–36.

65. S. Paterniti, M. Zureik, P. Ducimetiere, *et al.*, Sustained anxiety and 4-year progression of carotid atherosclerosis. *Arterioscler. Thromb. Vasc. Biol.* **21** (2001), 136–41.

66. B. Wolff, H. J. Grabe, H. Volzke, *et al.*, Relationship between psychological strain and carotid atherosclerosis in a general population. *Heart* **91** (2005), 460–64.

67. K. A. Matthews, J. F. Owens, L. H. Kuller, K. Sutton-Tyrrell, L. Jansen-McWilliams, Are hostility and anxiety associated with carotid atherosclerosis in healthy postmenopausal women? *Psychosom. Med.* **60** (1998), 633–8.

68. F. Lesperance, N. Frasure-Smith, M. Talajic, Major depression before and after myocardial infarction: its nature and consequences. *Psychosom. Med.* **58** (1996), 99–110.

69. C. M. Dickens, L. McGowan, C. Percival, *et al.*, Lack of a close confidant, but not depression, predicts further cardiac events after myocardial infarction. *Heart* **90** (2004), 518–22.

70. P. C. Strike, A. Steptoe, Behavioral and emotional triggers of acute coronary syndromes: a systematic review and critique. *Psychosom. Med.* **67** (2005), 179–86.

71. M. Naghavi, P. Libby, E. Falk, *et al.*, From vulnerable plaque to vulnerable patient: a call for new definitions and risk assessment strategies: part I. *Circulation* **108** (2003), 1664–72.

72. M. Maclure, M. A. Mittleman, Should we use a case-crossover design? *Ann. Rev. Public Health* **21** (2000), 193–221.

73. M. A. Mittleman, M. Maclure, J. B. Sherwood, *et al.*, Triggering of acute myocardial infarction onset by episodes of anger. *Circulation* **92** (1995), 1720–25.

74. S. N. Willich, M. Lewis, H. Lowel, *et al.*, Physical exertion as a trigger of acute myocardial infarction. *N. Engl. J. Med.* **329** (1993), 1684–90.

75. A. Steptoe, D. L. Whitehead, Depression, stress and coronary heart disease: the need for more complex models. *Heart* **91** (2005), 419–20.

76. A. K. Ferketich, J. A. Schwartzbaum, D. J. Frid, M. L. Moeschberger, Depression as an antecedent to heart disease among women and men in the NHANES I study. *Arch. Intern. Med.* **160** (2000), 1261–8.

77. S. A. Everson, G. A. Kaplan, D. E. Goldberg, J. T. Salonen, Hypertension incidence is predicted by high levels of hopelessness in Finnish men. *Hypertension* **35** (2000), 561–7.

78. R. Ross, Atherosclerosis: an inflammatory disease. *N. Engl. J. Med.* **340** (1999), 115–26.

79. M. J. Jarvisalo, A. Harmoinen, M. Hakanen, *et al.*, Elevated serum C-reactive protein levels and early arterial changes in healthy children. *Arterioscler. Thromb. Vasc. Biol.* **22** (2002), 1323–8.

80. O. T. Raitakari, M. Juonala, M. Kahonen, *et al.*, Cardiovascular risk factors in childhood and carotid artery intima-media thickness in adulthood: the Cardiovascular Risk in Young Finns Study. *J. Am. Med. Assoc.* **290** (2003), 2277–83.

81. W. E. Chrapko, P. Jurasz, M. W. Radomski, *et al.*, Decreased platelet nitric oxide synthase activity and plasma nitric oxide metabolites in major depressive disorder. *Biol. Psychiatry* **56** (2004), 129–34.

82. A. J. Broadley, A. Korszun, C. J. Jones, M. P. Frenneaux, Arterial endothelial function is impaired in treated depression. *Heart* **88** (2002), 521–3.

83. L. Ghiadoni, A. Donald, M. Cropley, *et al.*, Mental stress induces transient endothelial dysfunction in humans. *Circulation* **102** (2000), 2473–8.

84. M. Cesari, B. W. Penninx, A. B. Newman, *et al.*, Inflammatory markers and onset of cardiovascular events: results from the Health ABC study. *Circulation* **108** (2003), 2317–22.

85. L. Lind, Circulating markers of inflammation and atherosclerosis. *Atherosclerosis* **169** (2003), 203–14.

86. P. M. Ridker, C. H. Hennekens, J. E. Buring, N. Rifai, C-reactive protein and other markers of inflammation in the prediction of cardiovascular disease in women. *N. Engl. J. Med.* **342** (2000), 836–43.

87. G. E. Miller, C. A. Stetler, R. M. Carney, K. E. Freedland, W. A. Banks, Clinical depression and inflammatory risk markers for coronary heart disease. *Am. J. Cardiol.* **90** (2002), 1279–83.

88. E. C. Suarez, Joint effect of hostility and severity of depressive symptoms on plasma interleukin-6 concentration. *Psychosom. Med.* **65** (2003), 523–7.

89. A. N. Dentino, C. F. Pieper, M. K. Rao, *et al.*, Association of interleukin-6 and other biologic variables with depression in older people living in the community. *J. Am. Geriatr. Soc.* **47** (1999), 6–11.

90. B. W. Penninx, S. B. Kritchevsky, K. Yaffe, *et al.*, Inflammatory markers and depressed mood in older persons: results from the Health, Aging and Body Composition study. *Biol. Psychiatry* **54** (2003), 566–72.

91. D. B. Panagiotakos, C. Pitsavos, C. Chrysohoou, *et al.*, Inflammation, coagulation, and depressive symptomatology in cardiovascular disease-free people: the ATTICA study. *Eur. Heart J.* **25** (2004), 492–9.

92. W. J. Kop, J. S. Gottdiener, C. M. Tangen, *et al.*, Inflammation and coagulation factors in persons > 65 years of age with symptoms of depression but without evidence of myocardial ischemia. *Am. J. Cardiol.* **89** (2002), 419–24.

93. A. Steptoe, S. R. Kunz-Ebrecht, N. Owen, Lack of association between depressive symptoms and markers of immune and vascular inflammation in middle-aged men and women. *Psychol. Med.* **33** (2003), 667–74.

94. H. Tiemeier, A. Hofman, H. R. van Tuijl, *et al.*, Inflammatory proteins and depression in the elderly. *Epidemiology* **14** (2003), 103–7.

95. M. J. Davies, Stability and instability: two faces of coronary atherosclerosis. The Paul Dudley White Lecture 1995. *Circulation* **94** (1996), 2013–20.

96. W. Casscells, M. Naghavi, J. T. Willerson, Vulnerable atherosclerotic plaque: a multifocal disease. *Circulation* **107** (2003), 2072–5.

97. J. Danesh, R. Collins, R. Peto, G. D. Lowe, Haematocrit, viscosity, erythrocyte sedimentation rate: meta-analyses of prospective studies of coronary heart disease. *Eur. Heart J.* **21** (2000), 515–20.

98. J. Danesh, P. Whincup, M. Walker, *et al.*, Fibrin D-dimer and coronary heart disease: prospective study and meta-analysis. *Circulation* **103** (2001), 2323–7.

99. P. H. Whincup, J. Danesh, M. Walker, *et al.*, Von Willebrand factor and coronary heart disease: prospective study and meta-analysis. *Eur. Heart. J.* **23** (2002), 1764–70.

100. C. Monaco, A. Mathur, J. F. Martin, What causes acute coronary syndromes? Applying Koch's postulates. *Atherosclerosis* **179** (2005), 1–15.

101. R. von Kanel, P. J. Mills, C. Fainman, J. E. Dimsdale, Effects of psychological stress and psychiatric disorders on blood coagulation and fibrinolysis: a biobehavioral pathway to coronary artery disease? *Psychosom. Med.* **63** (2001), 531–44.

102. A. Steptoe, S. Kunz-Ebrecht, A. Rumley, G. D. Lowe, Prolonged elevations in haemostatic and rheological responses following psychological stress in low socioeconomic status men and women. *Thromb. Haemost.* **89** (2003), 83–90.

103. A. Steptoe, K. Magid, S. Edwards, *et al.*, The influence of psychological stress and socioeconomic status on platelet activation in men. *Atherosclerosis* **168** (2003), 57–63.

104. R. von Kanel, Platelet hyperactivity in clinical depression and the beneficial effect of antide-pressant drug treatment: how strong is the evidence? *Acta Psychiatr. Scand.* **110** (2004), 163–77.

105. R. von Kanel, J. E. Dimsdale, K. A. Adler, *et al.*, Effects of depressive symptoms and anxiety on hemostatic responses to acute mental stress and recovery in the elderly. *Psychiatry Res.* **126** (2004), 253–64.

106. T. Ljung, B. Andersson, B. A. Bengtsson, P. Bjorntorp, P. Marin, Inhibition of cortisol secretion by dexamethosone in relation to body fat distribution. *Obes. Res.* **4** (1996), 277–82.

107. R. Pasquali, B. Ambrosi, D. Armanini, *et al.*, Cortisol and ACTH response to oral dexametha-sone in obesity and effects of sex, body fat distribution, and dexamethasone concentrations: a dose–response study. *J. Clin. Endocrinol. Metab.* **87** (2002), 166–75.

108. V. Vicennati, R. Pasquali, Abnormalities of the hypothalamic-pituitary-adrenal axis in nondepressed women with abdominal obesity and relations with insulin resistance: evi-dence for a central and a peripheral alteration. *J. Clin. Endocrinol. Metab.* **85** (2000), 4093–8.

109. J. R. Seckl, N. M. Morton, K. E. Chapman, B. R. Walker, Glucocorticoids and 11beta-hydroxysteroid dehydrogenase in adipose tissue. *Recent Prog. Horm. Res.* **59** (2004), 359–93.

110. E. S. Epel, B. McEwen, T. Seeman, *et al.*, Stress and body shape: stress-induced cortisol secretion is consistently greater among women with central fat. *Psychosom. Med.* **62** (2000), 623–32.

111. A. Steptoe, S. R. Kunz-Ebrecht, L. Brydon, J. Wardle, Central adiposity and cortisol responses to waking in middle-aged men and women. *Int. J. Obes. Relat. Metab. Disord.* **28** (2004), 1168–73.

112. E. J. Brunner, H. Hemingway, B. R. Walker, *et al.*, Adrenocortical, autonomic, and inflamma-tory causes of the metabolic syndrome: nested case–control study. *Circulation* **106** (2002), 2659–65.

113. J. I. Hudson, M. S. Hudson, A. J. Rothschild, *et al.*, Abnormal results of dexamethasone suppression tests in nondepressed patients with diabetes mellitus. *Arch. Gen. Psychiatry* **41** (1984), 1086–9.

114. M. Roy, B. Collier, A. Roy, Hypothalamic-pituitary-adrenal axis dysregulation among dia-betic outpatients. *Psychiatry Res.* **31** (1990), 31–7.

115. R. Rosmond, S. Wallerius, P. Wanger, *et al.*, A 5-year follow-up study of disease incidence in men with an abnormal hormone pattern. *J. Intern. Med.* **254** (2003), 386–90.

116. D. I. Phillips, D. J. Barker, C. H. Fall, *et al.*, Elevated plasma cortisol concentrations: a link between low birth weight and the insulin resistance syndrome? *J. Clin. Endocrinol. Metab.* **83** (1998), 757–60.

117. H. W. Cohen, S. Madhavan, M. H. Alderman, History of treatment for depression: risk factor for myocardial infarction in hypertensive patients. *Psychosom. Med.* **63** (2001), 203–9.

118. D. A. Lawlor, G. D. Smith, S. Ebrahim, Association of insulin resistance with depression: cross sectional findings from the British Women's Heart and Health Study. *Br. Med. J.* **327** (2003), 1383–4.

119. B. A. Golomb, L. Tenkanen, T. Alikoski, *et al.*, Insulin sensitivity markers: predictors of accidents and suicides in Helsinki Heart Study screenees. *J. Clin. Epidemiol.* **55** (2002), 767–73.

120. S. A. Everson-Rose, P. M. Meyer, L. H. Powell, *et al.*, Depressive symptoms, insulin resistance, and risk of diabetes in women at midlife. *Diabetes Care* **27** (2004), 2856–62.

121. M. Timonen, M. Laakso, J. Jokelainen, *et al.*, Insulin resistance and depression: cross sectional study. *Br. Med. J.* **330** (2005), 17–18.

122. A. J. Dunn, A. H. Swiergiel, V. Palamarchouk, Brain circuits involved in corticotropin-releasing factor–norepinephrine interactions during stress. *Ann. N. Y. Acad. Sci.* **1018** (2004), 25–34.

123. W. R. Lovallo *Stress and Health: Biological and Psychological Interactions*, 2nd edn. (Thousand Oaks, CA: Sage, 2004).

124. M. A. Gimbrone, Jr, J. N. Topper, T. Nagel, K. R. Anderson, G. Garcia-Cardena, Endothelial dysfunction, hemodynamic forces, and atherogenesis. *Ann. N. Y. Acad. Sci.* **902** (2000), 230–39.

125. C. Cheng, R. de Crom, R. van Haperen, *et al.*, The role of shear stress in atherosclerosis: action through gene expression and inflammation? *Cell Biochem. Biophys.* **41** (2004), 279–94.

126. A. R. Dyer, V. Persky, J. Stamler, *et al.*, Heart rate as a prognostic factor for coronary heart disease and mortality: findings in three Chicago epidemiologic studies. *Am. J. Epidemiol.* **112** (1980), 736–49.

127. W. B. Kannel, C. Kannel, R. S. Paffenbarger, Jr, L. A. Cupples, Heart rate and cardiovascular mortality: the Framingham Study. *Am. Heart J.* **113** (1987), 1489–94.

128. M. P. Frenneaux, Autonomic changes in patients with heart failure and in post-myocardial infarction patients. *Heart* **90** (2004), 1248–55.

129. D. Liao, J. Cai, W. D. Rosamond, *et al.*, Cardiac autonomic function and incident coronary heart disease: a population-based case–cohort study. *Am. J. Epidemiol.* **145** (1997), 696–706.

130. M. T. La Rovere, J. T. Bigger, Jr, F. I. Marcus, A. Mortara, P. J. Schwartz, Baroreflex sensitivity and heart-rate variability in prediction of total cardiac mortality after myocardial infarction. *Lancet* **351** (1998), 478–84.

131. C. R. Lake, D. Pickar, M. G. Ziegler, *et al.*, High plasma norepinephrine levels in patients with major affective disorder. *Am. J. Psychiatry* **139** (1982), 1315–18.

132. R. C. Veith, N. Lewis, O. A. Linares, *et al.*, Sympathetic nervous system activity in major depression. Basal and desipramine-induced alterations in plasma norepinephrine kinetics. *Arch. Gen. Psychiatry* **51** (1994), 411–22.

133. J. W. Hughes, L. Watkins, J. A. Blumenthal, C. Kuhn, A. Sherwood, Depression and anxiety symptoms are related to increased 24-hour urinary norepinephrine excretion among healthy middle-aged women. *J. Psychosom. Res.* **57** (2004), 353–8.

134. I. T. Meredith, A. Broughton, G. L. Jennings, M. D. Esler, Evidence of a selective increase in cardiac sympathetic activity in patients with sustained ventricular arrhythmias. *N. Engl. J. Med.* **325** (1991), 618–24.

135. M. Moser, M. Lehofer, R. Hoehn-Saric, *et al.*, Increased heart rate in depressed subjects in spite of unchanged autonomic balance? *J. Affect. Disord.* **48** (1998), 115–24.

136. M. W. Agelink, C. Boz, H. Ullrich, J. Andrich, Relationship between major depression and heart rate variability: clinical consequences and implications for antidepressive treatment. *Psychiatry Res.* **113** (2002), 139–49.

137. A. C. Volkers, J. H. Tulen, W. W. van den Broek, *et al.*, Motor activity and autonomic cardiac functioning in major depressive disorder. *J. Affect. Disord.* **76** (2003), 23–30.

138. V. K. Yeragani, R. Pohl, R. Balon, *et al.*, Heart rate variability in patients with major depression. *Psychiatry Res.* **37** (1991), 35–46.

139. A. J. Broadley, M. P. Frenneaux, V. Moskvina, C. J. H. Jones, A. Korszun, Baroreflex sensitivity is reduced in depression. *Psychosom. Med.* **67** (2005), 648–51.

140. L. L. Watkins, P. Grossman, R. Krishnan, J. A. Blumenthal, Anxiety reduces baroreflex cardiac control in older adults with major depression. *Psychosom. Med.* **61** (1999), 334–40.

141. M. Horsten, M. Ericson, A. Perski, *et al.*, Psychosocial factors and heart rate variability in healthy women. *Psychosom. Med.* **61** (1999), 49–57.

142. C. K. Kim, S. P. McGorray, B. A. Bartholomew, *et al.*, Depressive symptoms and heart rate variability in postmenopausal women. *Arch. Intern. Med.* **165** (2005), 1239–44.

143. A. Gehi, D. Mangano, S. Pipkin, W. S. Browner, M. A. Whooley, Depression and heart rate variability in patients with stable coronary heart disease: findings from the Heart and Soul Study. *Arch. Gen. Psychiatry* **62** (2005), 661–6.

144. H. Hemingway, M. Marmot, Evidence based cardiology: psychosocial factors in the aetiology and prognosis of coronary heart disease – systematic review of prospective cohort studies. *Br. Med. J.* **318** (1999), 1460–67.

145. J. W. Lynch, G. A. Kaplan, R. D. Cohen, J. Tuomilehto, J. Salonen, Do cardiovascular risk factors explain the relation between socio-economic status, risk of all-cause mortality, cardiovascular mortality, and acute myocardial infarction? *Am. J. Epidemiol.* **144** (1996), 934–42.

146. F. J. Van Lenthe, E. Gevers, I. M. Joung, H. Bosma, J. P. Mackenbach, Material and behavioral factors in the explanation of educational differences in incidence of acute myocardial infarction: the Globe study. *Ann. Epidemiol.* **12** (2002), 535–42.

147. S. P. Wamala, M. A. Mittleman, K. Schenck-Gustafsson, K. Orth-Gomer, Potential explanations for the educational gradient in coronary heart disease: a population-based case–control study of Swedish women. *Am. J. Public Health* **89** (1999), 315–21.

148. M. Juonala, J. S. Viikari, T. Laitinen, *et al.*, Interrelations between brachial endothelial function and carotid intima-media thickness in young adults: the Cardiovascular Risk in Young Finns Study. *Circulation* **110** (2004), 2918–23.

149. A. M. Ostfeld, B. Z. Lebovits, R. B. Shekelle, O. Paul, A prospective study of the relationship between personality and coronary heart disease. *J. Chronic Dis.* **17** (1964), 265–76.

150. T. Hallstrom, L. Lapidus, C. Bengtsson, K. Edstrom, Psychosocial factors and risk of ischaemic heart disease and death in women: a twelve-year follow-up of participants in the population study of women in Gothenburg, Sweden. *J. Psychosom. Res.* **30** (1986), 451–9.

151. J. C. Barefoot, M. Schroll, Symptoms of depression, acute myocardial infarction, and total mortality in a community sample. *Circulation* **93** (1996), 1976–80.

152. S. W. Schwartz, J. Cornoni-Huntley, S. R. Cole, *et al.*, Are sleep complaints an independent risk factor for myocardial infarction? *Ann. Epidemiol.* **8** (1998), 384–92.

153. M. A. Whooley, W. S. Browner, Association between depressive symptoms and mortality in older women. *Arch. Intern. Med.* **158** (1998), 2129–35.

154. S. R. Cole, I. Kawachi, H. D. Sesso, R. S. Paffenbarger, I. M. Lee, Sense of exhaustion and coronary heart disease among college alumni. *Am. J. Cardiol.* **84** (1999), 1401–5.

155. M. Chang, R. A. Hahn, S. M. Teutsch, L. C. Hutwagner, Multiple risk factors and population attributable risk for ischemic heart disease mortality in the United States, 1971–1992. *J. Clin. Epidemiol.* **54** (2001), 634–44.

156. N. Yasuda, Y. Mino, S. Koda, H. Ohara, The differential influence of distinct clusters of psychiatric symptoms, as assessed by the general health questionnaire, on cause of death in older persons living in a rural community of Japan. *J. Am. Geriatr. Soc.* **50** (2002), 313–20.

157. S. A. Everson-Rose, J. S. House, R. P. Mero, Depressive symptoms and mortality risk in a national sample: confounding effects of health status. *Psychosom. Med.* **66** (2004), 823–30.

158. B. B. Gump, K. A. Matthews, L. E. Eberly, Y. F. Chang, Depressive symptoms and mortality in men: results from the Multiple Risk Factor Intervention Trial. *Stroke* **36** (2005), 98–102.

159. E. D. Eaker, J. Pinsky, W. P. Castelli, Myocardial infarction and coronary death among women: psychosocial predictors from a 20-year follow-up of women in the Framingham Study. *Am. J. Epidemiol.* **135** (1992), 854–64.

160. L. D. Kubzansky, I. Kawachi, A. Spiro, *et al.*, Is worrying bad for your heart? A prospective study of worry and coronary heart disease in the Normative Aging Study. *Circulation* **95** (1997), 818–24.

4

Depression and prognosis in cardiac patients

Heather S. Lett, Andrew Sherwood, Lana Watkins
and James A. Blumenthal

Coronary heart disease (CHD) is the leading cause of death in the USA and Europe [1,2]. In roughly half the cases, the first clinical manifestations of CHD – myocardial infarction (MI) or sudden death – are catastrophic. These events are sudden, unexpected and unpredictable. The economic cost of CHD is growing. For example, in the USA over $130 billion is spent on CHD each year in direct medical costs, disability payments and lost productivity [2]. Moreover, traditional risk factors such as cigarette smoking, hyperlipidaemia and hypertension do not account fully for the timing and occurrence of these events.

Depression is also a major health problem. It is associated with significant impairment of function, which may, at times, be worse than that of chronic medical disorders [3]. Depressive symptoms have been correlated with the presence of one or more chronic diseases [4,5], as well as inability to work [6], days in bed or days away from normal activities [4], increased mortality risk [7], increased use of medical services [8], and decreased wellbeing and lowered functioning [3]. Major depressive disorder (MDD) is the most prevalent of all psychiatric disorders, affecting up to 25% of women and 12% of men during their lifetime [9]. Since 1950, the prevalence of depression has increased significantly [10].

Depression is disproportionately prevalent among cardiac patients, with estimates of MDD of about 15% in patients following acute myocardial infarction (AMI) or coronary artery bypass graft (CABG), and an additional 20% with either minor depression or elevated levels of depressive symptoms as measured by questionnaires such as the Beck Depression Inventory (BDI) [11–17]. In addition, evidence has suggested that depression is a significant and independent risk factor for patients with CHD and may also be associated with increased 'cardiovascular vulnerability', a term that has been used to describe patients susceptible to acute coronary events based upon plaque, blood or myocardial characteristics [18,19]. Based on this evidence, there has been a great deal of interest into potential

Depression and Physical Illness, ed. A. Steptoe.
Published by Cambridge University Press. © Cambridge University Press 2006.

Table 4.1 Studies assessing the effect of depression on outcomes in coronary heart disease (CHD) Samples

Author	N/# events	Patients	Follow-up	Endpoint(s)	Adjusted RR
Carney et al. [27]	52/22 cardiac events	CHD	12 months	Cardiac event	RR = 2.2
Frasure-Smith et al. [145]	222/12 deaths	MI	6 months	Cardiac mortality	DIS : HR = 4.29
Frasure-Smith et al. [105]	222/21 deaths		18 months		DIS NS; BDI OR = 6.64
Frasure-Smith et al. [20]	896/39 deaths	MI	1 year	Cardiac mortality	Men OR = 3.05, women OR = 3.29
Lesperance et al. [146]	896/155 deaths		5 year		HR = 3.13–3.17
Lane et al. [22]	288/25 deaths	MI	4 months	Mortality	NS
Lane et al. [23]	288/28 deaths		1 year	Mortality	NS
Lane et al. [24]	288/31 deaths			CHD events	NS
Lane et al. [25]	288/38 deaths		3 years	Mortality	NS
Ahern et al. [147]	265/NA	MI	Varying	Mortality, cardiac arrest	RR = 1.38
Jenkinson et al. [148]	1376/247 deaths	MI	3 years	Mortality	NS
Ladwig et al. [149]	560/12 deaths, 17 arrythmic events	MI	6 months	Cardiac mortality Arrhythmic event	NS
Welin et al. [49]	275/167 deaths	MI	10 years	Cardiac mortality	RR = 3.16
Bush et al. [150]	144/17 deaths	MI	4 months	Mortality	RR = 3.5
Kaufmann et al. [151]	331/15 deaths	MI	6 months	Mortality	NS p = 0.04 (effect size not reported)
	331/33 deaths		12 months		

Study	Sample/events	Population	Follow-up	Outcome	Result
Irvine et al. [152]	318/number of events not reported	MI	2 years	Sudden cardiac death	RR = 2.45
Strik et al. [153]	318/25 cardiac events	MI	Mean 3.4 years	Mortality or reinfarction	HR = 2.32
Strik et al. [154]	206/16 events	MI	3 years	Mortality or AMI	NS
Horsten et al. [155]	292/81 deaths	Acute CHD event (MI or angina)	5 years	Mortality or cardiac event	RR = 1.9
Lesperance et al. [156]	430/16 deaths, 28 events	Unstable angina	1 year	Cardiac mortality or AMI	OR = 6.73
Connerney et al. [29]	309/8 deaths, 42 events	CABG	1 year	Cardiac event, mortality	Cardiac events, RR = 2.3; mortality NS; BDI = NS
Baker et al. [30]	158/6 deaths	CABG	Median 24 months	Mortality	OR = 6.24
Saur et al. [31]	416/NA	CABG	1 year	Mortality	NS
Blumenthal et al. [37]	817/122 deaths	CABG	Mean 5.2 years	Mortality	Moderate to severe depression, HR = 2.84; persistent depression, HR = 2.33
Burg et al. [36]	89/7 deaths	CABG	2 years	Cardiac mortality	OR = 23.16

BDI, Beck Depression Inventory; DIS, Diagnostic Interview Schedule; HR, hazard ratio; MI, myocardial infarction; NS, non-significant; OR, odds ratio; RR, relative risk.

Reprinted from Psychosom. Med. **66** (2004), 305–15, with permission from Lippincott Williams & Wilkins.

treatments for depression in cardiac patients, with the hope that successful mental health treatment might also have a favourable impact on cardiovascular and physical health outcomes (see Chapter 5). An understanding of the mechanisms underlying the relationship between depression and CHD will likely help to guide the most effective interventions. This chapter describes the evidence that depression is a risk factor in patients with established CHD and suggests potential mechanisms underlying the relationship between depression and adverse outcomes.

Depression and CHD outcomes

In this chapter, we focus on evidence that depression in patients with existing CHD poses a risk for increased morbidity and mortality. There is also evidence that depression is a primary risk factor for the onset of CHD in initially healthy patients. This research is summarised by Steptoe in Chapter 3. Studies providing the best evidence for depression as a secondary risk factor assess patients with existing CHD for depression and follow them over time in order to assess the extent to which depression predicts clinical outcomes over and above any association with other CHD risk factors such as disease severity and demographic risk factors. Such studies have been conducted in several CHD populations, including patients recovering from AMI, patients with stable CHD and patients awaiting CABG surgery. The design and results of these studies have been described previously by our group, and an updated summary is presented in Table 4.1 [11]. Studies that assessed the unique role of depression in predicting 'hard' endpoints such as death or reinfarction were included. Conclusions are drawn with particular emphasis placed on well-designed studies with adequate assessment of depression and sufficient statistical power.

The majority of the studies reporting a risk associated with depression have been conducted using patients hospitalised for MI. Most of these studies have reported large effect sizes, comparable to or greater in magnitude than traditional risk factors, suggesting that the presence of depression confers about 2.5 times the risk for mortality or non-fatal cardiac events. For example, Frasure-Smith et al. [20] followed 896 patients with a recent AMI for one year. The presence of elevated depressive symptoms on the BDI was a significant predictor of cardiac mortality after controlling for other multivariate predictors of mortality. Carney et al. [21] examined the effect of depression on prognosis in 358 depressed MI patients from the Enhancing Recovery in Clinical Heart Disease (ENRICHD) clinical trial and 408 non-depressed (BDI < 10) controls who met the ENRICHD medical inclusion criteria. There were 47 (6.1%) deaths and 57 (7.4%) non-fatal MIs over a follow-up period of up to 2.5 years. After adjusting for other risk factors, depressed patients had more than twice the risk for all-cause mortality compared with non-depressed patients, an effect that was not evident until more than six months after MI.

Although there have been some null findings for MI patients, most have been from small studies with methodological limitations such as limited follow-up or inadequate assessment of depression [14]. For example, in a series of studies assessing the relation of depression to outcome in 288 AMI patients at varying follow-up times, Lane et al. [22–25] reported that depression (assessed by the BDI) was not related to cardiac or all-cause mortality at 4 months', 1 year's or 3 years' follow-up; nor was it related to cardiac events at one year. However, a notable limitation of this series of studies is the small sample size and event rate, which can yield highly unstable estimates [26].

Studies of patients with stable CHD have reported significant associations of depression and clinical outcomes. Carney et al. [27] followed 52 patients for 12 months after catheterisation and found that a diagnosis of MDD was associated with more than twice the risk of having a cardiac event, even after controlling for other risk factors. Barefoot et al. [28] assessed 1250 patients with documented CHD using the Zung self-report depression scale at the time of diagnostic coronary angiography and followed patients for up to 19.4 years. Results showed that patients with moderate to severe depression were at 69% greater risk for cardiac death and 78% greater risk for all-cause death [28].

CABG surgery is a common surgical intervention for CHD patients. Depression rates are known to be particularly high in CABG patients, both before and immediately after surgery [29–35]. There has been an increase in studies assessing the possibility that CABG patients with depression incur an increased risk; however, to date there are relatively few prospective studies of this type [29–31,36,37]. Connerney et al. [29] followed 309 CABG patients for one year after surgery. Compared with non-depressed patients, depressed patients, as assessed by the Diagnostic Interview Schedule (DIS), were more than twice as likely to have a cardiac event within 12 months after surgery but were not at higher risk for mortality within the first year. In a more recent report from Duke University Medical Center [37], the effect of depression on mortality after CABG surgery was assessed in 817 patients followed for up to 12 years (mean = 5.2 years). On the day before surgery, the Center for Epidemiologic Studies Depression (CES-D) questionnaire [38] was used to categorise patients as having no depression (CES-D < 16), mild depression (CES-D = 16–26) or moderate to severe depression (CES-D $\geq$ 27). Results indicated that moderate to severe depression was independently associated with a two- to three-fold increased risk of mortality even after statistically controlling for age, gender, number of grafts, diabetes, smoking, left ventricular ejection fraction and history of AMI. Figure 4.1 depicts the unadjusted Kaplan–Meier survival curves for patients with no depression, mild depression and moderate to severe depression. Furthermore, as displayed in Figure 4.2, it was observed that even mild depression (CES-D > 16) that persisted for at least six months following CABG was associated with increased risk.

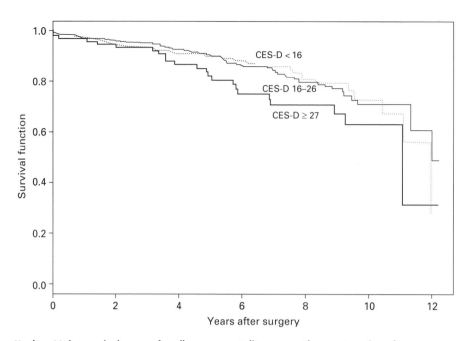

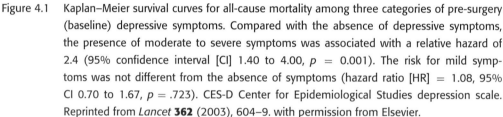

Figure 4.1   Kaplan–Meier survival curves for all-cause mortality among three categories of pre-surgery (baseline) depressive symptoms. Compared with the absence of depressive symptoms, the presence of moderate to severe symptoms was associated with a relative hazard of 2.4 (95% confidence interval [CI] 1.40 to 4.00, p = 0.001). The risk for mild symptoms was not different from the absence of symptoms (hazard ratio [HR] = 1.08, 95% CI 0.70 to 1.67, p = .723). CES-D Center for Epidemiological Studies depression scale. Reprinted from *Lancet* **362** (2003), 604–9. with permission from Elsevier.

Women are at increased risk after AMI [39] and CABG surgery [29,40,41] and are more likely to experience depression [35,42–44]. Therefore, researchers have theorised that elevated rates of depression may be responsible for the increased risk in women. However, evidence thus far has not provided support for this hypothesis. It is more likely that increased medical comorbidities might place women at greater risk for depression and adverse clinical outcomes, such as decreased functionality, older age at the time of surgery [44], increased angina, more severe hypertension and diabetes [45,46] and smaller coronary artery diameter [41,47]. Frasure-Smith *et al.* [20] investigated the possibility that the increased risk for women is due to higher rates of depression or gender differences in the impact of depression on clinical events, but they failed to find any evidence in support of these possibilities.

Depression is associated with several related psychosocial risk factors that have also been related to CHD outcomes such as negative affect, vital exhaustion [48], decreased social support [49,50], personality factors [51,52], anger expression [53], hostility [54], negative emotions [55,56] and anxiety [57]. The possibility that

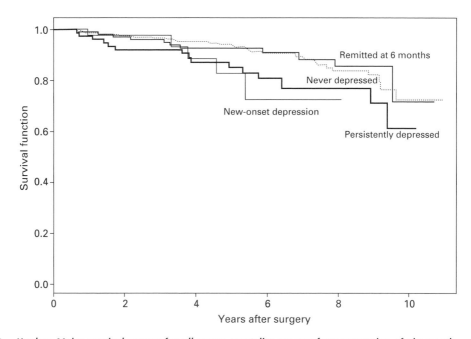

Figure 4.2   Kaplan–Meier survival curves for all-cause mortality among four categories of six-month course of depression. Using patients who were never depressed as the reference, the hazard ratio (HR) of persistent depression was 2.2 (95% confidence interval [CI] = 1.2 to 4.2, $p = 0.015$), the HR for new-onset depression was 2.2 (95% CI 0.8 to 5.8, $p = 0.121$) and the HR for remitted depression was 1.0 (95% CI 0.5 to 2.0, $p = 0.954$). Reprinted from *Lancet* **362** (2003), 604–9, with permission from Elsevier.

depression is also predictive of outcome via its association with these risk factors has been considered and is a source of controversy in the field today. For example, Denollet *et al.* [51,58] considered type D personality, defined as high negative affectivity and high social inhibition and marked by symptoms of depression, low emotional expression and low perceived social support. In a representative study [58], type D personality was assessed in patients (268 men, 35 women) with a recent coronary event. At five-year follow-up, type D personality was a significant predictor of all-cause mortality. Depression was a significant univariate predictor of mortality, but it was no longer associated with mortality when type D was added to the model. In a similar manner, Dickens *et al.* [50] provided preliminary evidence that social isolation, but not depression, uniquely predicts outcome for post-AMI patients. They reported that lack of a close confidant, but not a composite measure of depression and anxiety retrospectively reported for the week before AMI, was related to outcome. On the other hand, Frasure-Smith and Lesperance [56] compared measures of depression, anxiety, self-reported health, anger, stress, perceived social support and number of close friends and relatives in predicting mortality after

AMI. Exploratory factors analysis suggested that the various questionnaires tapped the underlying constructs of overt anger, social support and negative affect. Of these factors, only negative affect was uniquely predictive of outcome. Although few studies have conducted a comprehensive comparison of related psychosocial constructs, the majority that are available suggest that depression and negative affect are the factors that emerge as most predictive of increased risk [55].

Another controversy centres around the possibility that depression is merely a marker for disease severity, which ultimately is responsible for increased risk. In the studies presented in Table 4.1, the association between depression and measures of disease severity of risk is statistically controlled for in order to account for this possibility. However, as noted by Stewart *et al.* [59] and Lane *et al.* [60], it is almost impossible to statistically control for all measures of disease severity, risking the possibility of inflated estimates of association between depression and outcome. On the other hand, one must strike a balance with the possibility of overadjusting by including variables in the model that may mediate the relationship between depression and outcome. As shown in Table 4.1, the results of the majority of the well-designed studies suggest that depression confers a unique risk above and beyond any association with disease severity. In addition, studies thus far indicate that the cognitive and affective components of depression, rather than the somatic components, are associated most with increased risk for morbidity and mortality [56,61]. Thus, there is ample evidence that clinical depression is associated with risk for mortality and morbidity for patients with varying manifestations of CHD. Additionally, in a comprehensive review, Davidson *et al.* [12] noted that even minor elevations in depressive symptoms significantly increase the risk of CHD in healthy individuals and worsen the prognosis in patients with established CHD.

Biobehavioural mechanisms

A number of biobehavioural mechanisms have been hypothesised to underlie the relationship between depression and CHD. Thus far, most evidence for mechanisms comes from cross-sectional studies and prospective studies that track depression, the hypothesised mechanism, and CHD outcomes over time are needed to provide more conclusive support. Nonetheless, there is evidence that depression is associated with traditional risk factors for CHD such as hypertension, diabetes and insulin resistance [62,63] and markers of cardiac risk such as platelet activity [64], dysregulation of the autonomic nervous system [65,66], endothelial dysfunction, and alterations in the immune response/inflammation [67]. Depression is also associated with behavioural factors that are in turn associated with CHD risk, such as treatment adherence [68], smoking [69], heavy alcohol use and physical inactivity [70].

Traditional risk factors

Several risk factors for CHD, such as obesity, diabetes, hypertension and hyperlipidaemia, tend to occur together. Together, these risk factors have been described as the 'metabolic syndrome', which has been shown to contribute to the progression of CHD [71–73]. Diabetes and obesity in particular have been linked to depression [62,63], suggesting that they may link depression to adverse outcomes.

Platelet activity

Numerous pathological and clinical studies have shown that increased platelet activation plays a key role in the pathogenesis of CHD and acute coronary syndromes [74]. Furthermore, prospective data document a direct relationship between blood platelet concentration and aggregability and the long-term incidence of fatal CHD events in apparently healthy men [75]. Thus, it is no surprise that antiplatelet therapy with aspirin and thienopyridines has become the foundation for the treatment and prevention of CHD [76].

Several studies have demonstrated that platelet activation is increased in patients suffering from MDD [64,67,77], and it has been proposed that this phenomenon may be responsible for the increased risk of cardiovascular morbidity and mortality in depressed populations [78,79]. The role of serotonin in both platelet function [80] and depression [81] also provides suggestive evidence linking platelet activity and depression. Patients with MDD have been shown to exhibit alterations in multiple platelet parameters, including increases in serotonin receptor binding sites, glycoprotein 2B/3A and P-selectin receptors, as well as heightened levels of beta-thromboglobulin and platelet factor 4, which correspond with increased platelet activity [82]. Indeed, serotonin itself has been implicated as a significant contributor to the pathogenesis of acute coronary events and the conversion of chronic stable angina into an unstable coronary syndrome [83]. In animal models of CHD and endothelial injury, serotonin receptor antagonists provided potent protection against repetitive platelet aggregation even in the face of high levels of circulating catecholamines [83]. Thus, evidence suggests that platelet activity is likely to be a mechanism linking depression and CHD outcomes, a possibility warranting further research.

Autonomic nervous system functioning

Several measures of autonomic nervous system (ANS) functioning have been implicated in both CHD and MDD, including hypothalamic-pituitary-adrenocortical (HPA) axis functioning, baroreflex activity and heart-rate variability (HRV).

HPA axis functioning

Evidence that depressed patients often exhibit higher basal cortisol levels [66,84] and non-suppression of endogenous cortisol secretion following dexamethasone administration provides an overall picture of HPA axis hyperactivity in depression [85,86]. However, other research highlights the variability in HPA axis functioning in depressed samples, suggesting that HPA axis functioning in depression is better described as dysregulated [66,87,88]. HPA axis dysregulation is related to cardiovascular disease risk factors such as truncal obesity, hypercholesterolaemia, hypertriglyceridaemia, increased blood pressure and elevated heart rate [89,90].

Heart-rate variability

Reduced 24-hour HRV independently predicts mortality in patients with stable CHD [91] with a recent AMI [92] or with heart failure [93]. In each of these patient populations, depression is prevalent and is associated with abnormally low HRV, suggesting that low HRV may be involved in the increased risk of mortality in depressed cardiac patients [94–98]. In support of this notion, Carney *et al.* [99] found that including HRV as a co-variate in a model predicting depression-related risk for all-cause mortality significantly reduces the hazard ratio in AMI patients. This finding provides further evidence that low 24-hour HRV is involved in the relationship between depression and increased risk of mortality in cardiac patients.

Baroreceptor-mediated heart-rate control

Baroreceptor-mediated heart-rate control (BRC) provides a measure of the capacity of the vagus to modulate heart rate in response to blood-pressure changes and is an independent marker of mortality and of life-threatening ventricular arrhythmias [100–103]. Because BRC provides an index of myocardial stability, it may be particularly useful as a marker of vulnerable myocardium in depressed CHD patients. For example, CHD patients undergoing electrophysiological evaluation for arrhythmias and who report depressive symptoms exhibited a substantially higher mortality rate (75%) when compared with the overall mortality rate for the patient sample (14.5%) [104]. Similar findings were reported by Frasure-Smith and colleagues [105], who showed that AMI patients with both symptoms of depression and frequent premature ventricular contractions were at substantially greater risk of cardiac mortality compared with patients with symptoms of depression and without frequent premature beats.

Endothelial dysfunction

Endothelial dysfunction plays a vital role in the development, progression and clinical manifestations of atherosclerosis [106,107]. It has been related to a wide range of cardiovascular risk factors in both adults and children [108,109]. The clinical utility of peripheral vascular endothelial dysfunction assessment has been supported by the results of several prospective studies. Neunteufl *et al.* [110] studied 73 patients with angina undergoing cardiac catheterisation and found brachial artery flow-mediated dilation (FMD) to be an independent predictor of cardiovascular events, including death and MI, over a five-year follow-up period. Heitzer *et al.* [111] found that brachial artery assessment of endothelial dysfunction predicted cardio-vascular events (death, MI, stroke, coronary revascularisation) over a 4.5-year mean follow-up period in 281 patients with CHD. Perticone *et al.* [112] observed similar prediction of events in 225 untreated hypertensive patients over a two- to three-year follow-up period. Gokce *et al.* [113] found blunted FMD to be a predictor of events, including death, MI, unstable angina and ischaemic ventricular fibrillation during 30 days following vascular surgery in 187 patients with peripheral vascular disease. Although more prospective studies are needed [114], the emerging evidence has led to the suggestion that endothelial dysfunction provides a combined genetic/environmental 'barometer' of cardiovascular risk that has hitherto proven difficult to quantify by traditional risk assessment models [115].

Clinical depression and depressive symptoms may also convey CHD risk in part due to impairment of endothelial function. In a study reported by Rajagopalan and colleagues [116], FMD was significantly lower in 15 men and women diagnosed with MDD compared with 15 healthy controls. Similarly, Broadley *et al.* [117] observed impaired FMD in 12 patients who had been diagnosed with major depression compared with 10 healthy controls. Interestingly, in the latter study the patients had been treated successfully using a variety of antidepressant medications, suggesting that improvements in depressive symptomatology per se may not be a sufficient basis for ameliorating cardiovascular risk associated with depression. In the only other study of depression reported to date, Harris *et al.* [118] found depressive symptoms to be related inversely to FMD in a sample of healthy postmenopausal women.

Inflammation

A large body of experimental and clinical evidence suggests that inflammation plays a central role in the development and progression of atherosclerotic heart disease. C-reactive protein (CRP), an acute-phase reactant produced primarily in hepatocytes, is a highly sensitive marker of underlying systemic inflammation [119]. An elevated level of CRP is an independent risk factor for AMI and stroke, with some research showing that it may be a better predictor of a first cardiovascular event than low-density lipoprotein (LDL) cholesterol [120]. Several theories have been advanced to explain this relationship between elevated CRP levels and cardiovascular morbidity. Increased levels of CRP reflect low-grade inflammation in visceral adipose tissue and may simply be a marker for the dyslipidaemia and insulin resistance associated with the metabolic syndrome. Alternatively, increased levels of CRP may reflect a state of vascular or endothelial inflammation, which may predispose to atherogenesis and plaque rupture [121].

Several cross-sectional studies have demonstrated increased levels of CRP and other inflammatory markers in patients with depression [67,122,123] and with other CHD risk factors, such as the metabolic syndrome [124,125]. In an analysis of data describing 6914 men and women between the ages of 18 and 39 years from the National Health and Nutrition Examination Survey (NHANES) III, a history of MDD was associated strongly with elevated CRP. This association was present even after adjusting for potential confounders; it was strongest in men with recent or recurrent episodes of depression. However, there was no significant association between CRP and depression in women [126]. Depressed mood has also been associated with elevated levels of inflammatory markers in cohorts of elderly subjects. In the Health, Aging, and Body Composition study of well-functioning older people of 70–79 years of age, interleukin (IL)-6, tumor necrosis factor alpha (TNFα) and CRP were higher in individuals with depressed mood than in non-depressed individuals [127]. Similarly, in a subset of individuals aged 60 years or older from the Rotterdam study, IL-6 and CRP were higher in depressed people than in controls, although the findings for CRP were not significant after adjusting for confounding factors [128]. When considered in aggregate, these observational studies suggest that depression is characterised by elevated levels of CRP and other inflammatory markers. Whether depression causes elevated CRP or an inflammatory state causes the depression, or whether both depression and elevated CRP are due to an independent disease process, is unclear.

Behavioural and lifestyle risk factors

Many studies have shown that depression predicts poor adherence to prescribed regimens. In a meta-analysis, DiMatteo *et al.* [129] concluded that depressed patients are more than twice as likely to not adhere to prescribed therapies [68,130–132]. Non-adherence to recommended medication regimens and lifestyle changes is associated with decreased survival for CHD patients [133–135], suggesting that adherence may be a mechanism linking depression and CHD outcomes.

Smoking, very high levels of alcohol consumption and physical inactivity are important risk factors for CHD and are often targets for its prevention and treatment [136]. Depression is associated with increased rates of smoking [69] and appears to contribute to failure to adhere to smoking-cessation programmes [137]. Depression is also associated with increased alcohol use and physical inactivity [70]. Cross-sectional and longitudinal studies have shown that active individuals are less likely to be depressed and that inactive individuals who become active are at decreased risk for depression [70,138–144]. Furthermore, there is evidence that depression may potentiate other risk factors. Panagiotakos *et al.* [139] demonstrated that depression, especially when accompanied by alcohol use, physical inactivity and/or smoking, was associated with increased risk for the development of CHD.

Conclusions

There is considerable evidence that depression in CHD patients is associated with increased risk for cardiac morbidity and morbidity. However, as summarised by Carney and Freedland in Chapter 5, treatments thus far have been only moderately successful in improving depression in this population and have been largely unsuccessful in improving cardiac outcomes. Therefore, identifying effective treatments has become a priority.

A greater understanding of mechanisms linking depression and increased risk should guide selection of treatments and will provide the best chance of improving both depression and cardiac risk. Mechanisms for which promising evidence exists include traditional risk factors such as obesity, hypertension, diabetes and insulin resistance, markers of cardiac risk such as platelet activity, dysregulation of the autonomic nervous system, endothelial dysfunction and inflammation, and behavioural and lifestyle factors. Research on patient-treatment match is also likely to improve treatment efficacy. Ultimately, it may be possible to identify patients based on demographic, disease and psychological characteristics that are most likely to respond to particular treatments. Although it is not possible at this point to recommend any treatment for depression over another to reduce cardiac risk, depression is common in this population and certainly warrants treatment to improve quality of life.

REFERENCES

1. M. Rayner, S. Petersen, *European Cardiovascular Disease Statistics* (London: British Heart Foundation, 2000).
2. American Heart Association. *Heart Disease and Stroke Statistics: 2004 Update* (Dallas, TX; American Heart Association, 2003).
3. K. B. Wells, A. Stewart, R. D. Hays, *et al.*, The functioning and well-being of depressed patients: results from the Medical Outcomes Study. *J. Am. Med. Assoc.* **262** (1989), 914–19.
4. S. Murrell, S. Himmelfarb, K. Wright, Prevalence of depression and its correlates in older adults. *Am. J. Epidemiol.* **117** (1983), 173.
5. J. J. Schwab, N. D. Traven, G. J. Warheit, Relationships between physical and mental illness. *Psychosomatics* **19** (1978), 458–63.
6. S. Borson, R. A. Barnes, Symptomatic depression in elderly medical outpatients: I. Prevalence, demography, and health service utilization. *J. Am. Geriatr. Soc.* **34** (1986), 341–7.

7. B. W. Rovner, P. S. German, L. J. Brant, *et al.*, Depression and mortality in nursing homes. *J. Am. Med. Assoc.* **265** (1991), 993–6.

8. J. Johnson, M. M. Weissman, G. L. Klerman, Service utilization and social morbidity associated with depressive symptoms in the community. *J. Am. Med. Assoc.* **267** (1992), 1478–83.

9. R. C. Kessler, K. A. McGonagle, C. B. Nelson, *et al.*, Sex and depression in the National Comorbidity Survey: II. Cohort effects. *J. Affect. Disord.* **30** (1994), 15–26.

10. G. L. Klerman, M. M. Weissman, Increasing rates of depression. *J. Am. Med. Assoc.* **261** (1989), 2229–35.

11. H. Lett, J. Blumenthal, M. Babyak, *et al.*, Depression as a risk factor for coronary artery disease: evidence, mechanisms, and treatment. *Psychosom. Med.* **66** (2004), 305–15.

12. K. W. Davidson, N. Rieckman, F. Lesperance, Psychological theories of depression: potential application for the prevention of acute coronary syndrome recurrence. *Psychosom. Med.* **66** (2004), 165–73.

13. J. C. Barefoot, Depression and coronary heart disease. *Cardiologia* **42** (1997), 1245–50.

14. R. M. Carney, K. E. Freedland, Y. I. Sheline, E. S. Weiss, Depression and coronary heart disease: a review for cardiologists. *Clin. Cardiol.* **20** (1997), 196–200.

15. K. B. King, Psychologic and social aspects of cardiovascular disease. *Ann. Behav. Med.* **19** (1997), 264–70.

16. D. L. Musselman, D. L. Evans, C. B. Nemeroff, The relationship of depression to cardiovascular disease: epidemiology, biology, and treatment. *Arch. Gen. Psychiatry* **55** (1998), 580–92.

17. A. Rozanski, J. A. Blumenthal, J. Kaplan, Impact of psychological factors on the pathogenesis of cardiovascular disease and implications for therapy. *Circulation* **99** (1999), 2192–217.

18. M. Naghavi, P. Libby, E. Falk, *et al.*, From vulnerable plaque to vulnerable patient: a call for new definitions and risk assessment strategies: part I. *Circulation* **108** (2003), 1664–72.

19. M. Naghavi, P. Libby, E. Falk, *et al.*, From vulnerable plaque to vulnerable patient: a call for new definitions and risk assessment strategies: Part II. *Circulation* **108** (2003), 1772–8.

20. N. Frasure-Smith, F. Lesperance, M. Juneau, M. Talajic, M. G. Bourassa, Gender, depression, and one-year prognosis after myocardial infarction. *Psychosom. Med.* **61** (1999), 26–37.

21. R. M. Carney, J. A. Blumenthal, D. Catellier, *et al.*, Depression as a risk factor for mortality after acute myocardial infarction. *Am. J. Cardiol.* **92** (2003), 1277–81.

22. D. Lane, D. Carroll, C. Ring, D. G. Beevers, G. Y. Lip, Effects of depression and anxiety on mortality and quality-of-life 4 months after myocardial infarction. *J. Psychosom. Res.* **49** (2000), 229–38.

23. D. Lane, D. Carroll, C. Ring, D. G. Beevers, G. Y. Lip, Do depression and anxiety predict recurrent coronary events 12 months after myocardial infarction? *Q. J. Med.* **93** (2000), 739–44.

24. D. Lane, D. Carroll, C. Ring, D. G. Beevers, G. Y. Lip, Mortality and quality of life 12 months after myocardial infarction: effects of depression and anxiety. *Psychosom. Med.* **63** (2001), 221–30.

25. D. Lane, D. Carroll, C. Ring, D. G. Beevers, G. Y. Lip, In-hospital symptoms of depression do not predict mortality 3 years after myocardial infarction. *Int. J. Epidemiol.* **31** (2002), 1179–82.

26. P. Peduzzi, J. Concato, A. R. Feinstein, T. R. Holford, Importance of events per independent variable in proportional hazards regression analysis: II. Accuracy and precision of regression estimates. *J. Clin. Epidemiol.* **48** (1995), 1503–10.

27. R. M. Carney, M. W. Rich, K. E. Freedland, *et al.*, Major depressive disorder predicts cardiac events in patients with coronary artery disease. *Psychosom. Med.* **50** (1988), 627–33.

28. J. C. Barefoot, M. J. Helms, D. B. Mark, *et al.*, Depression and long-term mortality risk in patients with coronary artery disease. *Am. J. Cardiol.* **78** (1996), 613–17.

29. I. Connerney, P. A. Shapiro, J. S. McLaughlin, E. Bagiella, R. P. Sloan, Relation between depression after coronary artery bypass surgery and 12-month outcome: a prospective study. *Lancet* **358** (2001), 1766–71.

30. R. A. Baker, M. J. Andrew, G. Schrader, J. L. Knight, Preoperative depression and mortality in coronary artery bypass surgery: preliminary findings. *Aust. N. Z. J. Surg.* **71** (2001), 139–42.

31. C. D. Saur, B. B. Granger, L. H. Muhlbaier, *et al.*, Depressive symptoms and outcome of coronary artery bypass grafting. *Am. J. Crit. Care* **10** (2001), 4–10.

32. M. J. Underwood, R. K. Firmin, D. Jehu, Aspects of psychological and social morbidity in patients awaiting coronary artery bypass grafting. *Br. Heart. J.* **69** (1993), 382–4.

33. G. M. McKhann, L. M. Borowicz, M. A. Goldsborough, C. Enger, O. A. Selnes, Depression and cognitive decline after coronary artery bypass grafting. *Lancet* **349** (1997), 1282–4.

34. N. Timberlake, L. Klinger, P. Smith, *et al.*, Incidence and patterns of depression following coronary artery bypass graft surgery. *J. Psychosom. Res.* **43** (1997), 197–207.

35. E. J. Burker, J. A. Blumenthal, M. Feldman, *et al.*, Depression in male and female patients undergoing cardiac surgery. *Br. J. Clin. Psychol.* **34** (1995), 119–28.

36. M. M. Burg, C. Benedetto, R. Soufer, Depressive symptoms and mortality two years after coronary artery bypass graft surgery (CABG) in men. *Psychosom. Med.* **65** (2003), 508–10.

37. J. A. Blumenthal, H. Lett, M. Babyak, *et al.*, Depression as a risk factor for mortality after coronary artery bypass surgery. *Lancet* **362** (2003), 604–9.

38. M. Hautzinger, The CES-D scale: a depression-rating scale for research in the general population. *Diagnostica* **34** (1988), 167–73.

39. V. Vaccarino, H. M. Krumholz, J. Yarzebski, J. M. Gore, R. J. Goldberg, Sex differences in 2-year mortality after hospital discharge for myocardial infarction. *Ann. Intern. Med.* **134** (2001), 173–81.

40. R. V. Milani, C. J. Lavie, M. M. Cassidy, Effects of cardiac rehabilitation and exercise training programs on depression in patients after major coronary events 8. *Am. Heart J.* **132** (1996), 726–32.

41. G. T. O'Connor, J. R. Morton, M. J. Diehl, *et al.*, Differences between men and women in hospital mortality associated with coronary artery bypass graft surgery: the Northern New England Cardiovascular Disease Study Group. *Circulation* **88** (1993), 1–10.

42. A. L. Ai, C. Peterson, R. E. Dunkle, *et al.*, How gender affects psychological adjustment one year after coronary artery bypass graft surgery. *Women Health* **26** (1997), 45–65.

43. A. H. Con, W. Linden, J. M. Thompson, A. Ignaszewski, The psychology of men and women recovering from coronary artery bypass surgery. *J. Cardpulm. Rehabil.* **19** (1999), 152–61.

44. S. M. Czajkowski, M. Terrin, R. Lindquist, *et al.*, Comparison of preoperative characteristics of men and women undergoing coronary artery bypass grafting (the Post

Coronary Artery Bypass Graft [CABG] Biobehavioral Study). *Am. J. Cardiol.* **79** (1997), 1017–24.

45. E. D. Eaker, Psychosocial risk factors for coronary heart disease in women. *Cardiol. Clin.* **16** (1998), 103–11.

46. J. Z. Ayanian, E. Guadagnoli, P. D. Cleary, Physical and psychosocial functioning of women and men after coronary artery bypass surgery. *J. Am. Med. Assoc.* **274** (1995), 1767–70.

47. N. J. O'Connor, J. R. Morton, J. D. Birkmeyer, *et al.*, Effect of coronary artery diameter in patients undergoing coronary bypass surgery: Northern New England Cardiovascular Disease Study Group. *Circulation* **93** (1996), 652–5.

48. W. J. Kop, A. P. Appels, C. F. Mendes de Leon, H. B. de Swart, F. W. Bar, Vital exhaustion predicts new cardiac events after successful coronary angioplasty. *Psychosom. Med.* **56** (1994), 281–7.

49. C. Welin, G. Lappas, L. Wilhelmsen, Independent importance of psychosocial factors for prognosis after myocardial infarction. *J. Intern. Med.* **247** (2000), 629–39.

50. C. M. Dickens, L. McGowan, C. Percival, *et al.*, Lack of a close confidant, but not depression, predicts further cardiac events after myocardial infarction. *Heart* **90** (2004), 518–22.

51. J. Denollet, D. L. Brutsaert, Personality, disease severity, and the risk of long-term cardiac events in patients with a decreased ejection fraction after myocardial infarction. *Circulation* **97** (1998), 167–73.

52. I. Kawachi, D. Sparrow, L. D. Kubzansky, *et al.*, Prospective study of a self-report type A scale and risk of coronary heart disease: test of the MMPI-2 type A scale. *Circulation* **98** (1998), 405–12.

53. P. Angerer, U. Siebert, W. Kothny, *et al.*, Impact of social support, cynical hostility and anger expression on progression of coronary atherosclerosis. *J. Am. Coll. Cardiol.* **36** (2000), 1781–8.

54. L. A. Chaput, S. H. Adams, J. A. Simon, *et al.*, Hostility predicts recurrent events among postmenopausal women with coronary heart disease. *Am. J. Epidemiol.* **156** (2002), 1092–9.

55. L. D. Kubzansky, I. Kawachi, Going to the heart of the matter: do negative emotions cause coronary heart disease? *J. Psychosom. Res.* **48** (2000), 323–37.

56. N. Frasure-Smith, F. Lesperance, Depression and other psychological risks following myocardial infarction. *Arch. Gen. Psychiatry* **60** (2003), 627–36.

57. N. Frasure-Smith, F. Lesperance, M. Talajic, The impact of negative emotions on prognosis following myocardial infarction: is it more than depression? *Health Psychol.* **14** (1995), 388–98.

58. J. Denollet, J. Vaes, D. L. Brutsaert, Inadequate response to treatment in coronary heart disease: adverse effects of type D personality and younger age on 5-year prognosis and quality of life. *Circulation* **102** (2000), 630–35.

59. R. A. Stewart, F. M. North, T. M. West, *et al.*, Depression and cardiovascular morbidity and mortality: cause or consequence? *Eur. Heart J.* **24** (2003), 2027–37.

60. D. Lane, D. Carroll, G. Y. Lip, Anxiety, depression, and prognosis after myocardial infarction: is there a causal association? *J. Am. Coll. Cardiol.* **42** (2003), 1808–10.

61. J. C. Barefoot, B. H. Brummett, M. J. Helms, *et al.*, Depressive symptoms and survival of patients with coronary artery disease. *Psychosom. Med.* **62** (2000), 790–95.

62. R. J. Anderson, K. E. Freedland, R. E. Clouse, P. J. Lustman, The prevalence of comorbid depression in adults with diabetes: a meta-analysis. *Diabetes Care* **24** (2001), 1069–78.

63. J. H. Thakore, P. J. Richards, R. H. Reznek, A. Martin, T. G. Dinan, Increased intra-abdominal fat deposition in patients with major depressive illness as measured by computed tomography. *Biol. Psychiatry* **41** (1997), 1140–42.

64. D. L. Musselman, A. Tomer, A. K. Manatunga, *et al.*, Exaggerated platelet reactivity in major depression. *Am. J. Psychiatry* **153** (1996), 1313–17.

65. P. L. Delgado, F. A. Moreno, Role of norepinephrine in depression. *J. Clin. Psychiatry* **61** (2000), 5–12.

66. H. Akil, R. F. Haskett, E. A. Young, *et al.*, Multiple HPA profiles in endogenous depression: effect of age and sex on cortisol and beta-endorphin. *Biol. Psychiatry* **33** (1993), 73–85.

67. W. J. Kop, J. S. Gottdiener, C. M. Tangen, *et al.*, Inflammation and coagulation factors in persons > 65 years of age with symptoms of depression but without evidence of myocardial ischemia. *Am. J. Cardiol.* **89** (2002), 419–24.

68. R. M. Carney, K. E. Freedland, S. A. Eisen, M. W. Rich, A. S. Jaffe, Major depression and medication adherence in elderly patients with coronary artery disease. *Health Psychol.* **14** (1995), 88–90.

69. S. Lehto, H. Koukkunen, J. Hintikka, *et al.*, Depression after coronary heart disease events. *Scand. Cardiovasc. J.* **34** (2000), 580–83.

70. T. C. Camacho, R. E. Roberts, N. B. Lazarus, G. A. Kaplan, R. D. Cohen, Physical activity and depression: evidence from the Alameda County Study. *Am. J. Epidemiol.* **134** (1991), 220–31.

71. J. E. Roeters van Lennep, H. T. Westerveld, D. W. Erkelens, E. E. van der Wall, Risk factors for coronary heart disease: implications of gender. *Cardiovasc. Res.* **53** (2002), 538–49.

72. S. V. Rao, M. Donahue, F. X. Pi-Sunyer, V. Fuster, Results of expert meetings: obesity and cardiovascular disease – obesity as a risk factor in coronary artery disease. *Am. Heart J.* **142** (2001), 1102–7.

73. D. L. Sprecher, G. L. Pearce, How deadly is the 'deadly quartet'? A post-CABG evaluation. *J. Am. Coll. Cardiol.* **36** (2000), 1159–65.

74. C. Patrono, G. Renda, Platelet activation and inhibition in unstable coronary syndromes. *Am. J. Cardiol.* **80** (1997), 17–20E.

75. E. Thaulow, J. Erikssen, L. Sandvik, H. Stormorken, P. F. Cohn, Blood platelet count and function are related to total and cardiovascular death in apparently healthy men. *Circulation* **84** (1991), 613–17.

76. R. J. Gibbons, J. Abrams, K. Chatterjee, *et al.*, ACC/AHA 2002 guideline update for the management of patients with chronic stable angina: a report of the American College of Cardiology/American Heart Association Task Force on practice guidelines (Committee on the Mangament of Patients With Chronic Stable Angina). www.acc.org/clinical/guidelines/unstable/incorporated/index.htm.

77. F. Laghrissi-Thode, W. R. Wagner, B. G. Pollock, P. C. Johnson, M. S. Finkel, Elevated platelet factor 4 and beta-thromboglobulin plasma levels in depressed patients with ischemic heart disease. *Biol. Psychiatry* **42** (1997), 290–95.

78. V. L. Serebruany, P. A. Gurbel, C. M. O'Connor, Platelet inhibition by sertraline and *N*-desmethylsertraline: a possible missing link between depression, coronary events, and mortality benefits of selective serotonin reuptake inhibitors. *Pharmacol. Res.* **43** (2001), 453–62.

79. V. L. Serebruany, C. M. O'Connor, P. A. Gurbel, Effect of selective serotonin reuptake inhibitors on platelets in patients with coronary artery disease. *Am. J. Cardiol.* **87** (2001), 1398–400.

80. F. De Clerck, Effects of serotonin on platelets and blood vessels. *J. Cardiovasc. Pharmacol.* **17**: Suppl 5 (1991)

81. M. J. Owens, C. B. Nemeroff, Role of serotonin in the pathophysiology of depression: focus on the serotonin transporter. *Clin. Chem.* **40** (1994), 288–95.

82. P. Hrdina, D. Bakish, A. Ravindran, Platelet serotonergin indices in major depression: up-regulation of 5-HT2A receptors unchanged by antidepressant treatment. *Psychiatry Res.* **66** (1997), 73–85.

83. J. T. Willerson, J. F. Eidt, J. McNatt, *et al.*, Role of thromboxane and serotonin as mediators in the development of spontaneous alterations in coronary blood flow and neointimal proliferation in canine models with chronic coronary artery stenoses and endothelial injury. *J. Am. Coll. Cardiol.* **17**: Suppl (1991), 110B.

84. K. P. Lesch, G. Laux, H. M. Schulte, H. Pfuller, H. Beckmann, Corticotropin and cortisol response to human CRH as a probe for HPA system integrity in major depressive disorder. *Psychiatry Res.* **24** (1988), 25–34.

85. U. Ehlert, J. Gaab, M. Heinrichs, Psychoneuroendocrinological contributions to the etiology of depression, posttraumatic stress disorder, and stress-related bodily disorders: the role of the hypothalamus-pituitary-adrenal axis. *Biol. Psychol.* **57** (2001), 141–52.

86. P. W. Gold, F. K. Goodwin, G. P. Chrousos, Clinical and biochemical manifestations of depression. Relation to the neurobiology of stress (2). *N. Engl. J. Med.* **319** (1988), 413–20.

87. P. W. Gold, J. Licinio, M. L. Wong, G. P. Chrousos, Corticotropin releasing hormone in the pathophysiology of melancholic and atypical depression and in the mechanism of action of antidepressant drugs. *Ann. N. Y. Acad. Sci.* **771** (1995), 716–29.

88. J. W. Kasckow, D. Baker, T. D. Geracioti, Jr, Corticotropin-releasing hormone in depression and post-traumatic stress disorder. *Peptides* **22** (2001), 845–51.

89. R. Rosmond, P. Bjorntorp, The hypothalamic-pituitary-adrenal axis activity as a predictor of cardiovascular disease, type 2 diabetes and stroke. *J. Intern. Med.* **247** (2000), 188–97.

90. E. Agabiti-Rosei, C. Alicandri, M. Beschi, *et al.*, Relationships between plasma catecholamines, renin, age and blood pressure in essential hypertension. *Cardiology* **70** (1983), 308–16.

91. M. W. Rich, J. S. Saini, R. E. Kleiger, *et al.*, Correlation of heart rate variability with clinical and angiographic variables and late mortality after coronary angiography. *Am. J. Cardiol.* **62** (1988), 1–7.

92. R. E. Kleiger, J. P. Miller, J. T. Bigger, Jr, A. J. Moss, Decreased heart rate variability and its association with increased mortality after acute myocardial infarction. *Am. J. Cardiol.* **59** (1987), 256–62.

93. J. Nolan, P. D. Batin, R. Andrews, *et al.*, Prospective study of heart rate variability and mortality in chronic heart failure: results of the United Kingdom heart failure evaluation and assessment of risk trial (UK-heart). *Circulation* **98** (1998), 1510–16.

94. R. M. Carney, M. W. Rich, A. Tevelde, *et al.*, Major depressive disorder in coronary artery disease. *Am. J. Cardiol.* **60** (1987), 1273–5.

95. R. M. Carney, R. D. Saunders, K. E. Freedland, *et al.*, Association of depression with reduced heart rate variability in coronary artery disease. *Am. J. Cardiol.* **76** (1995), 562–4.

96. R. M. Carney, J. A. Blumenthal, P. K. Stein, *et al.*, Depression, heart rate variability, and acute myocardial infarction. *Circulation* **104** (2001), 2024–8.

97. G. Casolo, E. Balli, T. Taddei, J. Amuhasi, C. Gori, Decreased spontaneous heart rate variability in congestive heart failure. *Am. J. Cardiol.* **64** (1989), 1162–7.

98. E. P. Havranek, M. G. Ware, B. D. Lowes, Prevalence of depression in congestive heart failure. *Am. J. Cardiol.* **84** (1999), 348–50.

99. R. A. Carney, J. A. Blumenthal, K. E. Freedland, *et al.*, Low heart rate variability and the effect of depression on post-myocardial infarction mortality. *Arch. Intern. Med.* **165** (2005), 1486–91.

100. M. T. La Rovere, C. Bersano, M. Gnemmi, G. Specchia, P. J. Schwartz, Exercise-induced increase in baroreflex sensitivity predicts improved prognosis after myocardial infarction. *Circulation* **106** (2002), 945–9.

101. S. H. Hohnloser, T. Klingenheben, L. A. van de, *et al.*, Reflex versus tonic vagal activity as a prognostic parameter in patients with sustained ventricular tachycardia or ventricular fibrillation. *Circulation* **89** (1994), 1068–73.

102. G. M. De Ferrari, M. Landolina, M. Mantica, *et al.*, Baroreflex sensitivity, but not heart rate variability, is reduced in patients with life-threatening ventricular arrhythmias long after myocardial infarction. *Am. Heart J.* **130** (1995), 473-80.

103. G. E. Billman, P. J. Schwartz, H. L. Stone, Baroreceptor reflex control of heart rate: a predictor of sudden cardiac death. *Circulation* **66** (1982), 874–80.

104. G. J. Kennedy, M. A. Hofer, D. Cohen, R. Shindledecker, J. D. Fisher, Significance of depression and cognitive impairment in patients undergoing programed stimulation of cardiac arrhythmias. *Psychosom. Med.* **49** (1987), 410–21.

105. N. Frasure-Smith, F. Lesperance, M. Talajic, Depression and 18-month prognosis after myocardial infarction. *Circulation* **91** (1995), 999–1005.

106. G. Brevetti, A. Silvestro, V. Schiano, M. Chiariello, Endothelial dysfunction and cardiovascular risk prediction in peripheral arterial disease: additive value of flow-mediated dilation to ankle-brachial pressure index. *Circulation* **108** (2003), 2093–8.

107. P. O. Bonetti, L. O. Lerman, A. Lerman, Endothelial dysfunction: a marker of atherosclerotic risk. *Arterioscler., Thromb. Vasc. Biol.* **23** (2003), 168–75.

108. D. S. Celermajer, K. E. Sorensen, V. M. Gooch, *et al.*, Non-invasive detection of endothelial dysfunction in children and adults at risk of atherosclerosis. *Lancet* **340** (1992), 1111–15.

109. D. S. Celermajer, K. E. Sorensen, C. Bull, J. Robinson, J. E. Deanfield, Endothelium-dependent dilation in the systemic arteries of asymptomatic subjects relates to coronary risk factors and their interaction. *J. Am. Coll. Cardiol.* **24** (1994), 1468–74.

110. T. Neunteufl, S. Heher, R. Katzenschlager, *et al.*, Late prognostic value of flow-mediated dilation in the brachial artery of patients with chest pain. *Am. J. Cardiol.* **86** (2000), 207–10.

111. T. Heitzer, T. Schlinzig, K. Krohn, T. Meinertz, T. Munzel, Endothelial dysfunction, oxidative stress, and risk of cardiovascular events in patients with coronary artery disease. *Circulation* **104** (2001), 2673–8.

112. F. Perticone, R. Ceravolo, A. Pujia, *et al.*, Prognostic significance of endothelial dysfunction in hypertensive patients. *Circulation* **104** (2001), 191–6.

113. N. Gokce, J. F. Keaney, J., L. M. Hunter, *et al.*, Predictive value of noninvasively determined endothelial dysfunction for long-term cardiovascular events in patients with peripheral vascular disease. *J. Am. Coll. Cardiol.* **41** (2003), 1769–75.

114. G. B. Mancini, Vascular structure versus function: is endothelial dysfunction of independent prognostic importance or not? *J. Am. Coll. Cardiol.* **43** (2004), 624–8.

115. J. A. Vita, J. F. Keaney, Jr, Endothelial function: a barometer for cardiovascular risk? *Circulation* **106** (2002), 640–42.

116. S. Rajagopalan, R. Brook, M. Rubenfire, *et al.*, Abnormal brachial artery flow-mediated vasodilation in young adults with major depression. *Am. J. Cardiol.* **88** (2001), 196–8.

117. A. J. Broadley, A. Korszun, C. J. Jones, M. P. Frenneaux, Arterial endothelial function is impaired in treated depression. *Heart* **88** (2002), 521–3.

118. K. F. Harris, K. A. Matthews, K. Sutton-Tyrrell, L. H. Kuller, Associations between psychological traits and endothelial function in postmenopausal women. *Psychosom. Med.* **65** (2003), 402–9.

119. M. B. Pepys, G. M. Hirschfield, C-reactive protein: a critical update. *J. Clin. Invest.* **111** (2003), 1805–12.

120. P. M. Ridker, N. Rifai, L. Rose, J. E. Buring, N. R. Cook, Comparison of C-reactive protein and low-density lipoprotein cholesterol levels in the prediction of first cardiovascular events. *N. Engl. J. Med.* **347** (2002), 1557–65.

121. A. R. Tall, C-reactive protein reassessed. *N. Engl. J. Med.* **350** (2004), 1450–52.

122. M. Maes, W. J. Stevens, L. S. Declerck, *et al.*, Significantly increased expression of T-cell activation markers (interleukin-2 and HLA-DR) in depression: further evidence for an inflammatory process during that illness. *Prog. Neuropsychopharmacol. Biol. Psychiatry* **17** (1993), 241–55.

123. A. Appels, F. W. Bar, J. Bar, C. Bruggeman, M. de Baets, Inflammation, depressive symptomtology, and coronary artery disease. *Psychosom. Med.* **62** (2000), 601–5.

124. S. M. Haffner, Metabolic syndrome, diabetes and coronary heart disease. *Int. J. Clin. Pract. Suppl.* (2002) 31–7.

125. M. Frohlich, A. Imhof, G. Berg, *et al.*, Association between C-reactive protein and features of the metabolic syndrome: a population-based study. *Diabetes Care* **23** (2000), 1835–9.

126. D. E. Ford, T. P. Erlinger, Depression and C-reative protein in US adults. *Arch. Intern. Med.* **164** (2004), 1010–14.

127. B. Pennix, S. Kritchevsky, K. Yaffe, Inflammatory markers and depressed mood in older persons. *Biol. Psychiatry* **54** (2003), 566–72.

128. H. Tiemeier, A. Hofman, Inflammatory proteins and depression in the elderly. *Epidemiology* **14** (2003), 103–7.

129. M. R. DiMatteo, H. S. Lepper, T. W. Croghan, Depression is a risk factor for noncompliance with medical treatment: meta-analysis of the effects of anxiety and depression on patient adherence. *Arch. Intern. Med.* **160** (2000), 2101–7.

130. J. A. Blumenthal, R. S. Williams, A. G. Wallace, R. B. Williams, Jr, T. L. Needles, Physiological and psychological variables predict compliance to prescribed exercise therapy in patients recovering from myocardial infarction. *Psychosom. Med.* **44** (1982), 519–27.

131. R. M. Carney, K. E. Freedland, S. A. Eisen, *et al.*, Adherence to a prophylactic medication regimen in patients with symptomatic versus asymptomatic ischemic heart disease. *Behav. Med.* **24** (1998), 35–9.

132. R. C. Ziegelstein, J. A. Fauerbach, S. S. Stevens, *et al.*, Patients with depression are less likely to follow recommendations to reduce cardiac risk during recovery from a myocardial infarction. *Arch. Intern. Med.* **160** (2000), 1818–23.

133. Anonymous. Influence of adherence to treatment and response of cholesterol on mortality in the coronary drug project. *N. Eng. J. Med.* **303** (1980), 1038–41.

134. R. I. Horwitz, C. M. Viscoli, L. Berkman, *et al.*, Treatment adherence and risk of death after a myocardial infarction. *Lancet* **336** (1990), 542–5.

135. M. M. McDermott, B. Schmitt, E. Wallner, Impact of medication nonadherence on coronary heart disease outcomes: a critical review. *Arch. Intern. Med.* **157** (1997), 1921–9.

136. R. Danker, U. Goldbourt, V. Boyko, H. Reicher-Reiss, Predictors of cardiac and noncardiac mortality among 14,697 patients with coronary heart disease. *Am. J. Cardiol.* **91** (2003), 121–7.

137. A. H. Glassman, J. E. Helzer, L. S. Covey, *et al.*, Smoking, smoking cessation, and major depression. *J. Am. Med. Assoc.* **264** (1990), 1546–9.

138. A. L. Brosse, E. S. Sheets, H. S. Lett, J. A. Blumenthal, Exercise and the treatment of clinical depression in adults: recent findings and future directions. *Sports Med.* **32** (2002), 741–60.

139. D. B. Panagiotakos, C. Pitsavos, C. Chrysohoou, C. Stefanadis, P. Toutouzas, Risk stratification of coronary heart disease through established and emerging lifestyle factors in a Mediterranean population: CARDIO2000 epidemiological study. *J. Cardiovasc. Risk* **8** (2001), 329–35.

140. W. J. Strawbridge, S. Deleger, R. E. Roberts, G. A. Kaplan, Physical activity reduces the risk of subsequent depression for older adults. *Am. J. Epidemiol.* **156** (2002), 328–34.

141. D. Kritz-Silverstein, E. Barrett-Conno, C. Corbeau, Cross-sectional and prospective study of exercise and depressed mood in the elderly: the Rancho Bernardo study. *Am. J. Epidemiol.* **153** (2001), 596–603.

142. P. Hassmen, N. Koivula, A. Uutela, Physical exercise and psychological well-being: a population study in Finland. *Prev. Med.* **30** (2000), 17–25.

143. D. Scully, J. Kremer, M. M. Meade, R. Graham, K. Dudgeon, Physical exercise and psychological well being: a critical review. *Br. J. Sports Med.* **32** (1998), 111–20.

144. T. Stephens, Physical activity and mental health in the United States and Canada: evidence from four population surveys. *Prev. Med.* **17** (1988), 35–47.

145. N. Frasure-Smith, F. Lesperance, M. Talajic, Depression following myocardial infarction: impact on 6-month survival. *J. Am. Med. Assoc.* **270** (1993), 1819–25.

146. F. Lesperance, N. Frasure-Smith, M. Talajic, M. G. Bourassa, Five-year risk of cardiac mortality in relation to initial severity and one-year changes in depression symptoms after myocardial infarction. *Circulation* **105** (2002), 1049–53.

147. D. K. Ahern, L. Gorkin, J. L. Anderson, *et al.*, Biobehavioral variables and mortality or cardiac arrest in the Cardiac Arrhythmia Pilot Study (CAPS). *Am. J. Cardiol.* **66** (1990), 59–62.

148. C. M. Jenkinson, R. J. Madeley, J. R. Mitchell, I. D. Turner, The influence of psychosocial factors on survival after myocardial infarction. *Public Health* **107** (1993), 305–17.

149. K. H. Ladwig, M. Kieser, J. Konig, G. Breithardt, M. Borggrefe, Affective disorders and survival after acute myocardial infarction: results from the post-infarction late potential study. *Eur. Heart J.* **12** (1991), 959–64.

150. D. E. Bush, R. C. Ziegelstein, M. Tayback, *et al.*, Even minimal symptoms of depression increase mortality risk after acute myocardial infarction. *Am. J. Cardiol.* **88** (2001), 337–41.

151. M. W. Kaufmann, J. P. Fitzgibbons, E. J. Sussman, *et al.*, Relation between myocardial infarction, depression, hostility, and death. *Am. Heart J.* **138** (1999), 549–54.

152. J. Irvine, A. Basinski, B. Baker, *et al.*, Depression and risk of sudden cardiac death after acute myocardial infarction: testing for the confounding effects of fatigue. *Psychosom. Med.* **61** (1999), 729–37.

153. J. J. Strik, J. Denollet, R. Lousberg, A. Honig, Comparing symptoms of depression and anxiety as predictors of cardiac events and increased health care consumption after myocardial infarction. *J. Am. Coll. Cardiol.* **42** (2003), 1801–7.

154. J. J. Strik, R. Lousberg, E. C. Cheriex, A. Honig, One year cumulative incidence of depression following myocardial infarction and impact on cardiac outcome. *J. Psychosom. Res.* **56** (2004), 59–66.

155. M. Horsten, M. A. Mittleman, S. P. Wamala, K. Schenck-Gustafsson, K. Orth-Gomer, Depressive symptoms and lack of social integration in relation to prognosis of CHD in middle-aged women: the Stockholm Female Coronary Risk Study. *Eur. Heart. J.* **21** (2000), 1072–80.

156. F. Lesperance, N. Frasure-Smith, M. Juneau, P. Theroux, Depression and 1-year prognosis in unstable angina. *Arch. Intern. Med.* **160** (2000), 1354–60.

5

The management of depression in patients with coronary heart disease

Robert M. Carney and Kenneth E. Freedland

Introduction

Patients who survive an acute myocardial infarction (MI) often face a difficult period of psychological and social adjustment. During the weeks and months following an MI, survivors are confronted with the possibility of being physically incapacitated, of having another heart attack and of dying. Their usual roles and daily routines may be disrupted, their self-esteem may be injured, and some of their hopes and plans may be jeopardised. Even patients with stable coronary heart disease (CHD) who have never had an MI or other major cardiac event must live with the possibility that they might eventually have a heart attack, and many of them have to cope with angina pectoris, fatigue and other debilitating symptoms.

Given the stressors with which patients with CHD are confronted, it is not surprising that depression and anxiety are very common in these individuals. As many as 65% of post-MI patients are at least mildly anxious or depressed [1–3]. Although some patients return to their premorbid mood state within a few days or weeks after their MI, many have, or will develop, a more serious or persistent form of clinical depression.

Depressive disorders

The *Diagnostic and Statistical Manual of Mental Disorders*, 4th edn (DSM-IV-TR) of the American Psychiatric Association [4] defines the most widely used criteria for diagnosing psychiatric disorders. As described in DSM-IV-TR, *major depression* is a serious psychiatric disorder that tends to follow a chronic or recurrent course. A *major depressive episode* is present when five or more depressive symptoms, including dysphoric mood and/or loss of interest in usual activities, persist for at least two weeks and cause clinically significant distress or functional impairment. Approximately 16–22% of post-MI patients have a major depressive episode within a few

Depression and Physical Illness, ed. A. Steptoe.
Published by Cambridge University Press. © Cambridge University Press 2006.

weeks after the acute event [5–7], and about a third have an episode within a year. Many post-MI patients who meet the criteria for major depression were depressed before their MI [8].

Minor depression, a less severe depressive disorder, may be present if there are between two and four depressive symptoms. As with major depression, one of the symptoms must be either dysphoric mood or loss of interest in usual activities, the symptoms must be present for at least two weeks and the symptoms must cause distress or functional impairment. *Dysthymia* is a relatively mild depressive disorder. Unlike minor depression, dysthymia tends to be quite persistent and is often associated with chronically low self-esteem. Dysthymia is not diagnosed unless dysphoric mood and two or more other depressive symptoms have been present for at least two years [4]. About 25% of post-MI patients have either minor depression or dysthymia [5]. In some cases, a major depressive episode is superimposed on dysthymia, a condition known as 'double depression'.

Both major and minor depression are also common in patients who have not recently had an acute MI but who do have angiographically proven coronary artery disease (CAD). The prevalence of major depression is estimated to be between 17% and 23% in these patients [9–11], and about 17% have minor depression [11].

Patients with minor depression are at risk for developing the more serious major depressive disorder. In a study of patients with documented CAD but without a recent cardiac event, half of the patients who initially had minor depression developed major depression within the next 12 months [11]. Thus, although some cardiac patients with minor depression are experiencing nothing more than a mild transient emotional reaction that may not require any intervention other than support from family, friends and a trusted physician, many others will progress from minor to major depression, a condition that usually warrants treatment [11]. Minor depression is often treated for this reason, particularly in patients who have a prior history of major depressive episodes.

Effects of depression in cardiac patients

Patients who are depressed are more likely to experience social problems over the first year of post-MI recovery and are slower to return to work than are non-depressed patients [1,12–14]. In a study of the relationship between psychosocial functioning and a variety of chronic medical illnesses, heart disease and gastrointestinal disorders had the worst effects on patients' psychosocial functioning and quality of life [15]. However, depressed respondents reported worse psychosocial adjustment than their non-depressed counterparts across all chronic illnesses, including heart disease [16].

Depression has also been found to increase the risk of further medical morbidity and even mortality in CHD patients. Depression is associated with an increased risk for cardiac events, including cardiac mortality, in patients with recently diagnosed coronary disease [17,18] and following coronary artery bypass graft surgery [19–21]. The risk for mortality is especially high following an acute MI [7,22–27]. For example, Frasure-Smith *et al.* [7] found that depression was associated with a more than four-fold increased risk of mortality during the first six months following an acute MI, after adjusting for established prognostic variables including left ventricular dysfunction. Moreover, its prognostic significance was equivalent to that of left ventricular dysfunction and of a prior history of MI (see Chapter 4).

Treatments for depression

Pharmacotherapy

There are four major classes of antidepressant medications: tricyclic antidepressants (TCAs), monoamine oxidase inhibitors (MAOIs), selective serotonin reuptake inhibitors (SSRIs) and second-generation heterocyclic antidepressants. All have been shown to relieve depression in psychiatric patients. Although there is no reason to believe that antidepressants are less effective for depression in cardiac patients than in psychiatric patients, there has been relatively little efficacy research on antidepressants in cardiac populations. Furthermore, some antidepressants are contraindicated for many cardiac patients [28–30].

The TCAs and MAOIs are known to affect cardiac conduction, contractility, rate and rhythm, and may cause orthostatic hypotension [28–30]. These side effects are of special concern in patients with unstable angina, conduction disorders, heart failure or other complications of coronary disease. Orthostatic hypotension is of particular concern when treating older patients who are vulnerable to fall-related injuries, including life-threatening hip fractures. For these reasons, most experts caution against using any of the older antidepressants to treat cardiac patients.

SSRIs, on the other hand, are relatively free of cardiac side effects [31], but they pose a significant risk for drug–drug interactions [31]. Most cardiac patients take multiple medications for their disease and comorbid medical conditions, and so drug–drug interactions must always be considered when prescribing SSRIs for these patients. Nevertheless, SSRIs and other carefully selected antidepressants are believed to be reasonably safe when administered to cardiac patients with appropriate precautions [31,32]. Due to their relative safety, SSRIs are frequently selected to treat depression in patients with CHD.

However, there have been very few randomised controlled efficacy studies of any antidepressant in cardiac patients. Most of the existing studies have, understandably, focused on safety rather than efficacy. It is possible that depression in these patients may be qualitatively different from psychiatric depression and that it may not respond to the same kinds of treatment. Nevertheless, most clinical trials targeting depression in CHD patients have found that their depression can be treated successfully with conventional antidepressants [32], although few of these studies included a placebo control group. Shores and colleagues [32] published a comprehensive review of all published trials of pharmacological treatments for depression in patients with CHD. They concluded that more clinical trials of SSRIs are needed, as well as trials evaluating efficacy and safety of other types of antidepressant, such as nefazodone, venlafaxine and bupropion, in depressed patients with CHD.

The Sertraline Antidepressant Heart Attack Randomized Trial (SADHART) [33] was designed to evaluate the safety and efficacy of sertraline (an SSRI) in depressed patients hospitalised for an acute MI or unstable angina. SADHART was the first study to show that any antidepressant is safe for use early after an acute cardiac event. However, sertraline proved to be only modestly efficacious, and only in patients with relatively severe recurrent depression. Nevertheless, SADHART represents an important step towards improving the care of depressed cardiac patients following an acute cardiac event.

In summary, although there have been few trials of pharmacological treatment of depression in patients with stable CHD, and only one randomised controlled multicentre clinical trial in patients with a recent acute cardiac event, the existing evidence suggests that at least some of the available antidepressants are safe and effective in patients with CHD. Clearly, however, more clinical trials of antidepressants for depressed patients with CHD are needed.

Psychotherapy

Despite the availability of effective antidepressant medications, psychotherapy continues to play an important role in the treatment of depressive disorders. Some patients are unwilling to take psychotropic medications or do not comply with the prescribed regimen; also, as discussed in the preceding section, some medications are contraindicated for many cardiac patients. Regardless of whether they are taking psychotropic medications, many depressed cardiac patients need more emotional support and more intensive help with their personal adjustment problems than their physicians have the time or training to provide. Also, there is evidence that persistent depression may respond better to a combination of pharmacotherapy and psychotherapy than to either modality alone, at least for patients who are able to tolerate and cooperate with both forms of treatment [34].

A bewildering variety of psychotherapeutic interventions are used to treat depression in psychiatric patients, but they are not interchangeable. There is evidence that some psychotherapeutic interventions are more efficacious than others for these conditions. Of all the existing forms of psychotherapy for unipolar depression, cognitive–behavioural therapy (CBT) [35] and interpersonal psychotherapy (IPT) [36] are best supported by controlled clinical trials, e.g. [35]. Both CBT and IPT have been found to be significantly more effective than pill placebo plus clinical management and (depending upon the trial) nearly as effective as [37], as effective as [38] or more effective than [39] widely used antidepressant medications.

Cognitive–behavioural therapy

CBT is a structured short-term treatment that focuses on modifying depressogenic thoughts and beliefs, solving current problems and increasing the frequency of productive and pleasurable activities [34,35]. Patients undergoing CBT learn that their own thoughts govern their mood and behaviour, and that they can feel better by challenging and changing distorted, erroneous or otherwise maladaptive thoughts and then changing their behaviour accordingly. Most patients are not fully aware of their distressing thoughts and beliefs when they present for treatment.

Cognitive–behavioural therapists use a variety of techniques to help their patients identify and challenge maladaptive thoughts and replace them with more rational and adaptive thoughts. For example, a patient may be asked to use a 'dysfunctional thought record' (DTR) whenever he or she is feeling particularly discouraged, anxious or upset [35]. Depressed patients' DTR entries often reflect excessively pessimistic views of themselves, their future or the world in which they live. When feeling depressed, they may have such thoughts as 'My whole life is ruined', 'Nobody will ever want me again', or 'I can't take it any more'.

CBT helps patients to replace these ideas with more adaptive thoughts and to reinforce them with confirmatory behaviour change. For example, a depressed, socially isolated patient may progress from thinking 'I'll never meet anyone' and 'People will reject me if I try to be friendly' to 'It's not impossible to meet people, and it won't kill me even if some people don't respond to me the way in which I'd like them to.' To validate the patient's new way of thinking, the patient is given behavioural homework assignments such as attending social gatherings and initiating conversations and confirming that nothing terrible happens as a result. The behavioural assignments are made more challenging as the patient's confidence and skills increase, to ensure that most of his or her experiences are successful and encouraging. The patient's mood typically improves along with these developments. Furthermore, the patient can use the skills acquired in the process to cope more effectively with new problems that arise after the termination of therapy and to help prevent recurrent episodes of depression or anxiety.

Some of the cognitive aspects of CBT such as examining core beliefs may be difficult for medically ill, elderly or poorly educated patients, as well as for those with severe depression. In such cases, the behavioural components of CBT usually take precedence over the cognitive components, at least early in the course of treatment.

Behavioural activation techniques, for example, can be used to help the patient to resume normal activities without necessarily having to change the distorted pessimistic ideas that may be maintaining his or her inactivity (e.g. 'Now that I've had a heart attack, I'll never be able to play a round of golf again'). Resumption of activities (or, if the patient has acquired a physical disability, finding satisfying alternative activities) disconfirms such thoughts and usually has potent beneficial effects on the patient's mood.

Interpersonal psychotherapy

IPT was originally developed as a manualised short-term treatment for major depression for use in clinical research [36]. Its efficacy for major depression has been demonstrated in psychiatric patients, including in the National Institute of Mental Health (NIMH) Treatment of Depression Collaborative Research Program (TDCRP) [37]. Several studies have also shown that IPT can be used to treat both major and minor depression in medically ill patients [40–42].

IPT focuses on solving interpersonal problems as a way to overcome depression. During the initial evaluation, the therapist identifies social and interpersonal problems that appear to have played a role in the onset of the patient's depression. Typical problems include interpersonal losses (e.g. death of a close friend), role transitions (e.g. loss of employment due to medical illness) and role disputes (e.g. marital conflict). Social skills deficits that interfere with the ability to form relationships or to gain emotional support are also addressed in some cases.

Most of the subsequent sessions focus on strategies for overcoming the patient's most troubling social and interpersonal problems. For example, an elderly patient might become depressed after relocating in order to live closer to his or her children and grandchildren after undergoing coronary bypass surgery. Despite the advantages of living closer to the family, a patient in this situation might suffer from the loss of frequent contact with long-time friends. Consequently, the patient's interpersonal therapist might concentrate on helping the patient to mourn this loss and to develop friendships in his or her new home. Towards the end of successful treatment, the emphasis would shift toward consolidating and maintaining the gains that have been achieved and developing relapse prevention skills.

Psychotherapy for depression in CHD patients

Because depression has a major impact on psychosocial adjustment and medical outcomes in CHD patients, there is growing interest in its psychotherapeutic treatment. Numerous studies have tested psychological interventions that were designed to relieve various forms of emotional distress in this population. Several randomised controlled treatment trials have found that patients with CHD obtain significant psychosocial benefits from psychotherapeutic interventions, e.g. [43–45].

Unfortunately, the specific CBT or IPT interventions for depression and anxiety that have strong empirical support in psychiatric populations have not been systematically tested on cardiac patients. Other types of psychotherapeutic intervention have been tested instead, and many of these studies suffer from methodological shortcomings, including small samples, inadequate control groups, compromised randomisation procedures and inadequate assessment of psychological outcomes.

Most of these studies have evaluated the addition of psychosocial interventions to usual care or to a cardiac rehabilitation programme. A wide variety of psychotherapeutic and behavioural interventions have been tested, including traditional group psychotherapy and relaxation training. The principal targets of treatment have been equally diverse: depending upon the study, the intervention may have been intended to reduce anxiety or depression, to modify type A behaviour, or to otherwise promote psychosocial adjustment.

Although the patients in these studies generally become less depressed as a result of treatment, most of the randomised trials have failed to show a significantly greater reduction in depression in the intervention than in the control groups, e.g. [46–48]. However, as noted above, the majority of these studies have employed psychotherapeutic interventions that are not considered optimal treatments for depression. Thus, there is currently little evidence for the efficacy of the two standard depression interventions, or indeed for any psychotherapeutic intervention, for the treatment of depression in patients with CHD.

Other treatments

Exercise

Numerous controlled and uncontrolled studies have found certain types of exercise to effectively reduce depression [49]. Much of this work has been marred, however, by the lack of proper controls. In a meta-analysis of 14 randomised controlled clinical trials of exercise training as a treatment for depression, Lawlor and Hopker [49] reported that most of the studies suffer from significant methodological weaknesses, including non-blinded assessments, outcome analyses that included only protocol completers and inadequate follow-ups. They concluded that the efficacy of exercise in treating depression has not yet been firmly established.

Blumenthal and colleagues [50] enrolled 156 elderly patients with major depressive disorder in a randomised controlled clinical trial of exercise training or sertraline or sertraline plus exercise training. After 16 weeks of treatment, the groups did not differ significantly on any measure of depression. Without an untreated control group, there is no way to determine how many of the depressed patients would have improved without any form of treatment. Furthermore, although some of these patients had stable heart disease, having CHD was not an inclusion criterion.

Nevertheless, it appears that exercise training may be as effective as a widely used antidepressant in the treatment of depression in older patients, and possibly in carefully selected patients with stable CHD.

There have been several reports of uncontrolled studies of exercise and depression in patients with CHD. Many of these studies were of patients enrolled in cardiac rehabilitation, and most did not specifically target depressed patients, e.g. [51,52]. There have not been any randomised, controlled trials of exercise in CHD patients with depression.

Treating depression in order to reduce medical morbidity and mortality in CHD

Pharmacotherapy

Although there is at least limited evidence for the safety and efficacy of antidepressants for the treatment of depression in patients with CHD, little is known about the effects of treating depression on subsequent cardiac events. In one of the few relevant studies published to date, Avery and Winokur [53] found that non-suicidal deaths, especially deaths that were cardiac-related, occurred more frequently during a three-year follow-up among depressed patients who had received inadequate treatment for depression than among those whose treatment was considered adequate. Although this is an intriguing finding, alternative interpretations are possible. For example, it is possible that the patients who received inadequate treatment for their depression also received less than adequate care for other medical conditions. Additionally, the study was based on a small number of endpoints and did not focus on patients with established CHD.

The SADHART sample was not large enough to establish definitively whether treatment with sertraline reduces cardiac events in depressed patients. The authors did report, however, a non-significant trend towards fewer cardiac events among patients receiving sertraline compared with those in the placebo arm. The finding of a possible benefit from the SSRI is consistent with the results of epidemiological studies [54,55], and of laboratory studies showing that SSRIs act to inhibit platelet activation [56,57]. Depressed patients have been shown to have higher levels of platelet activation [58,59], which has been suggested as a possible mechanism for the increased risk of cardiac events in depressed patients [60]. The encouraging trend reported in the SADHART study suggests the need for a future study with a larger sample of patients with major depression after hospitalisation for an acute MI or unstable angina.

Psychotherapy

In a quantitative review of 16 randomised, controlled trials, Linden *et al.* [61] found that interventions for CHD patients that include a psychotherapeutic component are associated with significantly lower two-year rates of morbidity (odds ratio [OR] 1.84) and mortality (OR 1.70), compared with patients randomised to control groups. Although this is very encouraging, many of the studies included in the review had serious methodological limitations, and some had negative results. Furthermore, none of these studies specifically targeted depression or attempted to evaluate the efficacy of standard depression interventions.

The two largest trials accounted for 77% and 37% of the treated subjects included in the meta-analyses of mortality and morbidity outcomes, respectively, and both trials have been criticised for flawed randomisation procedures [61,62]. Many of the studies included in the review of Linden *et al.* [61] also combined psychotherapeutic with educational interventions without controlling for the possible interactions between them. If, for example, a study compared exercise training plus supportive psychotherapy versus exercise alone, and the former group was found to have a lower mortality rate, then this could have occurred because the supportive component of the psychotherapy improved adherence to the exercise protocol. Thus, the effect may have been due to differences in the level of exercise rather than to improved psychosocial functioning.

Four large randomised studies have been published since the Linden *et al.* [61] meta-analysis. The first was an attempt by Frasure-Smith *et al.* [63] to replicate their successful study, the Ischemic Heart Disease Life Stress Monitoring Program, using a more conventional random assignment procedure than was used in the first study. As in the first study, the 'distress levels' of those in the intervention arm were assessed by telephone beginning one week after discharge, and then monthly for one year, using the 20-item General Health Questionnaire (GHQ). Patients scoring 6 or more on this questionnaire and patients who were hospitalised were visited by a nurse, who offered an individually tailored intervention that could include emotional support, reassurance, education or referral to a mental health professional.

Although the patients were selected for 'non-specific distress' rather than for anxiety or depression, many of the participants were at least mildly depressed. However, the intervention had little effect on depression. Furthermore, unlike the original study, there was no difference in survival between the intervention and usual-care control group.

In a trial evaluating a psychological intervention for cardiac rehabilitation patients, Jones and West [64] randomised 1168 patients with a recent MI to receive a psychosocial intervention and 1160 patients to receive only usual care. The treatment consisted of seven two-hour out-patient sessions of a stress-management intervention, which included relaxation training, supportive counselling and education. The sessions were led by clinical psychologists and other medical personnel. Again, like the study of Frasure-Smith *et al.* [63], patients were not selected specifically for depression, and the intervention was not designed specifically to treat depression.

At six months, there were no significant differences between the treated and control patients in self-reported depression. Furthermore, by 12 months, 76 of the treated patients and 75 of the controls had died. Thus, no difference in mortality was found between the treated and control patients.

In a third study, Blumenthal and colleagues [65] randomly assigned 107 patients with documented CAD who developed myocardial ischaemia during a laboratory-based mental stress test either to exercise training or to a cognitive–behavioural stress-management group. Patients who lived too far away from the medical centre to conveniently return for follow-up visits were invited to participate as a usual-care comparison group.

Patients assigned to the stress-management intervention had significantly less severe wall-motion abnormalities on post-treatment mental stress testing, significantly fewer ischaemic episodes during ambulatory monitoring and fewer cardiac events compared with the usual-care participants. There were no significant differences between the stress-management and exercise groups at the end of the treatment. Unfortunately, a geographic criterion rather than random assignment was used to form the usual-care comparison group. Thus, although this was an otherwise excellent study with a very promising intervention, it cannot be concluded with confidence that the treatment was responsible for the outcome. Blumenthal *et al.* [65] argue against such interpretations, but it is possible that the usual-care patients may not have received the same quality of medical care as the patients who lived nearer to the medical centre. Blumenthal and colleagues are currently attempting to replicate their study, enrolling a larger sample and including a randomised usual-care control group. However, like the original study, this study does not focus exclusively on depressed patients.

The ENRICHD clinical trial

One randomised, controlled clinical trial did focus on depressed patients following a recent MI and utilised conventional depression treatments. The Enhancing Recovery in Coronary Heart Disease (ENRICHD) study was a multicentre clinical trial designed to determine whether treating depression and inadequate social support following acute MI reduces the risk of recurrent infarction and death [66]. A sample of 2481 patients (1084 women, 1397 men) with major or minor depression and/or low perceived social support were randomised to receive either usual care or an intervention that included individual and group CBT. In addition, sertraline or other appropriate antidepressants were given to those patients with severe depression at baseline (Hamilton Rating Scale for Depression [HRSD] score > 24) and to those patients who initially did not respond to CBT.

The intervention group showed a significantly greater improvement in depression after 6 months than the usual-care group, but the difference was only 1.7 points on the HRSD (-10.1 ± 7.8 vs. -8.4 ± 7.7, respectively) [67]. Although this represents a modest difference in depression between the intervention and the usual-care group, the trial was not designed to test the efficacy of the intervention for depression. Instead, the trial was designed to determine whether the intervention could reduce the rate of recurrent infarction or all-cause mortality. Thus, there was no attempt to control for non-specific treatment factors. Moreover, patients in the usual-care group were free to seek outside treatment for depression. About a fifth of the usual-care patients did so during the course of the trial.

Reinfarction-free survival during a mean follow-up of 29 months did not differ between the groups [67]. One of the explanations that the investigators offered for this null finding was that there was only a small difference between the groups in the depression outcomes. If their conclusion is correct, then more effective interventions for depression may be needed in order to affect medical outcomes.

The ENRICHD results are still being evaluated, and it is not yet certain why the trial failed or whether any form of depression treatment can improve survival. The depressed participants who were treated with antidepressants, with or without the addition of CBT, tended to survive longer than the patients who were not receiving any antidepressant. However, antidepressant therapy was not allocated by random assignment, and so this finding should be interpreted cautiously.

Another secondary analysis of the ENRICHD study sought to determine whether there was a relationship between improvement in depression and survival after the six-month intervention in patients who had a BDI score ≥ 10 and a past history of major depression and who completed the six-month post-treatment assessment [68]. Out of the 858 patients (409 usual care, 449 intervention) who met these criteria, the intervention-group patients whose depression did not improve were at higher risk for late mortality than were patients who responded to treatment. These results suggest that patients whose depression is refractory to CBT and sertraline, two standard treatments for depression, may be at higher risk for late mortality after an acute MI. This analysis was not planned before the trial, and so the results must be interpreted with caution. However, if the results are eventually replicated in a prospective study, then patients who are resistant to standard depression treatment should be followed more closely. More aggressive cardiological care may be warranted, including efforts to treat all other modifiable risk factors and all comorbid medical disorders to the fullest extent possible. More aggressive treatment for depression may also be warranted, but further research is needed to develop more effective ways to treat depression in patients with CHD who do not respond to first-line interventions.

Summary and conclusions

Although there is good evidence that depression is a risk factor for mortality and cardiac events in patients with CHD, there is not yet any evidence that psychotherapy and pharmacotherapy for depression improve survival in these patients or otherwise alter the course of their heart disease. On the other hand, there is evidence that a variety of pharmacological agents, especially in the SSRI class of antidepressants, can safely relieve depression in patients with CHD. Despite the growing popularity of psychosocial interventions to enhance psychosocial functioning and quality of life in cardiac patients, there is very little evidence that such treatments have a significant impact on depression in patients with CHD. Similarly, exercise training is used widely in cardiac rehabilitation programmes, and there is some evidence that it may improve depression as well as certain cardiac risk factors. However, there have not been any clinical trials of exercise training in depressed patients with CHD. Depressed CHD patients are likely to benefit from psychotherapy or exercise training as much as medically well, depressed patients. However, controlled clinical trials of recognised psychotherapeutic interventions for depression and clinical trials of exercise training that target depression in patients with CHD are needed. Moreover, additional clinical trials of other antidepressant medications are needed to provide evidence of their safety and efficacy.

Finally, despite the availability of safe and effective treatments, many depressed CHD patients do not receive any treatment for their depression. In one study, only 10% of CHD patients with major depression received treatment [5]. In a more recent study of patients with chronic heart failure, only 26% of depressed patients received treatment [69], even after their cardiologists and primary-care physicians were advised of their depression. Whether treating depression will improve medical outcomes remains to be seen. However, depressed patients should be identified and treated in order to improve their psychosocial adjustment, wellbeing and quality of life, regardless of whether such treatment can improve medical outcomes.

Acknowledgements

The preparation of this chapter was supported in part by grant no. RO-1HL58946 from the National Heart, Lung, and Blood Institute, and by the Lewis and Jean Sachs Charitable Lead Trust.

REFERENCES

1. E. L. Cay, N. Vetter, A. E. Philip, P. Dugard, Psychological status during recovery from an acute heart attack. *J. Psychosom. Res.* **16** (1972), 425–35.
2. S. H. Croog, S. Levine, *Life After Heart Attack* (New York: Human Sciences Press, 1982).
3. H. Cassem, T. P. Hackett, Psychiatric consultation in a coronary care unit. *Ann. Intern. Med.* **75** (1971), 9–14.

4. American Psychiatric Association. *Diagnostic and Statistical Manual of Mental Disorders*, 4th edn, text revision (Washington, DC: American Psychiatric Association, 2000).

5. S. J. Schleifer, M. M. Macari-Hinson, D. A. Coyle, *et al.*, The nature and course of depression following myocardial infarction. *Arch. Intern. Med.* **149** (1989), 1785–9.

6. R. M. Carney, K. E. Freedland, A. S. Jaffe, Insomnia and depression prior to myocardial infarction. *Psychosom. Med.* **52** (1990), 603–9.

7. N. Frasure-Smith, F. Lespérance, M. Talajic, Depression following myocardial infarction: impact on 6 month survival. *J. Am. Med. Assoc.* **270** (1993), 1819–25.

8. F. Lespérance, N. Frasure-Smith, M, Taljic, Major depression before and after myocardial infarction: its nature and consequences. *Psychosom. Med.* **58** (1996), 99–110.

9. R. M. Carney, M. W. Rich, A. J. Tevelde, *et al.*, Major depressive disorder in coronary artery disease. *Am. J. Cardiol.* **60** (1987), 1273–5.

10. M. B. Gonzalez, T. B. Snyderman, J. T. Colket, *et al.*, Depression in patients with coronary artery disease. *Depression* **4** (1997), 57–62.

11. M. Hance, R. M. Carney, K. E. Freedland, J. Skala, Depression in patients with coronary heart disease: a twelve month follow-up. *Gen. Hosp. Psychiatry* **18** (1995), 61–5.

12. M. J. Stern, L. Pascale, J. B. McLoone, Psychosocial adaption following an acute myocardial infarction. *J. Chronic. Dis.* **29** (1976), 213–26.

13. R. Mayou, A. Foster, B. Williamson, Psychosocial adjustment in patients one year after myocardial infarction. *J. Psychosom. Res.* **22** (1978), 447–53.

14. G. G. Lloyd, R. H. Cawley, Distress or illness? A study of psychosocial symptoms after myocardial infarction. *Br. J. Psychiatry* **142** (1983), 120–25.

15. A. L. Stewart, S. Greenfield, R. D. Hays, *et al.*, Functional status and well-being of patients with chronic conditions: results from the Medical Outcomes Study. *J. Am. Med. Assoc.* **262** (1989), 907–13.

16. K. B. Wells, A. Stewart, R. Hays, *et al.*, The functioning and well-being of depressed patients: results from the Medical Outcomes Study. *J. Am. Med. Assoc.* **262** (1989), 914–19.

17. R. M. Carney, M. W. Rich, K. E. Freedland, *et al.*, Major depressive disorder predicts cardiac events in patients with coronary artery disease. *Psychosom. Med.* **50** (1988), 627–33.

18. J. C. Barefoot, M. J. Helms, D. B. Mark, *et al.*, Depression and long-term mortality risk in patients with coronary artery disease. *Am. J. Cardiol.* **78** (1996), 613–17.

19. I. Connerney, P. Shapiro, J. S. McLaughlin, R. P. Sloan, In hospital depression after CABG surgery predicts 12-month outcome. *Psychosom. Med.* **62** (2000), 106.

20. M. M. Burg, C. M. Benedetto, R. Rosenberg, R. Soufer, Depression prior to CABG predicts 6-month and 2-year morbidity and mortality. *Psychosom. Med.* **63** (2001), 103.

21. J. A. Blumenthal, H. S. Lett, M. A. Babyak, *et al.*, Depression as a risk factor for mortality after coronary artery bypass surgery. *Lancet* **362** (2003), 604–9.

22. J. Irvine, A. Basinski, B. Baker, *et al.*, Depression and risk of sudden cardiac death after acute myocardial infarction: testing for the confounding effects of fatigue. *Psychosom. Med.* **61** (1999), 729–37.

23. D. K. Ahern, L. Gorkin, J. L. Anderson, *et al.*, Biobehavioral variables and mortality or cardiac arrest in the Cardiac Arrhythmia Pilot Study (CAPS). *Am. J. Cardiol.* **66** (1990), 59–62.

24. K. H. Ladwig, M. Kieser, J. Konig, G. Breithardt, M. Borggrefe, Affective disorders and survival after acute myocardial infarction. *Eur. Heart. J.* **12** (1991), 959–64.

25. R. M. Carney, J. A. Blumenthal, D. Catellier, *et al.*, Depression as a risk factor for mortality following acute myocardial infarction. *Am. J. Cardiol.* **92** (2003), 1277–81.

26. D. E. Bush, R. C. Ziegelstein, M. Tayback, *et al.*, Even minimal symptoms of depression increase mortality risk after acute myocardial infarction. *Am. J. Cardiol.* **88** (2001), 337–41.

27. M. W. Kaufmann, J. P. Fitzgibbons, E. J. Sussman, *et al.*, Relation between myocardial infarction, depression, hostility, and death. *Am. Heart. J.* **138** (1999), 549–54.

28. R. P. Pary, C. R. Tobias, S. Lippmann, Antidepressants and the cardiac patient: selecting an appropriate medication. *Postgrad. Med.* **85** (1989), 267–9.

29. A. H. Glassman, S. P. Roose, J. T. Bigger, The safety of tricyclic antidepressants in cardiac patients: risk/benefit reconsidered. *J. Am. Med. Assoc.* **269** (1993), 2673–5.

30. S. J. Warrington, C. Padgham, M. Lader, The cardiovascular effects of antidepressants. *Psychol. Med. Monogr. Suppl.* **16** (1989), 1–40.

31. Y. Sheline, K. E. Freedland, R. M. Carney, How safe are serotonin reuptake inhibitors for depression in patients with coronary heart disease? *Am. J. Med.* **102** (1997), 54–9.

32. M. M. Shores, M. Pascualy, R. C. Veith, Major depression and heart disease: treatment trials. *Semin. Clin. Neuropsychiatry* **3** (1998), 87–101.

33. A. H. Glassman, C. M. O'Connor, R. M. Califf, *et al.*, Sertraline treatment of major depression in patients with acute MI or unstable angina. *J. Am. Med. Assoc.* **288** (2002), 701–9.

34. M. B. Keller, J. P. McCullough, D. N. Klein, *et al.*, A comparison of nefazodone, the cognitive behavioral-analysis system of psychotherapy, and their combination for the treatment of chronic depression. *N. Engl. J. Med.* **342** (2000), 1462–9.

35. A. T. Beck, A. J. Rush, B. F. Shaw, G. Emery, *Cognitive Therapy of Depression* (New York: Guilford Press, 1979).

36. G. L. Klerman, M. M. Weissman, B. J. Rounsaville, E. S. Chevron, *Interpersonal Psychotherapy of Depression* (New York: Basic Books, 1984).

37. I. Elkin, M. T. Shea, J. T. Watkins, *et al.*, National Institute of Mental Health Treatment of Depression Collaborative Research Program: general effectiveness of treatments. *Arch. Gen. Psychiatry* **46** (1989), 971–82.

38. G. E. Murphy, A. D. Simons, R. D. Wetzel, P. J. Lustman, Cognitive therapy and pharmacotherapy, singly and together in the treatment of depression. *Arch. Gen. Psychiatry* **41** (1984), 33–41.

39. G. E. Murphy, R. M. Carney, R. D. Wetzel, M. Knesevitch, P. Whitworth, Cognitive therapy and depression: a controlled treatment outcome study. *Psychol. Rep.* **77** (1995), 403–20.

40. J. C. Markowitz, G, L. Klerman, S. W. Perry, K. F. Clougherty, A. Mayers, Interpersonal therapy of depressed HIV-seropositive patients. *Hosp. Community Psychiatry* **43** (1992), 885–90.

41. H. C. Schulberg, C. P. Scott, M. J. Madonia, S. D. Imber, Applications of interpersonal psychotherapy to depression in primary care practice. In *New Applications of Interpersonal Psychotherapy*, ed. G. L. Klerman, M. M. Weisman (Washington, DC: American Psychiatric Press, 1993), pp. 265–91.

42. J. M. Mossey, K. A. Knott, M. Higgins, K. Talerico, Effectiveness of a psychosocial intervention, interpersonal counseling, for subdysthymic depression in medically ill elderly. *J. Gerontol.* **51A** (1996), M172–8.

43. J. A. Blumenthal, C. F. Emery, Rehabilitation of patients following myocardial infarction. *J. Consult. Clin. Psychol.* **56** (1988), 374–81.

44. J. van Dixhoorn, H. J. Duivenvoorden, J. Pool, F. Verhage, Psychic effects of physical training and relaxation therapy after myocardial infarction. *J. Psychsom. Res.* **34** (1990), 327–37.

45. B. Oldenburg, R. J. Perkins, G. Andrews, Controlled trial of psychological intervention in myocardial infarction. *J. Consult. Clin. Psychol.* **53** (1985), 852–9.

46. R. H. Rahe, H. W. Ward, V. Hayes, Brief group therapy in myocardial infarction rehabilitation: three to four year follow-up of a controlled trial. *Psychosom. Med.* **41** (1979), 229–42.

47. A. W. Burgess, D. J. Lerner, R. B. D'Agostino, *et al.*, A randomized controlled trial of cardiac rehabilitation. *Soc. Sci. Med.* **24** (1987), 359–70.

48. N. B. Oldridge, G. Guyat, N. Jones, *et al.*, Effects on quality of life of comprehensive rehabilitation after acute myocardial infarction. *Am. J. Cardiol.* **67** (1991), 1084–9.

49. D. A. Lawlor, S. W. Hopker, The effectiveness of exercise as an intervention in the management of depression: systematic review and meta-regression analysis of randomised controlled trials. *Br. Med. J.* **322** (2001), 1–8.

50. J. A. Blumenthal, M. A. Babyak, K. A. Moore, *et al.*, Effects of exercise training on older patients with major depression. *Arch. Intern. Med.* **159** (1999), 2349–56.

51. R. V. Milani, C. J. Lavie, Prevalence and effects of cardiac rehabilitation on depression in the elderly with coronary heart disease. *Am. J. Cardiol.* **81** (1998), 1233–6.

52. C. J. Lavie, R. V. Milani, M. M. Cassidy, Y. E. Gilliland, Effects of cardiac rehabilitation and exercise training programs in women with depression. *Am. J. Cardiol.* **83** (1999), 1480–83.

53. D. Avery, G. Winokur, Mortality in depressed patients treated with electroconvulsive therapy and antidepressants. *Arch. Gen. Psychiatry* **33** (1976), 1029–37.

54. W. H. Sauer, J. A. Berlin, S. E. Kimmel, Effect of antidepressants and their relative affinity for the serotonin transporter on the risk of myocardial infarction. *Circulation* **108** (2003), 32–6.

55. W. H. Sauer, J. A. Berlin, S. E. Kimmel, Selective serotonin reuptake inhibitors and myocardial infarction. *Circulation* **104** (2001), 1894–8.

56. N. Hergovich, M. Aigner, H. G. Eichler, *et al.*, Paroxetine decreases platelet serotonin storage and platelet function in human beings. *Clin. Pharmacol. Ther.* **68** (2000), 435–42.

57. V. L. Serebruany, C. M. O'Connor, P. A. Gurbel, Effect of selective serotonin reuptake inhibitors on platelets in patients with coronary artery disease. *Am. J. Cardiol.* **87** (2001), 1398–400.

58. D. L. Musselman, U. M. Marzec, A. Manatunga, *et al.*, Platelet reactivity in depressed patients treated with paroxetine: preliminary findings. *Arch. Gen. Psychiatry* **57** (2000), 875–82.

59. F. Laghrissi-Thode, W. R. Wagner, B. G. Pollock, P. C. Johnson, M. S. Finkel, Elevated platelet factor 4 and β-thromboglobulin plasma levels in depressed patients with ischemic heart disease. *Biol. Psychiatry* **42** (1997), 290–95.

60. R. M. Carney, K. E. Freedland, G. E. Miller, A. S. Jaffe, Depression as a risk factor for cardiac mortality and morbidity: a review of potential mechanisms. *J. Psychosom. Res.* **53** (2002), 897–902.

61. W. Linden, C. Stossel, J. Maurice, Psychosocial interventions for patients with coronary artery disease: a meta-analysis. *Arch. Intern. Med.* **156** (1999), 745–52.

62. L. H. Powell, Unanswered questions in the Ischemic Heart Disease Life Stress Monitoring Program. *Psychosom. Med.* **51** (1989), 479–84.

63. N. Frasure-Smith, F. Lespérance, R. Prince, *et al.*, Randomized trial of home based psychosocial nursing intervention for patients recovering from myocardial infarction. *Lancet* **350** (1997), 473–9.

64. D. A. Jones, R. R. West, Psychological rehabilitation after myocardial infarction: multicentre randomized controlled trial. *Br. Med. J.* **313** (1996), 1517–21.

65. J. A. Blumenthal, W. Jiang, M. A. Babyak, *et al.*, Stress management and exercise training in cardiac patients with myocardial ischemia. *Arch. Intern. Med.* **157** (1997), 2213–23.

66. ENRICHD investigators. Enhancing Recovery in Coronary Heart Disease Patients (ENRICHD): study design and methods. *Am. Heart J.* **139** (2000), 1–9.

67. ENRICHD investigators. Effects of treating depression and low perceived social support on clinical events after a myocardial infarction: the Enhancing recovery in Coronary Heart Disease Patients (ENRICHD) randomized trial. *J. Am. Med. Assoc.* **289** (2003), 3106–16.

68. R. M. Carney, J. A. Blumenthal, K. E. Freedland, *et al.*, Depression and late mortality after myocardial infarction in the Enhancing Recovery in Coronary Heart Disease (ENRICHD) study. *Psychosom. Med.* **66** (2004), 466–74.

69. K. E. Freedland, M. W. Rich, J. A. Skala, *et al.*, Depression in hospitalized patients with congestive heart failure. *Psychosom. Med.* **63** (2001), 177.

6

Depression and physical disability

Brenda W. J. H. Penninx

This chapter describes the link between depression and disability. Disability can be defined as a restriction in or lack of ability to perform an activity because of impairment. These activities can include interpersonal relationships, work and school activities and physical activities; the latter is defined as 'physical disability'. In this chapter, the main focus is on physical disability, since this is the type of disability that has often been examined in relation to depression, especially in old age. However, when appropriate the chapter also elaborates on other types of disability.

The first section of this chapter describes the concept of disability in more detail. The next section provides an overview of research that examines the link between depression and disability. It then goes on to discuss underlying mechanisms that could explain the link between depression and disability. Subsequently, results of intervention studies that try to break the link between depression and disability are described. The chapter ends with some concluding remarks.

Disability: a functional indicator of physical health

Various chapters of this book demonstrate that the importance of chronic conditions for mental health is undisputed. These chapters show that conditions such as cardiovascular disease, diabetes, cancer and chronic fatigue are included among the strongest risk factors for depression, and that the presence of depression influences the course and management of these chronic illnesses. Especially in old age, individuals often have multiple chronic conditions, which may vary in their severity. Thus, in old age the complete picture of the link between depression and physical health cannot be portrayed by looking only at individual chronic diseases. Although individual diseases are important, and our system of modern medicine is often oriented toward the diagnosis and treatment of specific diseases, the consequences of single

Depression and Physical Illness, ed. A. Steptoe.
Published by Cambridge University Press. © Cambridge University Press 2006.

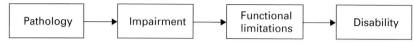

Figure 6.1   The disablement process.

and multiple diseases can be understood best by an evaluation of the functional status of the patient. Thus, to date, a functional assessment forms the hallmark of geriatric medicine and research.

Since about 1990, various assessments and concepts for functional status have been proposed and used in ageing studies. These generally fit into a conceptual model, called the disablement process [1], which uses concepts of the International Classification of Functioning, Disability and Health (ICF) provided by the World Health Organization WHO [2]. The disablement process model describes a pathway leading from pathology to impairment to functional limitations, and ultimately to disability (Figure 6.1). In this model, pathology refers to biochemical and physiological abnormalities that are detected and medically labelled as disease, injury or congenital or developmental conditions. Physical impairments are dysfunctions and structural abnormalities in specific body systems, such as conceptualised in poor muscle strength, poor balance or low walking speed. Functional limitations are experienced restrictions in performing fundamental physical actions used in daily life, e.g. the report of experiencing difficulty or inability with walking a quarter of a mile, climbing stairs or lifting 10 lbs., which can all be considered to be the building blocks of activities of daily life. Disability, the final stage of the disablement process, reflects how an individual's limitations interact with the demands of the environment. Disability indicates a restriction in or lack of ability to perform activities related to interpersonal relationships, work, school or physical activities. For the latter, also termed physical disability, various types can be distinguished, ranging in severity. Difficulty with essential activities of daily living (ADLs), such as eating, bathing, dressing and transferring from bed to chair, indicates severe disability, which usually identifies individuals who require extensive (institutional) help. Instrumental activities of daily living (IADLs), such as housekeeping tasks, paying bills and grocery shopping, are tasks that physically and cognitively are somewhat more complicated and more difficult than self-care tasks but are also necessary for independent living. Although (I)ADL disability is described as physical disability, it clearly has a mental component as well.

The number of older people living with physical disability increases dramatically with increasing age. Data from the US National Health Interview Survey of Disability show that in people aged 65 years and older, 18.8% of women and 10.9% of men need help with (I)ADL at home [3]. At 85 years or older, 54.8% of women and 36.9% of men need help with (I)ADL. One of the key paradoxes in gerontology is that although women live longer than men, women live with more physical disability at an older age. This is caused in large part by the prevalence of non-lethal but disabling chronic diseases generally being higher in older women than in older men. For instance, arthritis and joint symptoms such as pain and stiffness are typically higher in older women than older men; this is also the case for hearing and vision impairment, osteoporosis (with resulting falls and fractures) and obesity, which all have a marked adverse impact on disability levels.

Physical disability status has been demonstrated in epidemiological studies to be one of the most potent of all health status indicators in predicting adverse outcomes such as mortality, hospitalisation and nursing-home admission [4–6]. This is because disability measures are able to capture the impact of the presence and severity of multiple pathologies, including physical, cognitive and psychological conditions, and the potential synergistic effects of these conditions on overall health status. In line with this, older adults report that they often worry about their risk of disability more than about the disease itself, because function decline changes the scope of their daily life and threatens their ability to live independently. Since the adverse impact of disability on outcomes such as hospitalisation, healthcare utilisation and nursing-home admission is large, it is not surprising that physical disability has been associated with greatly increased health care costs. In a US study of 843 people aged 72 years or older, those with ADL disability were found to spend $10 000 more on 2-year costs for hospital, out-patient, nursing-home and home-care services than those without ADL disability [7].

Describing the link between disability and depression

There is an undisputed link between disability and depression. Many cross-sectional studies conducted among older and younger samples and in community-dwelling, clinical and institutionalised samples have demonstrated that physical disability is associated with increased depressive symptoms [8–12]. Depressed people were found to be more likely to report limitations in self-care tasks, (I)ADL and mobility. These observations have been confirmed for the presence of both significant depressive symptoms and syndromal depression that meets psychiatric criteria for major depressive disorder (MDD).

In more general definitions of functioning that include aspects such as psychosocial functioning, quality of life and wellbeing, depressed people have been shown to perform poorly compared with non-depressed people [13–16]. Depressed people report more disability days, more days lost from work [17], poorer physical and emotional health and increased use of general medical services and emergency care services [14]. The association with poorer functioning and disability is generally stronger for major depression than for depressive symptoms, which is in line with a dose–response association between depression and disability: the more depressed the individual, the more severely limited his or her functioning. However, since depressive symptoms are more prevalent in the general population (lifetime prevalence about 20–25%) than major depression (lifetime prevalence about 6%), the relative impact on functioning and service burden is at least as great for depressive symptoms compared with a psychiatric diagnosis of depression [14,15,17,18].

Disability levels among depressed people are not only significantly higher than those of non-depressed people but are also similar to or even greater than disability levels found among people with other chronic somatic conditions. Using data from 11 242 outpatients of the Medical Outcomes Study, Wells and Sherbourne [19] reported that the risk of poor functioning associated uniquely with depression (either symptoms or disorder) was comparable with or worse than that associated uniquely with eight major chronic medical conditions (hypertension, diabetes, advanced coronary artery disease, angina, arthritis, lung problems, back problems, gastrointestinal disorders). In a large community-based sample of people in late middle age and older, similar effects were found [15]. In the latter study, the poor functioning risk of depressive symptoms exceeded those of 16 of 18 medical somatic conditions because depressive symptoms combine a moderately large unique risk with a rather high prevalence.

The Global Burden of Disease Study points out that in economic terms, the cost of depression due to loss of productivity and wellbeing and use of health services ranks among the top five of all disorders [20]. Considering these data as well as its own projections, the WHO stated in 2000 that depression is the leading cause of disability, as measured in years lived with disability, and the fourth leading contributor to the global burden of disease, as indicated in terms of disability-adjusted life-years (DALYs). The WHO projects that in 2020, depression will reach second place behind cardiovascular disease in ranking of DALYs calculated for all ages and both sexes.

Considering these findings that depression and disability are connected, the question arises as to how this link should be interpreted. Is depression increasing disability? Is disability increasing depression levels? Or is the link due largely to other factors associated with both more disability and more depression? In the following sections, we further unravel the link between depression and disability by expanding more on prospective findings that examined a specific order in the link between depression and disability.

Disability increases the risk of depression

Several prospective studies have found that physical disability is a risk factor for the development of depression [21–24]. These studies controlled extensively for factors such as age, gender, medical conditions and income, but these could not take away the significant link. In a non-depressed sample of 680 older people, the presence of functional limitations (as assessed by vision, hearing or mobility problems) predicted the development of major depressive disorder [23]. Of the people without functional limitations, 11% developed depression during 4 years of follow-up compared with 21% of those in the high-limitations group. Among 889 older residents of London, the presence of ADL disability increased the risk of onset of significant depressive symptoms one year later by a factor of three [24]. In a Dutch study, depression and physical disability were measured at eight consecutive waves during three years of follow-up [25]. Using these data, the researchers found that physical disability was a predictor of both the onset and the persistence of depression.

This finding that disability increases the risk of depression is not surprising, since the onset of disability is a major stressor that leads to loss of perceived control, restriction of valued social or leisure activities, isolation and reduced quality of social support, all of which are psychosocial risk factors for depression. In addition, people with acquired physical disabilities inevitably encounter additional losses, such as the loss of function, role and body image, and may experience a greater dependency on others and a more negative view of themselves, their future and their world. Depression can occur as an outcome of certain somatic illnesses or medication, reflecting a biologically mediated process. For example, the structural and neurochemical changes involved in stroke and parkinsonism can lead to depression. Several factors that often co-occur with disability, such as arthritis, pain and cognitive and sensory impairment, can put older people at risk for late-life depression. It must be mentioned that certain symptoms of depression, especially somatic symptoms such as low energy levels and sleeping problems, may partly be a manifestation of disease [26].

It is interesting that several studies among older people have shown that symptoms of depression are predicted more strongly by the level of physical disability than by number or specific type of chronic conditions [23,27,28]. This indicates that the effect of chronic conditions on depressive symptomatology is mediated partly through the level of existing physical disability.

Depression increases the risk of disability

Several longitudinal studies have found evidence for a detrimental effect of depression on physical disability over time. Some of these studies used selected study samples of medical patients and/or did not exclude people with disability at baseline, which hampers the interpretation of whether disability is a cause rather than a consequence of depression [29–31]. However, other studies have examined the effect of depression on the onset of disability in a disability-free cohort at the start of the study, which rules out confounding by initial physical function and

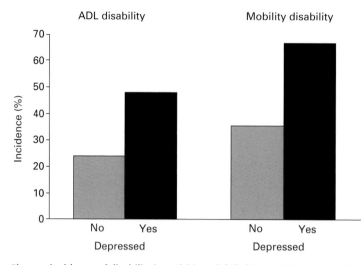

Figure 6.2   Six-year incidence of disability in activities of daily living (ADL) and mobility disability (disability in walking a quater of a mile or climbing stairs) among initially non-disabled people aged 65 years or older. Findings from the Establised Populations of the Epidemiologic Studies of the Elderly (EPESE) study [34].

consequently gives us a clearer picture of the causal role that depression appears to play in the development of disability [17,32–36]. The majority of these longitudinal studies have confirmed that people with depression have an increased risk of developing new disability in subsequent years. In general, the results of these studies indicate that in initially non-disabled populations, the existence of depression at baseline increases the risk for disability by 60% or more [37]. However, the estimated increased disability risks in the various studies range quite considerably. This wide range may be explained by the different types of disability outcome used (e.g. disability in less severe IADL versus disability in severe basic ADL), the type of depression assessment used (e.g. mild depressive symptoms versus psychiatric diagnosis of MDD) and the follow-up duration considered (one year versus six years). Although the effect of depression on disability has been confirmed for depressive symptoms and for a psychiatric diagnosis of MDD, it seems that the effect is somewhat larger for the most severe type of depression, which suggests the existence of a dose–response relationship between depression and subsequent disability.

In the Established Populations of the Epidemiologic Studies of the Elderly (EPESE) study, we explored the effect of significant depressive symptoms (as defined by a high score on the Center of Epidemiologic Studies Depression [CES-D] scale) on the onset of disability among more than 6000 initially non-disabled people aged 65 years or older [34]. We followed these people for six years and asked them every year about their disability levels. As shown in Figure 6.2, of the non-depressed people, 24% developed disability in ADL and 36% developed difficulty with walking a quarter of a mile or climbing stairs (mobility limitations). These percentages were significantly higher among depressed people (48% and 67%, respectively). The depressed people were 1.67 times more likely to develop new ADL disability and 1.73 times more likely to develop new mobility disability. When these risk estimates were adjusted for other variables that differed between depressed and non-depressed people, such as age, gender, education, income and medical conditions, the risk estimates decreased to 1.45 and 1.37, respectively. However, these risks were still considerable and remained highly significant. In various other studies, factors such as age, gender, education and medical conditions could not explain the link between depression and incident disability risk.

We may still wonder whether the interpretation of these disability studies is hampered by the possibility that depressed people may give overly pessimistic appraisals of their functioning and disability. Even when their functional status remains the same, people who are depressed tend to become more depressed over time and, therefore, may report more physical disabilities. However, the link between depression and functional decline is also observed for objectively assessed physical impairments, identifying an earlier stage of the disablement process (see Figure 6.1). Impairment assessments, e.g. walking speed or strength assessments, appear to be less influenced by personality, cognition and mood than self-reported measures of disability. In the EPESE study, we examined the link between depression at baseline (assessed by the CES-D score) and the four-year change in performance of standardised tasks, including a walking test, a standing balance test and a repeated chair–stand test. Depression was found to cause greater physical decline over four years [38]. Thus, the link between depression and incident disability is already present at earlier stages of the disablement process. More recently, we demonstrated with longitudinal data from the Dutch Longitudinal Aging Study Amsterdam that depression not only is associated with physical impairments but also accelerates the transition from physical impairments to disability [39]. In other words, these findings indicate that depression appears to accelerate the disablement process in older people.

Temporal sequence of the link between depression and disability

Most of the prospective studies discussed so far have examined the physical consequences of depression using a single assessment of depressed mood at one time point. Also, most studies that examined the effect of disability on depressive symptomatology have used only a single assessment of disability. Consequently, these studies do not tell us much about the temporal sequence of the link between depression and disability. Some questions remain unaddressed. For instance, what happens with disability patterns when a person recovers from depression? Do disability levels then return to normal? A few studies have examined depression and disability patterns at multiple periods over time and examined these questions. These studies were able to distinguish transient states of depression from more chronic depressive states.

Our data from the Longitudinal Aging Study Amsterdam conducted among community-dwelling older people provide strong evidence that the course of depression plays a differential role in the relationship of depression and physical decline over time [40]. About half (49.1%) of the people depressed at baseline (as defined by a CES-D score $\geq$ 16) were still depressed after 3 years. This percentage is similar to that in other studies [41], and illustrates the chronic nature of depression in old age. In this group of chronically depressed people, we found an increased risk for three-year physical decline. Subjects who remitted from their depression in three years did not show greater physical decline compared with people who had never been depressed. So, especially when chronically present, depression was found to have a substantial impact on physical decline over a longer period of time.

Synchrony of change over time between depression and disability levels has been described in other studies. For instance, in a study of 1994 primary-care patients and a study of 371 people with major depression, social disability levels improved when a depressed person became asymptomatic [42–44]. In a Dutch study, Ormel *et al.* [45] examined the extent to which psychosocial disability after remission from a major depressive episode was due to residual symptoms (state effect), the continuation of premorbid disability (trait effect) and disability that developed during the major depression episode and persisted beyond recovery (scar effect). Results showed that post-morbid psychosocial disability largely reflects continuation of premorbid psychosocial disability. Scarring did not occur routinely but was found in some people with a severe episode of depression. Again, these findings confirm synchrony of change between depressive symptoms and disability.

The finding of synchronous change of depression and disability in longitudinal studies indicates that, especially when chronically present, depression has a detrimental effect on functional status, which in turn could result in increased depressive symptoms. Such a situation could result in a process whereby depressive symptoms and physical dysfunctions interact to cause a progressive downward spiral in the health status of older people. It appears to be essential to break this downward spiral, e.g. through depression treatment, since observational longitudinal studies indicate that when mood is improved in depressed people this is likely associated with improved functional status. Later, this chapter presents results from some intervention studies that have tried to break the unfavourable link between depression and disability.

Explaining the link between depression and disability

Several mechanisms have been proposed to explain the detrimental effect of depression on physical function among older people. Subjects with depression are usually older, more often female, have a lower socioeconomic status and have worse health compared with their non-depressed peers. This leads to the hypothesis that age, sex, sociodemographics and baseline chronic conditions, rather than depression per se, might be responsible for the differential physical disability patterns between depressed and non-depressed subjects. This confounding hypothesis is likely to explain part of the link between depression and disability. In our EPESE analyses, for instance [34], the unadjusted ADL disability risk associated with depression declined by about 41% after taking into account age, sex, education and baseline chronic conditions (relative risk [RR] fell from 1.67 to 1.39). This large decline in risk indicates that unequal distributions of age, sex, education and physical health between depressed and non-depressed people add to the increased disability risk. However, after adjustment for these potential confounding variables in statistical analyses, the disability risk in depressed people remained significantly raised compared with that of non-depressed people, illustrating that the link is not due completely to simple confounding. Of course, it could be that in some cases depression may be a prodrome of not yet discovered or diagnosed (and, therefore, not measurable) medical conditions that affect physical disability. However, it is unlikely that this explains completely the increased disability risk for depression.

Therefore, other explanatory hypotheses should be considered as well. One of the first explanations could be sought in the nature of depression. Somatic symptoms of depression such as fatigue or sleeplessness may worsen health status in older people and may, therefore, contribute to the adverse physical consequences of depression. Studies have indicated, however, that the link between depression and increased disability risk continues to persist even if somatic symptoms are not considered in the assessment of depressive symptomatology [26]. Other possible mechanisms underlying the link between depression and increased disability risk have been described in the behavioural, psychosocial and biological areas.

Behavioural explanatory mechanisms

Certain behavioural risk profiles in depressed people may explain their higher risk for adverse health consequences (see Chapters 15–17). Behavioural risk factors appear to cluster in the same individuals. Increased smoking and alcohol consumption are well-documented in depression. Depressed people not only smoke more often but also are less likely to quit smoking, more likely to inhale more deeply and more likely to smoke more of each cigarette than non-depressed smokers [46]. In addition, the food intake of depressed people may be less adequate and nutritious than that of non-depressed people. It has been shown that some depressed people have a higher 24-hour caloric intake than non-depressed people [47]. On the other hand, certain vitamin deficiencies, such as vitamin B12 and folate deficiencies, are more prevalent in depressed older people [48], which illustrates that some depressed individuals may not get adequate nutrition.

Depressed people also engage less in physical activities such as walking, gardening and vigorous exercise activities such as sport. Physical inactivity thus is common among depressed people [34,49], partly because their attitudes towards exercise and exercise self-efficacy may be more negative. This can partly explain why depressed older individuals are more at risk for adverse health outcomes, since a sedentary lifestyle is one of the most important risk factors for the onset of disability in old age. This is an especially important observation, since the level of physical activity is potentially modifiable through an exercise regimen. Several clinical trials illustrate that when depressed older people are randomised to an exercise intervention, their depressed mood improves significantly.

Finally, depressed mood has shown to impede recovery processes by discouraging people from obtaining adequate medical attention and rehabilitation and following treatment regimens. It has been suggested that depressed people are generally less compliant in taking medications or following up on certain lifestyle regimens provided by healthcare professionals. This lower compliance could be due in part to lack of a supportive social network, which has been observed more often in depressed than in non-depressed people [50]. One study demonstrated that depressed cardiac patients received lower quality of care than their non-depressed peers, and this contributed to their higher mortality risk [51].

Psychosocial explanatory mechanisms

Depressed people differ from their non-depressed peers in various psychosocial factors. The social networks of depressed people are generally smaller and provide less instrumental and emotional support exchange [50] than those of non-depressed people. There is a downward spiral linking depression and low social support, with a small social network causing depression, and depression causing further social isolation. Therefore, it is not surprising that there is a strong association between depression and feelings of loneliness. Especially in old age, when social networks generally become smaller and people face losses of important others, loneliness becomes more prevalent and is often accompanied by depression. Loneliness and less emotional support have been linked directly with adverse health outcomes such as mortality and physical disability [52] and consequently may help to explain the unfavourable health outcomes of depression.

Depression is also associated with various psychological factors that have been related to poor health outcomes. For instance, a lower sense of control, lower feelings of (physical) self-efficacy and higher feelings of neuroticism have been observed consistently among depressed people [50]. In old age, feelings of losing control over one's life and low expectations regarding one's own physical abilities may have important consequences. Some researchers have proposed that depressed older people may experience motivational depletion and that they give up holding on to a healthy, active life, which ultimately leads to a worse health status.

Biological explanatory mechanisms

As described in more detail in other chapters of this book, the presence of depressive symptoms, and especially MDD, has physiological accompaniments, including altered autonomic balance, increased hypothalamic–pituitary–adrenal (HPA) axis function and altered immune function, all of which are biologically plausible contributors to pathogenesis. This section discusses how these biological mechanisms may relate to the link between depression and inflammation.

When depression is induced in laboratory studies, people show heightened sympathetic nervous-system-mediated cardiovascular responses. Depressive symptoms have been found to increase sympathetic nervous-system activation during everyday life, as documented by elevated resting heart rate and blood pressure, decreased heart-rate variability, increased ventricular arrhythmias, increased myocardial ischaemia and increased daytime urinary adrenaline excretion [53,54]. There is also evidence that parasympathetic nervous system function is reduced in depression. Altered autonomic nervous system function has been associated with cardiovascular disease prognosis and hypertension [55;56] and as a result could impact on a person's disability status. However, the link between nervous system function and disability has not yet been examined and confirmed in research studies, and so this explanatory mechanism is a hypothetical one.

Activation of the HPA axis may also play a key explanatory role in some of the health effects of depression. Hyperactivity of the HPA axis is caused by an enhanced cortisol response to adrenocorticotropic hormone (ACTH) and corticotropin-releasing hormone (CRH) as well as by a blunted feedback control by central glucocorticoid receptors [57]. Depressed people have been shown to exhibit hypersecretion of the adrenal steroid cortisol, adrenal hypertrophy and an increased cortisol response to ACTH [58]. Depression is also associated with a less efficient dexamethasone inhibition and less plasticity in the regulation of cortisol secretion. HPA axis hyperactivity has also been linked with various somatic health conditions, such as cardiovascular disease, obesity, hypertension, insulin resistance and diabetes. All of these conditions have been shown to be risk factors for physical disability, and so through these pathophysiological effects depression could impact on disability status. As yet, no studies have directly examined the link between HPA axis function and disability, and so this explanatory mechanism needs to be investigated in future research.

Inflammation, a chronic elevated immune response characterised by high levels of inflammatory cytokines, may also play a role in the pathophysiology of depression and disability. Cytokines are intracellular signalling polypeptides that determine host defence and regulate immune responses, the acute-phase reaction and haematopoiesis [59]. Depression can cause excess interleukin 6 (IL-6) production [60] through chronic glucocorticoid elevations [61], increased activity of the HPA axis [62], or central and peripheral catecholaminergic systems independent of the HPA axis [63]. Increased levels of inflammatory markers, e.g. IL-6, tumour necrosis factor alpha (TNF-α) and C-reactive protein (CRP), have been demonstrated among depressed psychiatric patients [64–67]. In our own work in a cohort of older people, a positive association was found between depressive symptomatology and plasma levels of IL-6 and TNF-α [68]. However, the association of depressive symptomatology with inflammation remains equivocal, since there have been some studies that could not confirm the link [69,70]. These inconsistent findings could indicate that the link between depression and inflammation is present only or more strongly for more severe depression and for older people, since inflammation levels are generally higher in older compared with younger people. Probably because inflammation is involved in many pathophysiological processes, including cardiovascular conditions, diabetes, osteoarthritis and lung disease, inflammation has been shown to be one of the strongest biological risk factors for physical disability in old age [71,72]. This indicates that inflammation could be a pathophysiological process that links depression to disability.

Intervening to break the link between depression and disability

Previous sections of this chapter have given strong evidence for a link between depression and disability. The question that arises is whether we can intervene to break this link. Would it, for instance, be possible to decrease disability burden by treating depression? Or would disability rehabilitation improve depressed mood? Fortunately, depression is a potentially modifiable and preventable condition. Prevention and treatment of depression may be one of the most effective targets for interventions aiming at reducing physical decline and increasing the number of years during which people maintain independence. Compared with the rather large number of observational studies in the area of depression and disability, not many studies have examined the potential effects of interventions on depression and disability. The intervention studies that do exist in this area of research have focused mainly on two types of intervention: pharmacotherapy and physical exercise.

Pharmacotherapy

The majority of intervention studies conducted in the area of depression involve pharmacotherapy, in which the primary aim has been to examine effects on depressed mood. The effect of pharmacotherapy on physical function has been much less studied. However, some trials also included an assessment of physical functioning, in most cases a rather broad measure, such as the Medical Outcomes Study 36-item short-form (SF-36) scale, which not only assesses aspects of disability but also incorporates concepts such as pain and social isolation. In a study by Lin *et al.* [73] conducted among 228 persistently depressed patients in primary care, those who received a collaborative care intervention that included psychiatric consultation, patient education and pharmacotherapy experienced significantly less limitations in their family, work and social activities compared with patients receiving usual primary care. Similar findings were observed in a study comparing pharmacotherapy and psychotherapy with usual care among 276 primary-care patients with major depression [74]. A few controlled trials have examined the effect of pharmacotherapy on a specific physical disability outcome measure. Overall, these studies indicate that the active treatment group showed greater improvement in physical functioning than did the placebo group [75–77]. For instance, in a six-week placebo-controlled study of nortriptyline in ambulatory depressed patients, subjects in the intervention group had significantly greater improved physical disability scores than did those in the placebo group [75]. This study also assessed objective measures of physical impairments, such as walking endurance. Although self-reported disability measures improved, the objective measures of physical impairments did not improve, which may suggest that the improvement in disability is relatively independent of improvement in physical impairment. In a randomised trial, 1801 older people were assigned to a care-management programme for depression (including antidepressant management) or to a usual-care control group. After 12 months of follow-up, those in the intervention group showed significantly greater improvement in functional impairment than those in the control group. This is one of the only studies to confirm the effectiveness of depression care management on a functional outcome over a long period of time [78].

Exercise interventions

Observational studies suggest that regular physical exercise may be one of the most important preventive factors for onset of late-life disability [79]. Clinical trials among older people have shown that exercise programmes improve self-reported functional scores and can prevent the onset of severe physical disability (ADL disability) [80,81]. These studies provide strong evidence for the benefits of physical exercise. However, benefits are not restricted to physical health alone but extend to the psychological domain of health as well. Longitudinal epidemiological studies have shown that a high level of physical activity reduces the risk of developing high depressive symptomatology over time [82], and that this effect is not limited to individuals who have been active throughout their adult life. In short, physical activity seems to be an effective form of prevention for depressive symptomatology among older adults, even when adopted later in life [83]. Physiological, biological and psychological mechanisms have been suggested to explain the antidepressive effects of exercise [84].

Evidence for a beneficial effect of exercise on psychological health is confirmed in several experimental studies, most of which have been conducted among clinically depressed people. For example, Greist *et al.* [85], McCann and Holmes [86] and Martinsen *et al.* [87] have shown that clinically depressed people randomised to an exercise programme were more likely to improve their depression status than those not receiving the exercise programme. Other experimental studies have shown that exercise programmes appear to be at least as effective in reducing clinical depression as more conventional treatment regimens such as antidepressant medication [88–90]. In clinically depressed patients, evidence for an antidepressive effect of exercise is provided by controlled trials involving resistance exercise [91] or aerobic exercise programmes [88,89].

In the Fitness, Arthritis and Senior Trial (FAST) involving 438 older participants with knee osteoarthritis, Penninx *et al.* [92] showed that aerobic exercise, but not resistance exercise, significantly lowered depression scores during an 18-month follow-up. The antidepressive effect of aerobic exercise was found for both people with initially high and with initially low depressive symptomatology and was the strongest for those who were the most compliant. It appeared that the antidepressive effect of exercise induced improvements in all subjects and did not normalise depressed mood only in those who had high initial depression levels. Both in initially depressed and non-depressed people, assignment to either aerobic or resistance exercise was associated with a significant improvement of physical disability levels during the 18-month follow-up. Overall, the results from this randomised controlled trial indicated that an exercise intervention among (mildly) depressed older people improved both mood and physical function.

Summary and conclusions

This chapter has reviewed the link between depression and physical disability. This link can best be described as a process whereby depressive symptoms and physical dysfunctions interact to cause a progressive downward spiral in health status. There is convincing evidence that depression increases the subsequent risk for physical disability and, in turn, physical disability results in increased depressive symptoms. The longitudinal associations between depression and physical disability appear to be independent of potentially confounding factors such as age, sex and medical comorbidity. The physical health deterioration associated with depression may be due to physiological changes induced by depression, the unhealthier behavioural and psychosocial risk profile of depressed older people, the somatic accompaniments of depression, and the decreased motivation of depressed older people for self-care. Both pharmacotherapy and exercise intervention have shown promising results in breaking the unfavourable link between depression and physical disability by improving depressive symptoms as well as disability levels.

REFERENCES

1. L. M. Verbrugge, A. M. Jette, The disablement process. *Soc. Sci. Med.* **38** (1994), 1–14.

2. World Health Organization. *International Classification of Functioning, Disability and Health.* (Geneva: WHO, 2001).

3. E. Kramarow, H. Lentzner, R. Rooks, J. Weeks, S. Saydah, *Health, United States, 1999: Health and Aging Chartbook* (Hyattsville, MD: National Center for Health Statistics, 1999).

4. J. M. Guralnik, L. Ferrucci, E. M. Simonsick, M. E. Salive, R. B. Wallace, Lower-extremity function in persons over the age of 70 years as a predictor of subsequent disability. *N. Engl. J. Med.* **332** (1995), 556–61.

5. B. W. Penninx, L. Ferrucci, S. G. Leveille, *et al.*, Lower extremity performance in nondisabled older persons as a predictor of subsequent hospitalization. *J. Gerontol. A Biol. Sci. Med. Sci.* **55** (2000), M691–7.

6. J. M. Guralnik, L. P. Fried, M. E. Salive, Disability as a public health outcome in the aging population. *Annu. Rev. Public Health* **17** (1996), 25–46.

7. T. R. Fried, E. H. Bradley, C. S. Williams, M. E. Tinetti, Functional disability and health care expenditures for older persons. *Arch. Intern. Med.* **161** (2001), 2602–7.

8. A. T. Beekman, D. J. Deeg, A. W. Braam, J. H. Smit, W. van Tilburg, Consequences of major and minor depression in later life: a study of disability, well-being and service utilization. *Psychol. Med.* **27** (1997), 1397–409.

9. Y. Forsell, A. F. Jorm, B. Winblad, Association of age, sex, cognitive dysfunction, and disability with major depressive symptoms in an elderly sample. *Am. J. Psychiatry* **151** (1994), 1600–604.

10. H. G. Koenig, L. K. George, Depression and physical disability outcomes in depressed medically ill hospitalized older adults. *Am. J. Geriatr. Psychiatry* **6** (1998), 230–47.

11. J. M. Lyness, D. A. King, C. Cox, Z. Yoediono, E. D. Caine, The importance of subsyndromal depression in older primary care patients: prevalence and associated functional disability. *J. Am. Geriatr. Soc.* **47** (2001), 647–52.

12. P. A. Sinclair, J. M. Lyness, D. A. King, C. Cox, E. D. Caine, Depression and self-reported functional status in older primary care patients. *Am. J. Psychiatry* **158** (2001), 416–19.

13. K. B. Wells, A. Stewart, R. D. Hays, *et al.*, The functioning and well-being of depressed patients: results from the Medical Outcomes Study. *J. Am. Med. Assoc.* **262** (1989), 914–19.

14. J. Johnson, M. M. Weissman, G. L. Klerman, Service utilization and social morbidity associated with depressive symptoms in the community. *J. Am. Med. Assoc.* **267** (1992), 1478–83.

15. J. Ormel, G. I. Kempen, D. J. Deeg, *et al.*, Functioning, well-being, and health perception in late middle-aged and older people: comparing the effects of depressive symptoms and chronic medical conditions. *J. Am. Geriatr. Soc.* **46** (1998), 39–48.

16. B. G. Druss, S. C. Marcus, R. A. Rosenheck, *et al.*, Understanding disability in mental and general medical conditions. *Am. J. Psychiatry* **157** (2000), 1485–91.

17. W. E. Broadhead, D. G. Blazer, L. K. George, C. K. Tse, Depression, disability days, and days lost from work in a prospective epidemiologic survey. *J. Am. Med. Assoc.* **264** (1990), 2524–8.

18. J. Ormel, M. VonKorff, T. B. Ustun, *et al.*, Common mental disorders and disability across cultures: results from the WHO Collaborative Study on Psychological Problems in General Health Care. *J. Am. Med. Assoc.* **272** (1994), 1741–8.

19. K. B. Wells, C. D. Sherbourne, Functioning and utility for current health of patients with depression or chronic medical conditions in managed, primary care practices. *Arch. Gen. Psychiatry* **56** (1999), 897–904.

20. C. J. Murray, A. D. Lopez, Alternative projections of mortality and disability by cause 1990–2020: Global Burden of Disease Study. *Lancet* **349** (1997), 1498–504.

21. G. J. Kennedy, H. R. Kelman, C. Thomas, The emergence of depressive symptoms in late life: the importance of declining health and increasing disability. *J. Community Health.* **15** (1990), 93–104.

22. R. E. Roberts, G. A. Kaplan, S. J. Shema, W. J. Strawbridge, Prevalence and correlates of depression in an aging cohort: the Alameda County Study. *J. Gerontol. B. Psychol. Sci. Soc. Sci.* **52** (1997), S252–8.

23. A. M. Zeiss, P. M. Lewinsohn, P. Rohde, J. R. Seeley, Relationship of physical disease and functional impairment to depression in older people. *Psychol. Aging* **11** (1996), 572–81.

24. M. J. Prince, R. H. Harwood, A. Thomas, A. H. Mann, A prospective population-based cohort study of the effects of disablement and social milieu on the onset and maintenance of late-life depression: the Gospel Oak Project VII. *Psychol. Med.* **28** (1998), 337–50.

25. S. W. Geerlings, A. T. Beekman, D. J. Deeg, W. van Tilburg, Physical health and the onset and persistence of depression in older adults: an eight-wave prospective community-based study. *Psychol. Med.* **30** (2000), 369–80.

26. L. F. Berkman, C. S. Berkman, S. Kasl, *et al.*, Depressive symptoms in relation to physical health and functioning in the elderly. *Am. J. Epidemiol* **124** (1986), 372–88.

27. A. T. Beekman, D. J. Deeg, S. W. Geerlings, *et al.*, Emergence and persistence of late life depression: a 3-year follow-up of the Longitudinal Aging Study Amsterdam. *J. Affect. Disord.* **65** (2001), 131–8.

28. J. Ormel, G. I. Kempen, B. W. Penninx, *et al.*, Chronic medical conditions and mental health in older people: disability and psychosocial resources mediate specific mental health effects. *Psychol. Med.* **27** (1997), 1065–77.

29. R. J. Turner, S. Noh, Physical disability and depression: a longitudinal analysis. *J. Health. Soc. Behav.* **29** (1988), 23–37.

30. J. Ormel, T. Oldehinkel, E. Brilman, W. vanden Brink, Outcome of depression and anxiety in primary care: a three-wave 3 1/2-year study of psychopathology and disability. *Arch. Gen. Psychiatry* **50** (1993), 759–66.

31. M. von Korff, J. Ormel, W. Katon, E. H. Lin, Disability and depression among high utilizers of health care: a longitudinal analysis. *Arch. Gen. Psychiatry* **49** (1992), 91–100.

32. M. L. Bruce, T. E. Seeman, S. S. Merrill, D. G. Blazer, The impact of depressive symptomatology on physical disability: MacArthur Studies of Successful Aging. *Am. J. Public Health* **84** (1994), 1796–9.

33. J. J. Gallo, P. V. Rabins, C. G. Lyketsos, A. Y. Tien, J. C. Anthony, Depression without sadness: functional outcomes of nondysphoric depression in later life. *J. Am. Geriatr. Soc.* **45** (1997), 570–78.

34. B. W. Penninx, S. Leveille, L. Ferrucci, J. T. van Eijk, J. M. Guralnik, Exploring the effect of depression on physical disability: longitudinal evidence from the established populations for epidemiologic studies of the elderly. *Am. J. Public Health* **89** (1999), 1346–52.

35. D. Cronin-Stubbs, C. F. de Leon, L. A. Beckett, *et al.*, Six-year effect of depressive symptoms on the course of physical disability in community-living older adults. *Arch. Intern. Med.* **160** (2000), 3074–80.

36. H. K. Armenian, L. A. Pratt, J. Gallo, W. W. Eaton, Psychopathology as a predictor of disability: a population-based follow-up study in Baltimore, Maryland. *Am. J. Epidemiol.* **148** (1998), 269–75.

37. E. J. Lenze, J. C. Rogers, L. M. Martire, *et al.*, The association of late-life depression and anxiety with physical disability: a review of the literature and prospectus for future research. *Am. J. Geriatr. Psychiatry* **9** (2001), 113–35.

38. B. W. Penninx, J. M. Guralnik, L. Ferrucci, *et al.*, Depressive symptoms and physical decline in community-dwelling older persons. *J. Am. Med. Assoc.* **279** (1998), 1720–26.

39. C. H. van Gool, G. I. Kempen, B. W. Penninx, *et al.*, Impact of depression on disablement in late middle aged and older persons: results from the Longitudinal Aging Study Amsterdam. *Soc. Sci. Med.* **60** (2005), 25–36.

40. B. W. Penninx, D. J. Deeg, J. T. van Eijk, A. T. Beekman, J. M. Guralnik, Changes in depression and physical decline in older adults: a longitudinal perspective. *J. Affect. Disord.* **61** (2000), 1–12.

41. G. J. Kennedy, H. R. Kelman, C. Thomas, Persistence and remission of depressive symptoms in late life. *Am. J. Psychiatry* **148** (1991), 174–8.

42. J. Ormel, M. Von Korff, B. W. van den, *et al.*, Depression, anxiety, and social disability show synchrony of change in primary care patients. *Am. J. Public Health* **83** (1993), 385–90.

43. G. I. Kempen, N. Steverink, J. Ormel, D. J. Deeg, The assessment of ADL among frail elderly in an interview survey: self-report versus performance-based tests and determinants of discrepancies. *J. Gerontol. B Psychol. Sci. Soc. Sci.* **51** (1996), 254–60.

44. L. L. Judd, H. S. Akiskal, P. J. Zeller, *et al.*, Psychosocial disability during the long-term course of unipolar major depressive disorder. *Arch. Gen. Psychiatry* **57** (2000), 375–80.

45. J. Ormel, A. J. Oldehinkel, W. A. Nolen, W. Vollebergh, Psychosocial disability before, during, and after a major depressive episode: a 3-wave population-based study of state, scar, and trait effects. *Arch. Gen. Psychiatry* **61** (2004), 387–92.

46. R. F. Anda, D. F. Williamson, L. G. Escobedo, *et al.*, Depression and the dynamics of smoking: a national perspective. *J. Am. Med. Assoc.* **264** (1990), 1541–5.

47. C. U. Onyike, R. M. Crum, H. B. Lee, C. G. Lyketsos, W. W. Eaton, Is obesity associated with major depression? Results from the Third National Health and Nutrition Examination Survey. *Am. J. Epidemiol.* **158** (2003), 1139–47.

48. B. W. Penninx, J. M. Guralnik, L. Ferrucci, *et al.*, Vitamin B(12) deficiency and depression in physically disabled older women: epidemiologic evidence from the Women's Health and Aging Study. *Am. J. Psychiatry* **157** (2000), 715–21.

49. T. Stephens, Physical activity and mental health in the United States and Canada: evidence from four population surveys. *Prev. Med.* **17** (1988), 35–47.

50. B. W. Penninx, T. van Tilburg, A. J. Boeke, *et al.*, Effects of social support and personal coping resources on depressive symptoms: different for various chronic diseases? *Health Psychol.* **17** (1998), 551–8.

51. B. G. Druss, W. D. Bradford, R. A. Rosenheck, M. J. Radford, H. M. Krumholz, Quality of medical care and excess mortality in older patients with mental disorders. *Arch. Gen. Psychiatry* **58** (2001), 565–72.

52. B. W. Penninx, T. G. van Tilburg, D. M. Kriegsman, *et al.*, Effects of social support and personal coping resources on mortality in older age: the Longitudinal Aging Study Amsterdam. *Am. J. Epidemiol.* **146** (1997), 510–19.

53. C. B. Nemeroff, D. L. Musselman, D. L. Evans, Depression and cardiac disease. *Depress. Anxiety* **8** Suppl 1 (1998), 71–9.

54. D. L. Musselman, D. L. Evans, C. B. Nemeroff, The relationship of depression to cardiovascular disease: epidemiology, biology, and treatment. *Arch. Gen. Psychiatry* **55** (1998), 580–92.

55. M. T. La Rovere, J. T. Bigger, Jr, F. I. Marcus, A. Mortara, P. J. Schwartz, Baroreflex sensitivity and heart-rate variability in prediction of total cardiac mortality after myocardial infarction: ATRAMI (Autonomic Tone and Reflexes After Myocardial Infarction) investigators. *Lancet* **351** (1998), 478–84.

56. T. G. Vrijkotte, L. J. van Doornen, E. J. de Geus, Effects of work stress on ambulatory blood pressure, heart rate, and heart rate variability. *Hypertension* **35** (2000), 880–86.

57. R. Pasquali, V. Vicennati, Activity of the hypothalamic-pituitary-adrenal axis in different obesity phenotypes. *Int. J. Obes. Relat. Metab. Disord.* **24** Suppl 2 (2000), 47–9.

58. J. L. Abelson, G. C. Curtis, Hypothalamic-pituitary-adrenal axis activity in panic disorder: 24-hour secretion of corticotropin and cortisol. *Arch. Gen. Psychiatry* **53** (1996), 323–31.

59. J. Van Snick, Interleukin-6: an overview. *Annu. Rev. Immunol.* **8** (1990), 253–78.

60. M. Maes, A. H. Lin, L. Delmeire, *et al.*, Elevated serum interleukin-6 (IL-6) and IL-6 receptor concentrations in posttraumatic stress disorder following accidental man-made traumatic events. *Biol. Psychiatry* **45** (1999), 833–9.

61. R. M. Sapolsky, L. C. Krey, B. S. McEwen, The neuroendocrinology of stress and aging: the glucocorticoid cascade hypothesis. *Endocrinol. Rev.* **7** (1986), 284–301.

62. A. Arimura, A. Takaki, G. Komaki, Interactions between cytokines and the hypothalamic-pituitary-adrenal axis during stress. *Ann. N. Y. Acad. Sci.* **739** (1994), 270–81.

63. S. Reichlin, Neuroendocrine-immune interactions. *N. Engl. J. Med.* **329** (1993), 1246–53.

64. M. Maes, H. Y. Meltzer, E. Bosmans, *et al.*, Increased plasma concentrations of interleukin-6, soluble interleukin-6, soluble interleukin-2 and transferrin receptor in major depression. *J. Affect. Disord.* **34** (1995), 301–9.

65. A. Sluzewska, J. Rybakowski, E. Bosmans, *et al.*, Indicators of immune activation in major depression. *Psychiatry Res.* **64** (1996), 161–7.

66. M. Berk, A. A. Wadee, R. H. Kuschke, A. O'Neill-Kerr, Acute phase proteins in major depression. *J. Psychosom. Res.* **43** (1997), 529–34.

67. M. Hornig, D. B. Goodman, M. Kamoun, J. D. Amsterdam, Positive and negative acute phase proteins in affective subtypes. *J. Affect. Disord.* **49** (1998), 9–18.

68. B. W. Penninx, S. Kritchevsky, K. Yaffe, *et al.*, Inflammatory markers and depressed mood in older men and women: results from the Health ABC study. Biol Psychiatry **54** (2003), 566–72.

69. H. Tiemeier, A. Hofman, H. R. van Tuijl, *et al.*, Inflammatory proteins and depression in the elderly. *Epidemiology* **14** (2003), 103–7.

70. A. Steptoe, S. R. Kunz-Ebrecht, N. Owen, Lack of association between depressive symptoms and markers of immune and vascular inflammation in middle-aged men and women. *Psychol. Med.* **33** (2003), 667–74.

71. B. W. Penninx, S. B. Kritchevsky, A. B. Newman, *et al.*, Inflammatory markers and incident mobility limitation in the elderly. *J. Am. Geriatr. Soc.* **52** (2004), 1105–13.

72. L. Ferrucci, T. B. Harris, J. M. Guralnik, *et al.*, Serum IL-6 level and the development of disability in older persons. *J. Am. Geriatr. Soc.* **47** (1999), 639–46.

73. E. H. Lin, M. VonKorff, J. Russo, *et al.*, Can depression treatment in primary care reduce disability? A stepped care approach. *Arch. Fam. Med.* **9** (2000), 1052–8.

74. J. L. Coulehan, H. C. Schulberg, M. R. Block, M. J. Madonia, E. Rodriguez, Treating depressed primary care patients improves their physical, mental, and social functioning. *Arch. Intern. Med.* **157** (1997), 1113–20.

75. S. Borson, G. J. McDonald, T. Gayle, *et al.*, Improvement in mood, physical symptoms, and function with nortriptyline for depression in patients with chronic obstructive pulmonary disease. *Psychosomatics* **33** (1992), 190–201.

76. J. H. Heiligenstein, J. E. Ware, Jr, K. M. Beusterien, *et al.*, Acute effects of fluoxetine versus placebo on functional health and well-being in late-life depression. *Int. Psychogeriatr.* **7**: Suppl (1995), 125–37.

77. R. G. Robinson, S. K. Schultz, C. Castillo, *et al.*, Nortriptyline versus fluoxetine in the treatment of depression and in short-term recovery after stroke: a placebo-controlled, double-blind study. *Am. J. Psychiatry* **157** (2000), 351–9.

78. J. W. Williams, Jr, W. Katon, E. H. Lin, *et al.*, The effectiveness of depression care management on diabetes-related outcomes in older patients. *Ann. Intern. Med.* **140** (2004), 1015–24.

79. J. E. Carlson, G. V. Ostir, S. A. Black, *et al.*, Disability in older adults: 2. Physical activity as prevention. *Behav. Med.* **24** (1999), 157–68.

80. B. W. Penninx, S. P. Messier, W. J. Rejeski, *et al.*, Physical exercise and the prevention of disability in activities of daily living in older persons with osteoarthritis. *Arch. Intern. Med.* **161** (2001), 2309–16.

81. W. H. Ettinger, Jr, R. Burns, S. P. Messier, *et al.*, A randomized trial comparing aerobic exercise and resistance exercise with a health education program in older adults with knee osteoarthritis: the Fitness Arthritis and Seniors Trial (FAST). *J. Am. Med. Assoc.* **277** (1997), 25–31.

82. M. E. Farmer, B. Z. Locke, E. K. Moscicki, *et al.*, Physical activity and depressive symptoms: the NHANES I Epidemiologic Follow-up Study. *Am. J. Epidemiol.* **128** (1988), 1340–51.

83. T. C. Camacho, R. E. Roberts, N. B. Lazarus, G. A. Kaplan, R. D. Cohen, Physical activity and depression: evidence from the Alameda County Study. *Am. J. Epidemiol.* **134** (1991), 220–31.

84. T. C. North, P. McCullagh, Z. V. Tran, Effect of exercise on depression. *Exerc. Sport. Sci. Rev.* **18** (1990), 379–415.

85. J. H. Greist, M. H. Klein, R. R. Eischens, *et al.*, Running as treatment for depression. *Compr. Psychiatry* **20** (1979), 41–54.

86. I. L. McCann, D. S. Holmes, Influence of aerobic exercise on depression. *J. Pers. Soc. Psychol.* **46** (1984), 1142–7.

87. E. W. Martinsen, A. Medhus, L. Sandvik, Effects of aerobic exercise on depression: a controlled study. *Br. Med. J. (Clin. Res. Ed.)* **291** (1985), 109.

88. J. A. Blumenthal, M. A. Babyak, K. A. Moore, *et al.*, Effects of exercise training on older patients with major depression. *Arch. Intern. Med.* **159** (1999), 2349–56.

89. M. Babyak, J. A. Blumenthal, S. Herman, *et al.*, Exercise treatment for major depression: maintenance of therapeutic benefit at 10 months. *Psychosom. Med.* **62** (2000), 633–8.

90. J. K. McNeil, E. M. LeBlanc, M. Joyner, The effect of exercise on depressive symptoms in the moderately depressed elderly. *Psychol. Aging* **6** (1991), 487–8.

91. N. A. Singh, K. M. Clements, M. A. Fiatarone, A randomized controlled trial of progressive resistance training in depressed elders. *J. Gerontol. A Biol. Sci. Med. Sci.* **52** (1997), M27–35.

92. B. W. Penninx, W. J. Rejeski, J. Pandya, *et al.*, Exercise and depressive symptoms: a comparison of aerobic and resistance exercise effects on emotional and physical function in older persons with high and low depressive symptomatology. *J. Gerontol. B Psychol. Sci. Soc. Sci.* **57** (2002), 124–32.

7

Chronic pain and depression: twin burdens of adaptation

Christina M. Van Puymbroeck, Alex J. Zautra
and Peter-Panagioti Harakas

Introduction

It is estimated that chronic pain afflicts between 50 and 80 million people in the USA [1]. Adding to this burden of pain, feelings of depression frequently accompany the pain [2]. These depressive symptoms include feelings of sadness, loss of pleasure and fatigue and range in severity from transient malaise to persistent and debilitating episodes. For many people, it is common sense that negative feelings would follow painful experiences, but a number of researchers have noted that depressed patients frequently report high levels of pain as well. Not only is pain a common somatic complaint in individuals suffering from depressive disorders [3], but also, according to some accounts, more than 50% of clinically depressed patients report pain as a symptom [4]. Not all investigators use the same criteria to determine the presence of depression, and so the exact prevalence of depression among patients with chronic pain is not easy to estimate [5]. Banks and Kerns [6] reviewed only studies that used standardised criteria to diagnose depressive disorders and estimated that at any given point 30–54% of clinic-based patients suffer from major depressive disorder (MDD), a rate substantially higher than that found in the general population [7] and higher than in out-patients of other medical conditions[1].

Thus, there appears to be a strong association between depressive symptoms and persistent pain, but the underlying causal mechanisms remain poorly understood. Nevertheless, our conceptualisations of both pain and depression are evolving at a rapid pace, offering the possibility of a full accounting of the complex relationships between depression, pain, illness and immune functioning.

---

[1] In an effort to compare rates of depressive symptomatology across different pain conditions, Hawley and Wolfe [8] reported the results of a longitudinal study of 6153 pain patients: depression scores among various chronic pain groups, such as rheumatoid arthritis, osteoarthritis and low back pain, were not significantly different, but in fibromyalgia patients depression scores were elevated in comparison with other chronic pain conditions.

Depression and Physical Illness, ed. A. Steptoe.
Published by Cambridge University Press. © Cambridge University Press 2006.

For centuries, pain was understood as a sensation arising from underlying tissue damage. In 1965, this bottom-up (stimulus-response) model of pain was challenged by Melzack and Wall's [9] gate-control theory of pain, which emphasised a top-down multidimensional conceptualisation of pain. The gate-control theory posited three dimensions of pain: a sensory-physiologic dimension, a motivational-affective dimension and a cognitive-evaluative dimension. A number of psychosocial models of the pain–depression relationship followed in the footsteps of gate-control theory and further emphasised the importance of psychological processes in the experience of chronic pain. Nonetheless, despite numerous studies conducted in this area over the past decades, the causal relationship between pain and depression remains controversial [10]. For this reason, we believe it is instructive to briefly review the historically dominant hypotheses formulated about the nature of the pain–depression relationship.

Antecedent hypothesis

The first proposed pathway for the relationship between depression and chronic pain is that depression is responsible for the onset or maintenance of pain in individuals who suffer from both sets of symptoms. This hypothesis, often termed the 'antecedent hypothesis' [2], posits that depression precedes pain. Early studies used psychogenic conceptualisations of pain to suggest that chronic pain was potentially a variant of depressive disorder [11], a form of 'masked' depression characterised by continuous pain, denial of emotional and interpersonal difficulties and inability to tolerate success and happiness [12]. This research has been criticised widely on both methodological [13] and theoretical [14] grounds. Despite the repudiation of much of the early research, several more recent studies still suggest that depression plays a significant role in the aetiology of chronic pain and often precedes the development of chronic pain [15,16].

Consequence hypothesis

The consequence hypothesis views depression as secondary to chronic pain. According to this view, depressive symptoms follow the onset of pain. This reactive depression is often seen as the result of an incapacitating physical condition that arises from the sustained reduction in physical and social activities [17].

Common pathogenesis

The common pathogenesis model assumes that depression and pain, although clearly distinct conditions, have a shared aetiology. The proposed mechanisms include key neurotransmitters such as serotonin, noradrenaline, substance P and corticotropin-releasing factor (CRF) [18]. In a similar fashion, other researchers have proposed that chronic inescapable stress might be the link between chronic pain and depression, and that the hypothalamic-pituitary-adrenocortical (HPA) axis might be specifically involved in the aetiology of both [19]. Thus, depressive symptoms may manifest in patients with chronic pain because of long-term stress activation of the HPA axis as a result of chronic pain.

Other researchers view the effects of stress as having an even more prominent role in explaining the pain–depression association. One of the theories developed to explain medically unexplained chronic pain such as found in fibromyalgia focuses on dysregulation of the human stress response as a result of central nervous system processes [20]. This view is consistent with research findings that stressors perceived as inescapable, unavoidable or unpredictable evoke strong biological reactions [21] and with findings from animal studies that early life stressors may permanently biologically impact animals' responses to stressors [22]. The proposed mechanisms involve disturbances in CRF production, which affect the HPA axis by producing central effects on nociceptive processing, leading to abnormalities in autonomic function [20].

Cognitive–behavioural theories

The relationship between chronic pain and depression has often been explained within a cognitive–behavioural framework. Here, coping beliefs and behaviours are considered to play important roles in the patient's adjustment. In this vein, thoughts that sustain the 'illness role', or the belief that medications and solicitous responses from others are necessary, have been shown to co-vary with depression. One frequently discussed set of cognitions in patients with pain is referred to as 'catastrophising'. Patients who catastrophise expect the worse outcome and worry excessively about possible negative consequences of events in an effort to defend against pain exacerbations. These cognitions have been found to be associated with depression [23]. In the cognitive–behavioural mediation model of depression [24], the direct relationship between pain and depressed mood is influenced by cognitive appraisal variables such as perceived interference and lack of self-control. Patients' judgements of the extent to which pain affects their ability to participate in social, recreational, vocational, family and domestic activities, and the satisfaction they derive from such activities, is referred to as perceived interference [24]. The cognitive–behavioural mediation model challenged the notion of pain as a variant of depression and appeared to offer a parsimonious integration of earlier cognitive and behavioural theories on the relationship of pain and depression [25–28].

Psychoneuroimmunological developments

A comprehensive review of current research provides strong evidence that depressive symptoms can also be conceived of as affective, behavioural and cognitive responses to immune activation. Profound immune activation can occur due to internal (e.g. bacterial) or external (e.g. grief) stressors that also activate the HPA axis. At the heart of this argument is the increasingly well-articulated relationship between pro-inflammatory cytokines and the symptoms of depression. In this view, depressive symptoms are seen as evolutionarily valuable responses, i.e. responses intended to conserve energy for survival in the face of an internal or external threat. Similarly, neuroimaging studies have provided evidence that pain is also a homeostatic response predicated on the need to avoid further harm by energy conservation and withdrawal.

We may thus surmise that depressed mood and chronic pain are distinct but related responses to underlying physiological events driven by mechanisms that evolved because they promoted survival. When these responses are not regulated properly by countervailing homeostatic processes, however, they become self-propagating, pathological and chronic.

Depression and the immune system

Although the relationship between depressive symptoms and immune regulation is complex [29], accumulating evidence suggests that depressive symptoms are related to the action of several cytokines (see Chapters 12 and 14). Cytokines are signalling proteins that facilitate communication between immune cells and that play a key function in the regulation of the immune response [30]. It is these cytokines that induce the functional changes in the brain characteristic of the non-specific symptoms of infection. These symptoms, termed 'sickness behaviours' [31], are comprised of behavioural (restlessness, reduced activity, hypersomnia, social withdrawal), cognitive (lack of concentration, loss of interest) and affective (depressed mood, anhedonia) components that match closely the criteria for depression as defined by the *Diagnostic and Statistical Manual of Mental Disorders*, 4th edn (DSM-IV) [32]. These behaviours may be considered to be part of a homeostatic process used to conserve energy to fight infection [33] and may represent a motivational state that promotes resistance to pathogens by resetting an organism's priorities [34].

Evidence for the association between depressive symptoms and cytokines comes from both animal and human studies. Experimental studies have shown that the administration of proinflammatory cytokines to animals induces sickness behaviours [35,36], whereas administration of the respective cytokine antagonists reverses some of these depressive-like symptoms [37]. In humans, increased plasma concentrations of cytokines such as interleukin 6 (IL-6) have been observed in depressed patients [38,39], and pro-inflammatory cytokines have been associated with the development of feelings of distress, despair and hopelessness expressed by many cancer patients [30]. Furthermore, cytokines such as interferon alpha

(IFN-α) appear to be implicated in depressive states experienced by patients receiving cytokine therapy. For example, people with cancer or hepatitis who are administered purified or recombinant cytokines develop flu-like neurovegetative symptoms, followed after several weeks by the onset of psychiatric disorders, with depression being the most prevalent [30,40–42]. Three of these symptoms have been identified as particularly destructive to the patient's quality of life: anhedonia (loss of pleasure), alterations in cognitions and changes in responses to pain. The implication of cytokines in the expression of depressive symptoms appears to be so strong that some authors have proposed that these depressive effects of cytokines during cytokine therapy constitute the basis of a 'cytokine-associated depressive syndrome' [43].

Depressive symptoms are also highly prevalent in chronic inflammation associated with autoimmune diseases such as systemic lupus erythematosus (SLE) and multiple sclerosis (MS) [44–46]. To illustrate this, MS-associated depressive symptoms have been shown to correlate with tumour necrosis factor alpha (TNF-α) and interferon gamma (IFN-γ) mRNA expression in patients during acute episodes [47]. Accordingly, a number of researchers now suggest that at least some of these symptoms are not simply reactions to the suffering caused by the specific medical condition but may be associated with immune changes that precede the development of the clinical symptoms of the autoimmune disease [48,49].

Evolving understanding of pain

Early thinking about pain emphasised the specificity viewpoint – the idea that pain is a distinct sensation represented by specific elements in both the central and the peripheral nervous system. The current perspective is one of convergence, where pain is conceived as an integrated state caused by a pattern of convergent somatosensory activity (that arises from perceptions of sensory stimulation on or in the body) within the neuromatrix. This perspective is typified by Melzack and Wall's [50] gate-control theory, which posits that both small- and large-diameter afferent nerve fibres converge on the primary somatosensory cortex via the somatosensory thalamus, where they produce the feeling of pain through activation of wide-dynamic-range (WDR) cells [50,51].

However, more recent evidence obtained using functional neuroimaging techniques has provided a profoundly different picture of the neurological substrate of pain. Providing strong support for the early proponents of the specificity perspective, Craig [52,53] has identified specific labelled lines as well as convergent somatic activity in an organised hierarchical system in the brain that serves the purpose of maintaining the body's homeostasis. The system includes a spino-thalamo-cortical pathway that provides a neural representation of the state of the body and leads to a subjective meta-representation of feelings from the body that are associated with emotion, such as feelings of exhaustion or malaise, and the corresponding negative affect. These pathways are present in only a few primate species and are developed to a high degree in humans. In this view, pain is a feeling from the body transmitted by lamina I neurons first to the homeostatic system in the spinal cord and hindbrain, and then on to the forebrain, where they provide a cortical image of the afferent representation of interoception (or the perceived physiological state of the body). In the forebrain, these afferent signals also activate the limbic motor cortex, which motivates a behavioural response. In the case described above (exhaustion, malaise, negative affect), the likely response is to shut down; in the case of pain, the likely response is withdrawal. Thus, pain is demonstrated to be a homeostatic emotion akin to temperature or itch, with a line-dedicated pathway that maps on to interoceptive systems in the forebrain and activates a motivational system. Put simply, the feeling of pain, like depression, is both a distinct sensation and a motivation.

Pain, depression and the immune system

Equally important as the evidence that pain and depression are both motivational processes is the mounting evidence that pain can also be a product of immune activation and subsequent inflammatory processes. Maier and colleagues [54] demonstrated that products of immune activation, such as the cytokine interleukin 1 beta (IL-β), increase pain sensitivity. Another cytokine, TNF-α, can also produce hyperalgesia. Watkins and Maier [55] suggest that hyperalgesia serves an adaptive function in that it discourages movement, conserves energy and promotes wound healing.

Abramov and colleagues [56] propose that the immune system necessarily participates in nociception in a variety of diseases and probably has a role in the development of chronic pain syndromes. Animal studies in their laboratory demonstrate that immune activation leads to hyperalgesia and, more importantly, that in stress-sensitive animals this hyperalgesia is significantly stronger and leads to increased vocalisation. They suggest that the response of stress-sensitive animals with activated immune systems is akin to the facilitation of emotional response components of pain in humans under conditions of immune stimulation.

In studies of patients with and without autoimmune disease, Zautra and colleagues [57] have found that the presence of depression amplifies the relationship between disease activity and stress. Zautra *et al.* found that stress leads to predictable increases in disease activity both in individuals with rheumatoid arthritis (an autoimmune disease) and with osteoarthritis (a non-immune-related disease). However, only participants with rheumatoid arthritis had an increase in IL-6 during and after stress; depression amplified this difference, with depressed participants with rheumatoid arthritis showing the highest levels of immune activation in response to stress. This relationship was particularly strong for stressors of an interpersonal nature, which makes sense considering the survival value of maintaining intimate relationships among the chronically ill. Indeed, cross-sensitisation between cytokines and stressors has been demonstrated in several studies, suggesting that cytokines might change brain circuitry, making it more responsive to stress [30]. In another study that supports the relationship between cytokines and stress sensitivity, Zautra and Smith [58] showed that depressive symptoms led to increases in perceived stress and pain in patients with rheumatoid arthritis. However, for patients with osteoarthritis, who do not have the same level of circulating cytokines as those with rheumatoid arthritis, depression was related only to pain and not to stress. Depression was a risk factor for pain in both samples of patients, but only in patients with rheumatoid arthritis did depression predict stress-reactive pain.

The link between immune activation and pain has been explored further by Watkins and colleagues [59], who noted that peripheral events that induce hyperalgesia also activate immune cells, which in turn activate peripheral nerves that terminate in the brain or dorsal horn of the spinal cord. Experimental studies have shown that hyperalgesia can be elicited by direct administration of substances known to evoke the release of pro-inflammatory cytokines [60]. Watkins *et al.* concluded that pain facilitation is part of the larger set of adaptive sickness behaviours mediated by cytokines that also serve the purpose of conserving energy for essential functions when the immune system signals to the brain that a threat is present.

Role and function of antidepressants

If depression and pain are processes induced by immune activation and dysregulation, then one would expect that antidepressant medications act directly or indirectly on the immune system and not only on the monoamine systems through which these drugs have long been thought to exert their effects. Antidepressant medication would also be expected to cause a decrease in pain as the pro-inflammatory immune products are down-regulated. This in fact appears to be the case. Capuron and Dantzer [30], Castanon and colleagues [61] and Yirmiya and colleagues [62] point out that all antidepressant drugs, regardless of their pharmacological class, attenuate the behavioural and neuroendocrine effects of immune activation. In addition, it has been demonstrated that antidepressant treatment causes a shift in the balance between pro- and anti-inflammatory cytokine production in the brain [61].

Musselman and colleagues [63] demonstrated that paroxetine reduces the incidence of major depression by 34% in melanoma patients treated with interferon-α. Clomiprimine, imipramine and citalopram were likewise shown to suppress the secretion of interleukin 2 (IL-2) by activated T-lymphocytes and of IL-1β and TNF-α by stimulated monocytes [64]. Maes and colleagues [65] provided additional evidence for the immunoregulatory effects of tricyclic and selective serotonin reuptake inhibitor (SSRI) antidepressants through the inhibition of IFN-γ and stimulation of an anti-proinflammatory cytokine, interleukin 10 (IL-10).

Antidepressant medications are used widely in chronic and neuropathic pain conditions for their antinociceptive effects, even in the absence of depressive symptomatology [66]. Sawynok *et al.* [67] note that antidepressants exhibit analgesic properties in multiple systems, including inflammatory, nociceptive and neuropathic test systems. Support for the analgesic qualities of tricyclic antidepressants comes from both human and animal models [68], and these medications are increasingly being used in the management of headaches, arthritis, cancer pain and other types of chronic and neurogenic pain [69,70]. In a review of 59 randomised placebo-controlled trials, Lynch [71] found that the data in support of the use of tricyclic antidepressant for analgesia were undisputed, but studies of the newer antidepressant class of SSRIs yielded conflicting results.

Chronicity: the role of sensitisation

Up to this point, we have outlined the evidence that both depression and pain are sickness behaviours provoked by pro-inflammatory cytokines and comprising an adaptation designed to minimise harm and maximise recovery when a threat to the organism is perceived. However, both depression and pain symptoms may become chronic through processes of sensitisation, which allow the symptoms to self-propagate, requiring less and less stimulation (perceived threat) to set them into motion.

Central sensitisation is a well-known and oft-studied mechanism, whereby the neurochemical substrate that facilitates the sensation continues to fire in the absence of objective stimuli. Central pain sensitisation occurs as low-threshold afferents that normally do not transmit pain signals become recruited through persistent central nervous system activation to transmit pain signals. This state of hyperexcitability includes the temporal summation of repetitive C-fibre stimulation, amplification of the pain response, spinal neurons behaving as wide-ranging dynamic cells, and the spread of pain sensitivity to non-injured areas [72,73]. Winkelstein [74] suggests that cytokines released upon initial insult (injury- or inflammation-induced) affect the electrophysiological responses of pain and help to establish a continuous feedback loop. She found that not only are cytokines such as IL-1, IL-6 and TNF up-regulated in persistent pain, but also they induce the expression of multiple pain mediators, such as prostaglandins and substance P, which leads to further spinal sensitisation. In addition, neuroinflammation occurs, in which immune cells migrate from the periphery into the central nervous system, leading directly to central sensitisation.

A review of the clinical presentation of depressive disorder suggests that central sensitisation processes may underlie depressed affect as well as pain. Depression is persistent within episodes and typically recurrent throughout the lifespan. The DSM-IV Mood Disorders field trials found that the most frequent course was 'recurrent, with antecedent dysthymia, without full interepisode recovery' [75]. Two related hypotheses have been offered to account for the chronicity of the disorder: the kindling and scar hypotheses.

The scar hypothesis suggests that a depressive episode wears away personal resources, leaving in its wake a relatively more vulnerable psyche to protect against future depressions [76]. One area on which a scar is most evident is that of cognitive attributions. Children who have been depressed show a deterioration of attributional styles that does not remit, even when the depressive episode has ended [77].

The kindling hypothesis proposes that changes in information processing potentiates depressive processes so that where a stressor may have been present to evoke the first depressive episode, each new episode is more and more autonomous and less related to external stimuli [78]. Indeed, the neurochemical changes provoked by stressors are typically fairly short-lived. However, these changes can be re-elicited by mild stressor conditions that would have only minor impact on their own [79]. In 2000, Joiner [76] offered an integrative model in which he argued that depression is characterised by both erosive processes, which corrode psychological resources, and self-propagating processes, which serve to prolong or exacerbate symptoms and leave the individual more vulnerable to recurrences.

There is now evidence that cytokines provoke a sensitisation response that can exert a proactive influence on the development of depression and other forms of psychopathology. IL-1β has been shown to elicit sensitisation effects in animal studies, increasing the coexpression of the stress hormones CRF and arginine-vasopressin (AVP). Upon initial administration of IL-1β, increased levels of CRF and AVP became evident after 4 days and peaked on day 11, although the phenotypic change was present for several weeks following administration. If the rats were subject to an additional stressor, in this case foot-shock, then the stress hormone levels were significantly enhanced, providing support for the hypothesis that peptide coexpression makes the HPA system more responsive to all sorts of challenges [80]. Administration of TNF-α has also been shown to elicit sickness behaviours at a much lower dosage than is typically required to evoke such behaviours if the second administration follows the first by 14–28 days. This sensitisation has a specific timeframe in which it can occur: sensitisation was not evident when the second TNF-α dosage was within seven days of the first [81]. Typically, psychological stressors have been considered 'processive', as they involve the cognitive processing of a situation and require higher cortical functioning. The category of stressor has now been broadened to include 'systemic' or metabolic insults, such as viral and bacterial infections, which may evoke many of the same neurochemical changes as the processive stressors. Interestingly, sensitisation occurs when the initial and subsequent stressors are the same (e.g. instances of loss) and when the stressors are of different classes (e.g. initial stressor, loss; second stressor, virus). Thus, cross-sensitisation can occur between stressors and cytokine challenges [79]. In fact, when systemic stressors occur on a backdrop of processive stress, a synergistic effect may occur.

Thus, the following picture emerges: When a stressor occurs in sufficient strength, regardless of whether it is a psychosocial or physiological threat, the organism mounts a vigorous defence through the immune system, leading to high levels of circulating cytokines, which can evoke both depressive symptoms and pain as part of the array of sickness behaviours designed to protect and defend the individual. In this view, the frequent comorbidity of depression and pain arises because each symptom is a manifestation of the same homeostatic drive to conserve energy for survival. This cascade of events may be highly adaptive following an acute stressor but may become chronic and maladaptive. Central sensitisation processes may sustain and reinstigate these sickness behaviours in a positive-feedback loop that, over time, can give rise to depression and pain even without a precipitating threat.

Resilience

If pain and depressive symptoms both originate as processes of adaptation that are vulnerable to becoming chronic and debilitating when dysregulated, then it behoves us to consider what can be done to support and restore the self-regulation of such processes. What do the aforementioned relationships suggest about potential models of resilience and, relatedly, methods of prevention and intervention? Two pathways seem particularly critical to the discussion of resilience in the face of most types of pathology: the preservation of homeostatic boundaries and restoration of equilibrium. The first pathway, preservation, can be thought of as a mechanism of primary prevention: how can we preserve the self-regulation of these systems in order to facilitate a response to threat of sufficient intensity and length to ward off the danger while retaining the necessary homeostatic elements that bring our physiology and psychology back to their baseline states? In particular, how do we sustain the fine distinctions that individuals must make, particularly once the context itself has become the cue for arousal? For instance, a child growing up in an abusive environment shows resilience when, having few other options, he or she can transport him- or herself out of the situation through fantasy and daydreaming. However, when the child grows up, he or she may no longer be adaptive to resort to fantasy in the face of conflict. Here, the adult's nervous and immune systems are forced to make clear distinctions between past and present threats, between his or her generalised learned fear of conflict and actual danger to the self. Charney [82] makes the suggestion that resilience may in fact be characterised by an ability to avoid overgeneralising conditioned stimuli to the larger context, having reversible storage of emotional memories and being able to facilitate extinction of learned responses. Psychophysiological flexibility built on complexity and a capacity for variability in responding may hold the key.

The question of how to facilitate the extinction of learned responses leads us directly to the second pathway, restorative processes, which allow a system to return to normal functioning after a period of heightened responsiveness, sensitization, and maladaption. McEwen and Stellar [83] identify allostatic load as the cumulative impact that substantially raises health risk due to chronic dysregulations in multiple systems. Considering how to reduce allostatic load is a preventive intervention as well, but at a different stage of adaptation. Here we need to identify the ingredients of recovery as well as the mechanisms for their appropriate utilisation.

Charney [82] offers one framework for the psychobiological mechanisms of resilience and vulnerability in which he identifies 11 potential mediators of the psychobiological response to extreme stress. Each of these 11 mediators offers the possibility of a treatment target, either alone or in functional interactions. Charney suggests that the psychobiological profile of a resilient individual is characterised by high relative levels of dehydroepiandrasterone (DHEA), neuropeptide Y, galanin, testosterone, and 5-hydroxytryptamine 1a (5-HT_{1a}) and benzodiazepine receptor function, and low relative levels of HPA axis activation, CRF, and locus coeruleus-noradrenaline activity. Based on the mounting evidence that there may be an endophenotype for resistance to hopelessness and anhedonia in the face of stress, Charney suggests the potential utility of a wide array of biochemical agents, including psychostimulants, dopamine reuptake inhibitors, dopamine receptor agonists and N-methyl-D-aspartate (NMDA) receptor antagonists to treat the symptoms of anhedonia and hopelessness in the face of traumatic stress for individuals with a more vulnerable endophenotype. Future research will continue to elucidate how the restoration of balance in the hormonal and endocrine systems can alleviate the negative consequences of stress-related systemic activation.

Emotion complexity

Work in emotional regulation is another promising avenue for interventions to support and restore homeostatic functioning. At its foundation this work derives from an understanding of emotions as complex motivational systems of approach and avoidance that govern cognition and behaviour. Unlike Charney [82], here the emphasis is on cognitive and affective systems of regulation rather than the associated physiological substrates. Positive emotions and negative emotions, for example, have been shown to behave as independent affect systems rather than as opposite ends of a single affective continuum [84–86].

This distinction between affective states has important ramifications for regulation of the stress response. Zautra [87] has reviewed a number of studies showing that positive emotions play an important role in promoting resilience in the face of a variety of stress-producing and negative experiences. One well-established consequence of pain is an increase in negative affect during the pain event [88,89], which over time (in the condition of chronic pain) leads to stable elevations in negative affect [90]. Positive emotions can play a pivotal role in undoing these negative affective states and improving health risks associated with negative affect. They appear to serve a restorative function in the face of stress [87].

Research in our laboratory with arthritis patients has led to the development of a dynamic affect (DA) model [86,91,92] that may help guide further research in this area. The model predicts changes in affective complexity as a function of stress. While positive and negative affects are independent factors under ordinary circumstances, under conditions of pain and stress affective space is compressed towards a more bipolar state. The uncertainty inherent in stressors provokes this simplification of complex emotional systems because of increased demand on information processing to resolve the uncertainty and reduce threat. In times when uncertainty is high, such as under conditions of stress or pain, the additional demands of maintaining a complex emotional framework would tax the system's capacity, leading to a simpler 'black-versus-white' structure of affective experience. This collapse to a one-dimensional affective system is evident in the increasingly inverse relationship between positive and negative affects during times of stress [87]. The consequences for people in chronic pain and, by extension, for those who suffer from long-term depression, are considerable. With worsening pain, affective complexity is compromised, leading the individual to adopt increasingly simple representations of his or her emotional states and less flexibility in response to challenge. Since it is stressful circumstances that lead to this representational simplification, in these instances negative affect crowds out positive affect. Mood clarity is one factor that the DA model predicts will support the maintenance of independent systems even under stress, and, indeed, our data bear this out. Arthritis patients with greater mood clarity retained more independence in their ratings of positive and negative mood states [86]. Furthermore, the presence of positive affect diminished the extent of the strong positive relationship between negative affect and pain [93]. The DA model lends itself to testable hypotheses regarding interventions intended to increase the ability to maintain emotional complexity and enhance opportunities for positive affect during times of stress. In our view, facilitating the retention of the independent affective structure through interventions focused on emotional regulation among people who are ill, in pain or otherwise under chronic stress will lead to greater flexibility in coping responses and better functional outcomes.

Negative emotions also have adaptive significance, as they narrow the thought–action repertoire in response to threat, and thus allowing for a rapid corrective response. However, positive emotions are necessary to rebound from negative experiences and return to a more regulated state. In a study demonstrating the relationship between physiological and psychological resilience, Tugade and Frederickson [94] found that positive emotions and cognitive appraisals contributed to the ability of resilient individuals to regulate their cardiovascular reactivity quickly in response to negative emotional arousal. Furthermore, they found that resilience can be taught to individuals who show greater stress reactivity for a longer duration than people who return to homeostatic functioning more easily after a threat. Tugade and Frederickson suggest that an intervention that promotes positive appraisal styles might prove especially useful for building resilience. This is particularly important in light of a recent study that provided evidence that people who are dysphoric demonstrate a reduced ability to use mood-incongruent recall to repair sad moods, even when instructed to do so [95]. Indeed, it has been shown that people who report higher daily positive mood have more responsive immune systems than those that report lower positive mood [96], and that people who are able to regain and maintain positive emotional states are less likely to show symptoms of ill-health or use medical services during stressful periods [97].

As predicted by the dynamic model of affect [86], the ability to focus inwards and to identify complex emotions has been shown to increase the ability to regulate mood [98]. Likewise, greater emotional knowledge, in particular the ability to discriminate among negative emotions, was associated with larger repertoires of emotional regulation strategies in a experience-sampling study [99].

Cognitive–behavioural therapy (CBT) is commonly used in pain-management programmes to assist patients in changing maladaptive ways of thinking and feeling in response to pain and illness. These therapies encompass a variety of techniques, including biofeedback, autogenic training, relaxation training, cognitive restructuring, distraction and activity pacing. An extensive literature on the use of CBT for rheumatoid arthritis has confirmed the utility of CBT for increasing adaptive pain-coping responses and self-efficacy expectations [100,101] as well as reducing inflammatory processes [100] and joint pain and swelling [102]. However, a comprehensive review of studies of CBT for rheumatoid arthritis has demonstrated one area of weakness, namely that CBT has not been shown to reduce depression in patients with pain [103]. In fact, in a well-controlled study by Bradley *et al.* [100], depression worsened while pain and disease indices improved as a result of CBT. The current focus on pain management in these CBT programmes limits their effectiveness by relative inattention to deficits in positive affect resources that appear critical to enhancing physical and psychological functioning in patients with pain and sustaining health and wellbeing over the long term. Ongoing clinical trials research in our laboratory is currently testing the hypothesis that adding an emotion-regulation emphasis to traditional CBT for pain management will improve a wide array of outcomes, including both pain and depression.

To summarise, resilience in the face of negative events allows the system to respond flexibly and to restore homeostasis promptly following activation. Traditional pain-management protocols targeting pain exclusively show little effect on improving depression. Including depression as an additional therapeutic target in pain-management programmes may foster resilience by preserving emotional complexity and maintaining independently functioning positive and negative affective systems. This allows positive emotions to restore balance after negative emotional experiences.

Conclusion

Depression and pain can be conceived of as two different, but closely related, sets of symptoms that co-vary with immune activation in response to harm or threat of harm. When these processes become dysregulated, the physiological, cognitive and emotional changes engendered by neuroendocrine immune activation can become chronic and systemic, leading to the maintenance of alarm responses long after their utility has ended. Overactivation of the HPA axis and monoamine systems as a result of these alarm responses is particularly implicated in the aetiology of syndromes of both chronic pain and depression and may maintain these conditions after the immune system itself has been quieted.

The mounting evidence for the implication of multiple systems in the experience of and recovery from depression and pain provides a wide array of intervention possibilities. Depression, pain and immune responses to a perceived threat may initiate elevations in one another, potentially leading to the dysregulation in multiple systems. Targets for intervention are diverse, including physiological, cognitive and emotional regulation. Furthermore, a consideration for the interconnectivity of the systems in the human body urges the adoption of a multifaceted approach to restoration of homeostasis. Emotional complexity is one such approach that has shown promise in regulating cognitive, affective and behavioural manifestations of allostatic load.

REFERENCES

1. B. Fox, Pain and its magnitude. In *Pain Management: A Practical Guide for Clinicians*, ed. R. S. Weiner (New York: CRS Press, 2002), pp. 3–8.

2. D. A. Fishbain, R. Cutler, H. L. Rosomoff, R. S. Rosomoff, Chronic pain associated depression: antecedent or consequence of chronic pain? A review. *Clin. J. Pain* **13** (1997), 116–37.

3. R. Wörz, Pain in depression – depression in pain. *Pain Clin. Updates* **11** (2003), 1–4.

4. L. von Knorring, C. Perris, M. Eisemann, U. Eriksson, H. Perris, Pain as a symptom in depressive disorders: II. Relationship to personality traits as assessed by means of KSP. *Pain* **17** (1983), 377–84.

5. J. M. Romano, J. A. Turner, Chronic pain and depression: does the evidence support a relationship? *Psych. Bull.* **97** (1985), 18–34.

6. S. M. Banks, R. D. Kerns, Explaining high rates of depression in chronic pain: a diathesis-stress framework. *Psych. Bull.* **119** (1996), 95–110.

7. D. G. Blazer, R. C. Kessler, K. A. McGonagle, M. S. Swartz, The prevalence and distribution of major depression in a national community sample: the National Comorbidity Survey. *Am. J. Psychiatry* **151** (1994), 979–86.

8. D. J. Hawley, F. Wolfe, Depression is not more common in rheumatoid arthritis: a 10-year longitudinal study of 6,153 patients with rheumatic disease. *J. Rheumatol.* **20** (1993), 2025–31.

9. R. Melzack, P. D. Wall, Pain mechanisms: a new theory. *Science* **50** (1965), 971–9.

10. R. H. Dworkin, What do we really know about the psychological origins of chronic pain? *Am. Pain Soc. Bull.* **1** (1991), 7–11.

11. G. Engel, 'Psychogenic' pain and the pain-prone patient. *Am. J. Med.* **26** (1959), 899–918.

12. D. Blumer, H. Heilbronn, Chronic pain as a variant of depressive disease: the pain-prone disorder. *J. Nerv. Ment. Dis.* **170** (1982), 425–8.

13. D. C. Turk, P. Salovey, Chronic pain as a variant of depressive disease: a critical reappraisal. *J. Nerv. Ment. Dis.* **172** (1984), 398–404.

14. J. B. W. Williams, R. L. Spitzer, Idiopathic pain disorder: a critique of pain-prone disorder and a proposal for a revision of the DSM-III category psychogenic pain disorder. *J. Nerv. Ment. Dis.* **170** (1982), 415–19.

15. P. Leino, G. Magni, Depressive and distress symptoms as predictors of low back pain, neck-shoulder pain, and other musculoskeletal morbidity: a 10-year follow-up of metal industry employees. *Pain* **53** (1993), 89–94.

16. G. Magni, C. Moreschi, S. Rigatti-Luchini, H. Merskey, Prospective study on the relationship between depressive symptoms and chronic musculoskeletal pain. *Pain* **56** (1994), 289–97.

17. R. A. Sternbach, *Pain Patients: Traits and Treatments* (New York, Academic Press, 1974).

18. L. C. Campbell, D. J. Clauw, F. J. Keefe, Persistent pain and depression: a biopsychosocial perspective. *Biol. Psychiatry* **54** (2003), 399–409.

19. G. Blackburn-Munro, R. Blackburn-Munro, Chronic pain, chronic stress and depression: coincidence or consequence? *J. Neuroendocrinol.* **13** (2001), 1009–23.

20. D. J. Clauw, G. P. Chrousos, Chronic pain and fatigue syndromes: overlapping clinical and neuroendocrine features and potential pathogenic mechanisms. *Neuroimmunomodulation* **4** (1997), 134–53.

21. G. P. Chrousos, P. W. Gold, The concepts of stress and stress system disorders. Overview of physical and behavioral homeostasis. *J. Am. Med. Assoc.* **267** (1992), 1244–52.

22. R. M. Sapolsky, Why stress is bad for your brain. *Science* **273** (1996), 749–50.

23. F. G. Keefe, G. K. Brown, K. S. Wallston, D. S. Caldwell, Coping with rheumatoid arthritis pain: catastrophizing as a maladaptive strategy. *Pain* **37** (1989), 51–6.

24. T. E. Rudy, R. D. Kerns, D. C. Turk, Chronic pain and depression: toward a cognitive-behavioral mediation model. *Pain* **35** (1988), 129–40.

25. A. T. Beck, *Cognitive Therapy and the Emotional Disorders* (New York: Harper & Row, 1967).

26. L. P. Rehm, A self-control model of depression. *Behav. Ther.* **8** (1977), 787–804.

27. C. B. Ferster, A functional analysis of depression. *Am. Psychol.* **28** (1973), 857–70.

28. P. M. Lewinsohn, Clinical and theoretical aspects of depression. In *Innovative Treatment Methods in Psychopathology*, ed. K. S. Calhoun, H. E. Adams, K. M. Mitchell (New York: John Wiley & Sons, 1974), pp. 121–43.

29. E. P. Zorrilla, L. Luborsky, J. R. McKay, *et al.*, The relationship of depression and stressors to immunological assays: a meta-analytic review. *Brain Behav. Immun.* **15** (2001), 199–226.

30. L. Capuron, R. Dantzer, Cytokines and depression: the need for a new paradigm. *Brain Behav. Immun.* **17** (2003), S119–24.

31. S. Kent, R. M. Bluthe, K. W. Kelley, R. Dantzer, Sickness behavior as a new target for drug development. *Trends Pharmacol. Sci.* **13** (1992), 24–8.

32. American Psychiatric Association. *Diagnostic and Statistical Manual of Mental Disorders*, 4th edn, text revision (Washington DC: American Psychiatric Association, 2000).

33. B. L. Hart, Biological basis of the behavior of sick animals. *Neurosci. Biobehav. Rev.* **12** (1988), 123–7.

34. K. W. Kelley, R. M. Bluthe, R. Dantzer, *et al.*, Cytokine-induced sickness behavior. *Brain Behav. Immun.* **17**: Suppl 1 (2003), 112–18.

35. H. Anisman, L. Kokkinidis, Z. Merali, Further evidence for the depressive effects of cytokines: anhedonia and neurochemical changes. *Brain Behav. Immun.* **16** (2002), 544–56.

36. R. M. Bluthé, S. Layé, B. Michaud, *et al.*, Role of interleukin-1β and tumor necrosis factor-α in lipopolysaccharide-induced sickness behaviour: a study with interleukin-1 type I receptor deficient mice. *Eur. J. Neurosci.* **12** (2000), 4447–56.

37. S. F. Maier, L. R. Watkins, Intracerebroventricular interleukin-1 receptor antagonist blocks the enhancement of fear conditioning and interference with escape produced by inescapable shock. *Brain Res.* **695** (1995), 279–82.

38. M. Maes, H. Y. Meltzer, E. Bosmans, *et al.*, Increased plasma concentrations of interleukin-6, soluble interleukin-6, soluble interleukin-2, and transferrin receptor in major depression. *J. Affect. Disord.* **34** (1995), 301–9.

39. A. Sluzewska, J. Rybakowski, E. Bosmans, *et al.*, Indicators of immune activation in major depression. *Psychiatry Res.* **64** (1996), 161–7.

40. M. Malaguarnera, I. Di Fazio, S. Restuccia, *et al.*, Interferon alpha-induced depression in chronic hepatitis C patients: comparison between different types of interferon alpha. *Neuropsychobiology* **37** (1998), 93–7.

41. M. Malaguarnera, I. Di Fazio, B. A. Trovato, G. Pistone, G. Mazzoleni, Alpha-interferon (IFN-α) treatment of chronic hepatitis C: analysis of some predictive factors for the response. *Int. J. Clin. Pharmacol. Ther.* **39** (2001), 239–45.

42. S. Bonaccorso, V. Marino, A. Puzella, *et al.*, Increased depressive ratings in patients with hepatitis C receiving interferon-alpha based immunotherapy are related to interferon-alpha-induced changes in the serotonergic system. *J. Clin. Psychopharmacol.* **22** (2002), 86–90.

43. R. de Beaurepaire. Questions raised by the cytokine hypothesis of depression. *Brain Behav. Immun.* **16** (2002), 610–17.

44. M. G. Cavallo, P. Pozzilli, R. Thorpe, Cytokines and autoimmunity. *Clin. Exp. Immunol.* **96** (1994), 1–7.

45. G. A. Hutchinson, J. E. Nehall, D. T. Simeon, Psychiatric disorders in systemic lupus erythematosus. *West Indian Med. J.* **45** (1996), 48–50.

46. T. Pincus, J. Griffith, S. Pearce, D. Isenberg, Prevalence of self-reported depression in patients with rheumatoid arthritis. *Br. J. Rheumatol.* **35** (1996), 879–83.

47. K. G. Kahl, N. Kruse, H. Faller, H. Weiss, P. Rieckmann, Expression of tumor necrosis factor-α and interferon-γ mRNA in blood cells correlates with depression scores during an acute attack in patients with multiple sclerosis. *Psychoneuroendocrinology* **27** (2002), 671–81.

48. Y. Pollak, E. Orion, I. Goshen, H. Ovadia, R. Yirmiya, Experimental autoimmune encephalomyelitis-associated behavioral syndrome as a model of 'depression due to multiple sclerosis.' *Brain Behav. Immun.* **16** (2002), 533–43.

49. Y. Pollak, H. Ovadia, E. Orion, R. Yirmiya. The EAE-associated behavioral syndrome II. Modulation by anti-inflammatory treatments. *J. Neuroimmunol.* **137** (2003), 100–108.

50. P. D. Wall, Dorsal horn electrophysiology. In *Handbook of Sensory Physiology: Somatosensory System* ed. A. Igg. (Berlin: Springer-Verlag, 1973), pp. 253–70.

51. D. D. Price, *Psychological and Neural Mechanisms of Pain* (New York, Raven, 1988).

52. A. D. Craig, The functional anatomy of lamina I and its role in post-stroke central pain. In *Nervous System Plasticity and Chronic Pain*, ed. J. Sandkuhler, B. Bromm, G. F. Gebhart (Amsterdam: Elsevier, 2000), pp. 137–51.

53. A. D. Craig, Pain mechanisms: labeled lines versus convergence in central processing. *Annu. Rev. Neurosci.* **26** (2003), 1–30.

54. S. F. Maier, E. P. Wiertelak, D. Martin, L. R. Watkins, Interleukin-1 mediates behavioral hyperalgesia produced by lithium chloride and endotoxin. *Brain Res.* **623** (1993), 321–4.

55. L. R. Watkins, S. F. Maier, Beyond neurons: evidence that immune and glial cells contribute to pathological pain states. *Physiol. Rev.* **82** (2002), 981–1011.

56. Y. B. Abramov, A. Y. Kozlocv, O. S. Sinel'shchikova, G. V. Torgovanova, Nociceptive reactions during stimulation of immunity in rats with different individual sensitivities to stress. *Neurosci. Behav. Physiol.* **33** (2003), 821–6.

57. A. J. Zautra, D. C. Yocum, I. Villanueva, *et al.*, Immune activation and depression in women with rheumatoid arthritis. *J. Rheumatol.* **31** (2004), 457–63.

58. A. J. Zautra, B. W. Smith, Depression and reactivity to stress in older women with rheumatoid arthritis and osteoarthritis. *Psychosom. Med.* **63** (2001), 687–96.

59. L. R. Watkins, S. F. Maier, L. E. Goehler, Cytokine-to-brain communication: a review and analysis of alternative mechanisms. *Life Sci.* **57** (1995), 1011–26.

60. L. R. Watkins, S. F. Maier, Implications of immune-to-brain communication for sickness and pain. *Proc. Natl. Acad. Sci. U. S. A.* **96** (1999), 7710–13.

61. N. Castanon, R. M. Bluthe, R. Dantzer, Chronic treatment with the atypical antidepressant tianeptine attenuates sickness behavior induced by peripheral but not central lipopolysaccharide and interleukin-1β in the rat. *Psychopharmacology* **154** (2001), 50–60.

62. R. Yirmiya, Y. Pollak, O. Barak, *et al.*, Effects of antidepressant drugs on the behavioral and physiological responses to lipopolysaccharide (LPS) in rodents. *Neuropsychopharmacology* **24** (2001), 531–44.

63. D. L. Musselman, D. H. Lawson, J. F. Gumnick, *et al.*, Paroxetine for the prevention of depression induced by high-dose interferon-α. *N. Engl. J. Med.* **344** (2001), 961–6.

64. Z. Xia, J. W. DePierre, L. Nässberger, Tricyclic antidepressants inhibit IL-6, IL-1β and TNF-α release in human blood monocytes and IL-2 and interferon-γ in T-cells. *Immunopharmacology* **34** (1996), 27–37.

65. M. Maes, C. Song, A. H. Lin, *et al.*, Negative immunoregulatory effects of antidepressants inhibition of interferon-gamma and stimulation of interleukin-10 secretion. *Neuropsychopharmacology* **20** (1999), 370–79.

66. J. Sawynok, Antidepressants as analgesics: an introduction. *J. Psychiatry. Neurosci.* **26** (2001), 20.

67. J. Sawynok, M. J. Esser, A. R. Reid, Antidepressants as analgesics an overview of central and peripheral mechanisms of action. *J. Psychiatry Neurosci* **26** (2001), 21–9.

68. R. Lee, P. S. Spencer, Antidepressants and pain: a review of the pharmacological data supporting the use of certain tricyclics in chronic pain. *J. Int. Med. Res.* **5**: Suppl 1 (1977), 146–56.

69. A. E. Panerai, M. Bianchi, P. Sacerdote, *et al.*, Antidepressants in cancer care. *J. Palliat. Care* **7** (1991), 42–4.

70. J. S. McDaniel, D. L. Musselman, M. R. Porter, D. A. Reed, C. B. Nemeroff, Depression in patients with cancer diagnosis, biology, and treatment. *Arch. Gen. Psychiatry* **52** (1995), 88–99.

71. M. E. Lynch, Antidepressants as analgesics a review of randomized controlled trials. *J. Psychiatry Neurosci.* **26** (2001), 30–36.

72. A. J. Cook, C. J. Woolf, P. D. Wall, S. B. McMahon, Dynamic receptive field plasticity in rat spinal cord dorsal horn following C-primary afferent input. *Nature* **325** (1987), 151–3.

73. J. Ru-Rong, T. Kohno, K. A. Moore, C. J. Woolf, Central sensitization and LTP do pain and memory share similar mechanisms? *Trends Neurosci.* **26** (2003), 696–705.

74. B. A. Winkelstein, Mechanisms of central sensitization, neuroimmunology and injury biomechanics in persistent pain: implications for musculoskeletal disorders. *J. Electromyogr. Kinesiol.* **14** (2004), 87–93.

75. M. B. Keller, D. N. Klein, R. M. A. Hirshfeld, *et al.*, Results of the DSM-IV mood disorders field trial. *Am. J. Psychiatry* **152** (1995), 843–9.

76. T. E. Joiner, Depression's vicious scar self-propagating and erosive processes in depression chronicity. *Clin. Psychol. Sci. Pract.* **7** (2000), 203–18.

77. S. Nolen-Hoeksema, J. S. Girgus, M. E. P. Seligman, Learned helplessness in children: a longitudinal study of depression, achievement, and explanatory style. *J. Pers. Soc. Psychol.* **51** (1986), 435–42.

78. K. S. Kendler, L. M. Thornton, C. O. Gardner, Stressful life events and previous episodes in the etiology of major depression in women: an evaluation of the 'kindling' hypothesis. *Am. J. Psychiatry* **157** (2000), 1243–51.

79. H. Anisman, Z. Merali, S. Hayley, Sensitization associated with stressors and cytokine treatments. *Brain Behav. Immun.* **17** (2003), 86–93.

80. F. J. H. Tilders, E. D. Schmidt, Cross-sensitization between immune and non-immune stressors: a role in the etiology of depression? *Adv. Exp. Med. Biol.* **461** (1999), 179–97.

81. S. Hayley, K. Brebner, S. Lacosta, Z. Merali, H. Anisman, Sensitization to the effects of tumor necrosis factor-α: neuroendocrine, central monoamine and behavioral variations. *J. Neurosci.* **19** (1999), 5654–65.

82. D. S. Charney, Psychobiological mechanisms of resilience and vulnerability: implications for successful adaptation to extreme stress. *Am. J. Psychiatry* **161** (2004), 195–216.

83. B. S. McEwen, E. Stellar, Stress and the individual: mechanisms leading to disease. *Arch. Intern. Med.* **153** (1993), 2093–101.

84. E. Diener, R. A. Emmons, The independence of positive and negative affect. *J. Pers. Soc. Psychol.* **47** (1984), 1105–17.

85. D. Watson *Mood and Temperment* (New York: Guilford Press, 2000).

86. A. Zautra, B. Smith, G. Affleck, H. Tennen, Examinations of chronic pain and affect relationships: applications of a dynamic model of affect. *J. Consult. Clin. Psychol.* **69** (2001), 786–95.

87. A. J. Zautra *Emotions, Stress, and Health* (New York: Oxford University Press, 2003).

88. G. Affleck, H. Tennen, S. Urrows, P. Higgins, Individual differences in the day-to-day experience of chronic pain: a prospective daily study of rheumatoid arthritis patients. *Health Psychol.* **10** (1991), 419–26.

89. A. J. Zautra, M. H. Burleson, C. A. Smith, *et al.*, Arthritis and perceptions of quality of life: an examination of positive and negative affect in rheumatoid arthritis patients. *Health Psychol.* **14** (1995), 399–408.

90. A. J. Zautra, J. J. Marbach, K. G. Raphael, *et al.*, The examination of myofascial face pain and its relationship to psychological distress among women. *Health Psychol.* **14** (1995), 223–31.

91. M. C. Davis, A. J. Zautra, B. W. Smith, Chronic pain, stress and the dynamics of affective differentiation. *J. Person.* **72** (2004), 1133–59.

92. J. W. Reich, A. J. Zautra, M. C. Davis, Dimensions of affect relationships: models and their integrative implications. *Rev. Gen. Psychol.* **7** (2003), 66–83.

93. A. J. Zautra, L. Johnson, M. C. Davis, Positive affect as a source of resilience for women in chronic pain. *J. Consult. Clin. Psychol.* **73** (2005), 212–20.

94. M. M. Tugade, B. L. Frederickson, Resilient individuals use positive emotions to bounce back from negative emotional experiences. *J. Pers. Soc. Psychol.* **86** (2004), 320–33.

95. J. Joorman, M. Siemer, Memory accessibility, mood regulation, and dysphoria: difficulties in repairing sad mood with happy memories? *J. Abnorm. Psychol.* **113** (2004), 179–88.

96. A. A. Stone, J. M. Neale, D. S. Cox, *et al.*, Daily events are associated with a secretory immune response to an oral antigen in men. *Health Psychol.* **13** (1994), 440–46.

97. S. L. Goldman, D. T. Kraemer, P. Salovey, Beliefs about mood moderate the relationship of stress to illness and symptom reporting. *J. Psychosom. Res.* **41** (1996), 115–28.

98. C. McFarlan, R. Buehler, The impact of negative affect on autobiographical memory: the role of self-focused attention to moods. *J. Pers. Soc. Psychol.* **75** (1998), 1424–40.

99. L. Felman Barrett, J. Gross, T. C. Christensen, M. Benvenuto, Knowing what you're feeling and knowing what to do about it: mapping the relation between emotion differentiation and emotion regulation. *Cogn. Emotion* **15** (2001), 713–24.

100. L. A. Bradley, L. D. Young, K. O. Anderson, *et al.*, Effects of psychological therapy on pain behavior or rheumatoid arthritis patients. *Arthritis Rheum.* **30** (1987), 1105–14.

101. J. C. Parker, K. L. Smarr, S. P. Buckelew, *et al.*, Effects of stress management on clinical outcomes in rheumatoid arthritis. *Arthritis Rheum.* **38** (1995), 1807–18.

102. V. Radojevic, P. Nicassio, M. Weisman, Behavior therapy with and without family support for rheumatoid arthritis. *Behavi. Ther.* **2** (1992), 13–30.

103. P. M. Nicassio, M. A. Greenberg, Psychosocial management of chronic pain in arthritis. In *Treatment of Rheumatic Diseases, 2nd edn*, ed. M. H. Weisman, M. Weinblatt, J. Louie (Orlando, FL: William Saunders, 2001), pp. 147–61.

8

The interrelationship of depression and diabetes

Dominique L. Musselman, Angela Bowling, Natalie Gilles, Hannah Larsen, Ephi Betan and Lawrence S. Phillips

> …in the pre-war literature, diminished glucose tolerance was frequently reported to be statistically demonstrable in patients with melancholia.
>
> H. M. Von Praag (1965)

Introduction: diabetes

The worldwide prevalence of diabetes is increasing at an alarming rate. According to the World Health Organization (WHO), approximately 150 million people worldwide have diabetes mellitus. Due to the combined impact of sedentary lifestyles, increased prevalence of obesity, and the rising age of the population, this number may double by 2025. In developed countries, people aged 65 or older will be at highest risk; however, most new cases in developing countries will be individuals between 45 and 64 years of age. Countries reporting the largest number of cases are India, followed (in order) by China, the USA, Indonesia, Japan, Pakistan, Russia, Brazil, Italy and Bangladesh [1]

Diabetes mellitus is a heterogeneous metabolic disease in which hyperglycaemia is a central feature. Diabetes is the world's leading cause of non-traumatic limb amputation, new cases of end-stage renal disease [2] and blindness in adults [1,3]. Nearly 50% of the 18 million diabetes patients in the USA are unaware of their diabetes [4]; in some countries, that number may be as high as 80% [5]. Other debilitating consequences of diabetes include diabetic neuropathy and foot ulcers. Diabetes is the fourteenth leading cause of death worldwide and also contributes to cardiac and stroke-related morbidity and mortality. The actual number of deaths per year attributed to diabetes is difficult to ascertain but is estimated to be approximately four million [1].

Type 2 diabetes dwarfs the prevalence of type 1 and other types of diabetes. In addition to hyperglycaemia, diabetes is also associated with abnormalities in

Depression and Physical Illness, ed. A. Steptoe.
Published by Cambridge University Press. © Cambridge University Press 2006.

protein, carbohydrate and fat metabolism. These metabolic perturbations result from insufficient insulin action on peripheral target tissues, due to insufficient insulin secretion (type 1), diminished tissue response to insulin (type 2) or some combination of both. Some beta-cell loss is required for the development of type 1 diabetes, which manifests in most individuals by age 20 years. Type 1 diabetes is thought to result from a genetic susceptibility together with an autoimmune reaction stimulated by an environmental stimulus. Although debate continues, type 2 diabetes likely stems from inadequate insulin secretion, increased insulin resistance or a combination of both. Patients with type 2 diabetes exhibit insulin levels that are considerably higher than in patients with type 1 diabetes, but the circulating insulin is insufficient to overcome the insulin resistance involving the adipose tissue, muscle and liver. In type 2 diabetes, the defect in insulin action occurs largely at the post-receptor level, although exact mechanisms remain poorly understood. The genetic contribution to type 2 diabetes is more remarkable than in type 1, with a concordance rate over 90% in identical twins [6].

As studies have indicated, depression constitutes a major risk factor in the development of type 2 diabetes and likely accelerates the onset of diabetes complications. This chapter reviews the pathophysiological alterations related to glucose intolerance in depressed patients and the beneficial effects of depression treatment upon glycaemic control. Understanding the bidirectional relationship between depression and diabetes, including the sociocultural, biological and psychological pathways of influence, is ultimately critical to the treatment and prevention of diabetes.

Epidemiology

Diagnosis of depression in patients with diabetes

In contrast to the debate regarding criteria for the diagnosis of major depression in patients with cancer [7], scrutiny of the depression symptom patterns in diabetic patients has been less controversial [8,9]. One of the many screening tools for depression, the Beck Depression Inventory (BDI) [10], has been utilised in many studies of medically ill patients. Although the BDI cannot provide a formal diagnosis of major depression, it has been demonstrated to distinguish accurately between diabetic patients with and without major depression. Even though diabetic patients may experience neurobehavioural depressive symptoms attributable to their underlying diabetes, such as weight loss, diminished appetite, hypersomnia, psychomotor retardation and loss of libido, attention to the neurocognitive symptoms of depression (depressed mood, diminished interest or enjoyment, poor concentration, feelings of worthlessness, excessive or inappropriate guilt, recurrent thoughts of death or suicide) allows clinicians to identify easily major depression in diabetic patients [11–13]. Of note is the observation that the presence of major depression in diabetic

Table 8.1 Prevalence of unipolar depression in patients with diabetes

Ref.	No. and type of patients	Methods	Prevalence of depression in individuals with diabetes
Gavard et al. [16]	20 studies with adults; at least 25 study subjects per study	Meta-analysis of 9 controlled and 11 uncontrolled studies of patients with type 1 or type 2 diabetes, or both	*Controlled studies:* Diagnostic interview: 8.5–27% (mean 14%) Self-report symptom scales: 22–60% (mean 32%) *Uncontrolled studies:* Diagnostic interview: 11.0–19.9% (mean 15.4%) Self-report symptom scales: 10.0–28.0% (mean 19.6%)
Anderson et al. [17]	42 studies with adults; at least 25 study subjects per study; total subjects 21 351	Meta-analysis of 20 controlled and 22 uncontrolled studies of patients with type 1 or type 2 diabetes, or both	*Controlled studies:* Diagnostic interview: 9% (aggregate mean) Self-report symptom scales: 26% *Uncontrolled studies:* Diagnostic interview: 14% Self-report symptom scales: 35% *All studies:* Diagnostic interview: 11% Self-report symptom scales: 31%

*Aggregate mean = weighted by number of subjects per study.

patients results in symptom amplification; that is, even when accounting for the severity of diabetes, diabetic patients with comorbid depression experience more symptoms associated with their diabetes than do their non-depressed counterparts [14]. Nevertheless, the increasing recognition of the negative impact of depression upon the quality of life of those who suffer from diabetes has led to the development of organisations such as the European Depression in Diabetes Research Consortium (EDID), which conducts research regarding the most prevalent and costly mental health problem associated with diabetes – depression [15].

Prevalence of depression in diabetic patients

Since the 1980s, many researchers have attempted to determine the prevalence rates of major depression or the severity of depressive symptoms in patients with diabetes. Table 8.1 shows a relatively large range across controlled and uncontrolled studies, likely due to methodological differences. Some studies include both type 1 and type 2 diabetes patients without distinguishing between the types. Other studies do not specify the duration of depression, the extent of diabetes-related complications or the time since the most recent diabetes-related hospitalisation. Most of the studies relied on self-report questionnaires to ascertain the dimensional severity of depressive symptoms, while some of the studies used observer-administered structured clinical interviews to provide the categorical diagnosis of major depression. The earlier meta-analysis by Gavard *et al.* [16] of studies of diabetic patients with comorbid depression, and the more recent one by Anderson *et al.* [17] (which included the studies analysed by Gavard) reveal a mean of 14% (range 9–27%), or an aggregate mean (weighted by the number of subjects in a study) of 9%, of studies using diagnostic interviews. The studies that utilised self-reporting depressive symptom scales reported a higher prevalence rate of moderate to severe depressive symptoms ranging from 22 to 60% (mean 32%) [16] and an aggregate mean of 26% [17]. This almost two-fold difference in prevalence rates of depression between formal diagnostic assessment and self-reporting of diabetic patients underscores the importance of structured psychiatric diagnostic interviews in obtaining a conservative estimate of the prevalence of depression in diabetic patients.

Another major limitation in these studies of the rates of depression in diabetic patients is the lack of information with regard to ethnic minority populations. Despite the fact that prevalence of diabetes in certain minority populations is nearly twice that in white populations, there is relatively little information regarding the prevalence of depression in these minority groups [18–20], including Native Americans [21] and African Americans.

Sociocultural risk factors for depression in diabetes

Critical to understanding the relationship between depression and diabetes is examining the contributions of socioeconomic status [22,23], given the studies documenting the association of socioeconomic hardship and poor health, irrespective of race [24–26]. As summarised by Fisher and colleagues [27], diabetic patients at higher risk for depression have less education, are unmarried or have poor social support, and experience more chronic stressors or negative life events [27,28]. Education, functional impact of diabetes and financial stress may contribute the most to depression and anxiety in patients with diabetes early in their disease [27]. Gender differences also exist, which may interact with socioeconomic factors. Women with diabetes appear twice as likely as men to experience psychological distress [29–31].

Impact of diabetes on depression

In an attempt to understand the interrelationship between diabetes and depressive symptoms, a number of researchers have scrutinised the severity of diabetes and associated extent and character of depressive symptomatology. Lustman and colleagues [32] conducted a meta-analysis of multiple controlled cross-sectional studies of diabetic patients (type 1 and type 2) and determined that the severity of depressive symptoms was correlated with the magnitude of glycated haemoglobin (HbA1c) ($r = 0.28$, 95% confidence interval [CI] 0.2 to 0.36). Unfortunately, as in other medical diseases, patients who suffer complications of their diabetes, e.g. painful neuropathy, report more depression [28,33–35]. Studies that examine the temporal relationship between perturbations in depressive symptoms and fluctuations in glycaemic control are rare, even over a six-month period, the time arguably needed for diabetic patients to inculcate healthy self-care behaviours and improve their metabolic status. For example, during an eight-month-long study, a group of type 1 diabetic patients ($n = 55$) who enhanced their metabolic control exhibited significant reductions in depression and anxiety symptoms and an improvement in their quality of life [36]. The notion that improved glycaemic control may exert its own antidepressive effect is suggested by a relatively large ($n = 569$), although short-term (three months), randomised double-blind treatment of type 2 diabetic patients treated with either placebo or the oral hypoglycaemic agent glipizide. In this study population, increased glycaemic control in the glipizide-treated patients was associated with better quality of life and self-reported mental health, although the improvements were not statistically significant [37].

Impact of depression on diabetes

Similarly to non-depressed individuals, many patients with psychiatric disorders are physically inactive and obese, and these are risk factors for the development of type 2 diabetes [38]. Although certain sociocultural factors and diabetes-related medical complications may increase the risk of depression in diabetic patients, gradually accumulating data (see Table 8.2) indicate that major depression or clinically significant levels of depressive symptoms contribute to the development of type 2 diabetes.

Even after controlling for potential confounding factors such as age, gender, race, education, body weight, socioeconomic status, other psychiatric disorders and use of health services, these studies indicate that depression remains a significant risk factor for development of diabetes [39,42,44]. Thus, rather than being only a secondary emotional response to diabetic complications, depression may be an independent risk factor in initiating type 2 diabetes. After a patient is diagnosed with diabetes, increased levels of depressive symptoms are associated not only with a decreased ability to regularly continue prescriptions of oral hypoglycaemic medications and decreased adherence to a diabetic diet [45] but also with functional impairment and increased healthcare costs (including use of prescriptions and ambulatory care) [45–47]. A meta-analysis of multiple cross-sectional

Table 8.2 Antecedent depression and subsequent risk of type 2 diabetes

Study	Number of subjects	Diagnostic method	Duration of follow-up (years)	Findings	Comments
East Baltimore site of the Epidemiologic Catchment Area Survey [39]	1715 men and women	DIS [40]	13	RR: 2.23 (95% CI 0.90 to 5.55)	
Kawakami et al. [44]	2764 male employees	Zung Depression Rating Scale [41]	8	HR = 2.31 (95% CI 1.03 to 5.20)	
Study of Women's Health Across the Nation (SWAN) [42]	2254 premenopausal, middle-aged women from ethnically diverse backgrounds	CES-D [43]	2	OR = 2.81 (95% CI 1.22 to 6.45) for depressed African American women	Too few cases of diabetes developed in the other ethnic groups to reliably examine depression in other ethnic groups

CES-D, Center for Epidemiological Studies Depression Scale; CI, Confidence interval; DIS = Diagnostic Interview Schedule; OR, odds ratio; RR, relative risk.

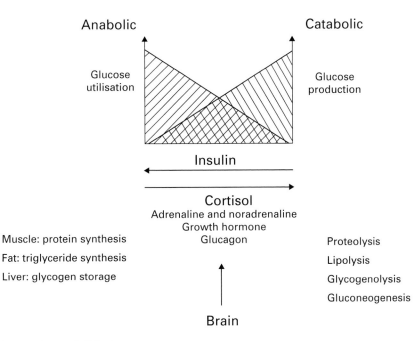

Figure 8.1   Depression and diabetes.

studies by de Groot and colleagues [34] has confirmed that patients with diabetes and comorbid depression exhibit poorer glycaemic control and greater prevalence of multiple diabetes complications (sexual dysfunction, neuropathy, retinopathy, nephropathy, macrovascular disease). In a ten-year study of women ($n = 76$) with type 1 or type 2 diabetes, development of coronary heart disease (CHD) was significantly more rapid in the women with depression, even after adjusting for other risk factors for CHD (age, duration of diabetes, body mass index, hypertension, hyperlipidaemia) [48]. Whether depression acts as a major risk factor or a predictor for diabetes-related mortality will likely be determined in the near future [49].

Biology

The central nervous system syndrome of major depression is associated with myriad pathophysiological abnormalities, including increased release and action of counter-regulatory hormones, perturbations in glucose transport function and increased secretion of pro-inflammatory cytokines. Such abnormalities may contribute to insulin resistance and/or pancreatic beta-islet cell dysfunction (Figure 8.1, Table 8.3).

Increased release of counter-regulatory hormones in depression

Psychological stress, defined here as a perceived challenge to wellbeing, may be accompanied by increased release of counter-regulatory hormones such as

Table 8.3 Organs and related hormones necessary for glucose homeostasis

Brain (hypothalamus)
   Corticotropin-releasing factor

Anterior pituitary
   Adrenocorticotropin
   Growth hormone

Adrenal gland
   Adrenal cortex: cortisol
   Adrenal medulla: adrenaline and noradrenaline

Autonomic nervous system
   adrenaline and noradrenaline
   Acetylcholine

Gut
   Cholecystokinin
   Glucagon-like peptide 1

Pancreas
   Alpha-islet cell: glucagon
   Beta-islet cell: insulin

Adipose organ
   Leptin
   Adiponectin

catecholamines, glucagon, glucocorticoids and growth hormone (GH). These counter-regulatory hormones serve to raise blood levels of glucose [50] and thus act in a delicate balance with insulin and other insulin-like factors to maintain a critical physiological variable, the level of blood glucose. For normal brain function, the blood glucose level must be prevented from falling below a certain threshold; moreover, blood glucose levels may have to be increased rapidly in order to satisfy a sudden need for energy. Major depression, sometimes described as 'a stress response gone awry', is often associated with sympathoadrenal activation, hypothalamic–pituitary–adrenocortical (HPA) hyperactivity and alterations in activity of the hypothalamic-GH axis [51]. Adrenaline and glucagon initiate the quick acute elevation in blood glucose in response to stress; GH and glucocorticoid action prolong the increase in blood glucose over subsequent hours [52]. Stress-induced elevations of glucocorticoids induce elevations of glucose concentrations, largely through synergy with other counter-regulatory hormones, to stimulate gluconeogenesis, glycogenolysis, lipolysis and inhibition of peripheral glucose transport and utilisation [52–57].

Congruent with the above components of the stress response are the observations that, in comparison with controls, depressed patients exhibit insulin resistance during intravenous [58,59] or oral [60] glucose tolerance tests (GTTs) and insulin tolerance tests [61,62]. This evidence of impaired glycaemic control in patients with major depression may be the consequence, at least in part, of increased release of counter-regulatory hormones. Unfortunately, despite hundreds of studies in which counter-regulatory hormone physiology has been scrutinised in patients with mood disorders, concomitant glucoregulatory dysfunction has been largely unexplored. An exception is a study performed by Winokur and colleagues [60]. During an oral GTT, depressed patients without any other diabetes risk factors exhibited a greater decrement in glucagon plasma concentrations compared with controls. This was likely a compensatory response to the increased glucose concentrations during the GTT. Enhanced release of counter-regulatory hormones in patients with depressive disorders may be a critical link between depression and diabetes and certainly warrants continued investigation.

Alterations in glucose transport in depression

Glucose is a necessary metabolic substrate of all mammalian cells, and its influx into cells is mediated by glucose transporters. Facilitative glucose transporters exist in six isoforms; GLUT1 facilitates the entry of glucose into endothelial cells and astrocytes, and GLUT3 entry into neurons [63].

Glucose utilisation is used as an index of neuronal activity, which can be quantified using functional magnetic resonance imaging (fMRI) and non-invasive positron-emission tomography (PET). In PET, GLUT1 and GLUT3 carry the radio-labelled tracer $[^{18}F]$-fluorodeoxyglucose (FDG) across the blood–brain barrier. In comparison with non-depressed controls, the PET scans of individuals with major depression reveal reduced glucose utilisation in the left lateral prefrontal cortex. Furthermore, severity of depressive symptoms is often correlated significantly to the decrement in left frontal cortical function. After clinical response to somatic depression treatment, glucose metabolism improves within the cingulate cortex, prefrontal cortex and/or basal ganglia [64–66]. However, whether glucoregulatory function in the periphery normalises remains to be investigated [52]. Moreover, the regional decrements in neuronal activity in depression could plausibly result from perturbations of GLUT, as has been observed in Alzheimer's disease [67] and Huntington's disease [68,69].

Alterations in peripheral GLUT function may also exist in patients with depression. An insulin-sensitive glucose transporter, GLUT4, exists in its highest concentrations in fat (brown or white), heart and muscle (red or white). Under usual conditions, glucose consumption in the brain does not affect glucose transport; however, glucose transport in the periphery is affected by plasma concentrations of glucose [70]. Only relatively recently has ^{13}C-magnetic resonance spectroscopy (MRS) revealed that the reduced sensitivity to insulin of diabetic patients includes defects in glucose transport across plasma membranes [71] and an element of abnormal glycogen synthesis in muscle [72]. Whether such glucoregulatory perturbations are due to abnormalities in the GLUT4 transporter, and whether similar abnormalities of glucose handling and glycogen storage exist in depressed patients with and without diabetes, remain to be investigated.

Increased immuno-inflammatory activation in depression

An underlying link between depression and diabetes may be the enhanced secretion of pro-inflammatory cytokines, intercellular signalling polypeptides produced by activated cells [73]. The pro-inflammatory cytokines interleukin (IL)-1, IL-6 and tumour necrosis factor alpha (TNF-α) are elevated in many patients with diabetes due to secretion by adipose tissue [74] and, with increasing age, increased production by monocytes and macrophages [75,76]. The overexpression of TNF-α in adipose and muscle tissue of obese individuals may not only interfere with insulin action [75,77–83] but also increases susceptibility to "sickness behaviour". Among their multiple actions, the pro-inflammatory cytokines also induce sickness behaviour, a constellation of non-specific symptoms including anorexia, anhedonia, fatigue, decreased psychomotor activity and disappearance of body-care activities [84,85], which overlap with the symptoms of major depression. Perhaps not surprisingly, IL-6 is elevated in many patients with major depression [86–92]; whether significant elevations in these inflammatory mediators presage development of depression, or specific depressive symptoms such as fatigue, is currently a focus of active research.

Treatment of depression in patients with diabetes

Critique of the empirical literature

Despite the adverse impact of major depression in patients with diabetes, there have been only three studies (one controlled study of psychotherapy, two controlled studies of antidepressant medication) in diabetic patients with depression (Table 8.4) [93]. All three studies demonstrated the effectiveness of antidepressive treatment on depressive symptoms of patients with either type 1 or type 2 diabetes. A major finding was that nortriptyline decreased depression but had an adverse

Table 8.4 Treatment of depression in diabetes: results of double-blind controlled randomised trials

Treatment	Type of diabetes, n	Effect on depression	Effect of depression treatment on HbA1c or compliance with blood glucose monitoring
Nortriptyline vs. placebo × 8 weeks [13]	Type 1: 14 Type 2: 14	Effective (nortryptiline dosed to achieve plasma concentrations of 50–150 ng/ml)	No statistically significant difference in HbA1c between groups No effect on BGM
CBT + diabetes education programme vs. diabetes education programme alone × 10 weeks [94]	Type 2: 51	Effective (individual CBT once/week in 1-h sessions)	CBT + diabetes education programme associated with ↓d HbA1c by 0.7% at 6 months CBT + diabetes education programme associated with ↓d BGM post-treatment vs. pre-treatment
Fluoxetine vs. placebo × 8 weeks [148]	Type 1: 26 Type 2: 34	Effective (fluoxetine in doses ≤ 40 mg/day)	No statistically significant difference in HbA1c between groups BGM not assessed

BGM, blood glucose monitoring; CBT, cognitive–behavioural therapy; ↓d, decrease; HbA1c, haemoglobin A1c.

effect on glucose control, whereas fluoxetine improved depression and tended to improve glucose regulation (-0.4% in HbA1c; $p = 0.24$).

These relatively small studies lacked sufficient sampling power (i.e. too few patients) to identify other potential benefits of clinically effective treatment of depression, e.g. enhancement of overall function, relief of diabetic symptom burden or reduction of healthcare utilisation. Furthermore, the presence or absence of underlying neurohormonal perturbations was not assessed before treatment; thus, whether normalisation of these pathways is associated with a reduction of HbA1c is not known. Interestingly, as these studies lacked a uniform intervention algorithm of diabetes treatment, this deficiency may have contributed to the lack of significant reduction of HbA1c during the active treatment period of these studies. A reduction of HbA1c by 0.5% or more is considered the minimally clinically significant improvement in glucose control [95].

A third related consideration was the variable chosen to assess adherence to diabetes treatment, i.e. blood glucose monitoring, assessed in two of the three studies [13,94]. Although this is a standard element of diabetes education programmes, many patients do not monitor their glucose regularly or accurately [96]. Treatment with nortriptyline was associated with no effect [97] upon glucose monitoring;

moreover, less glucose monitoring was reported by the depressed patients who received cognitive–behavioural therapy (CBT) than those patients who received diabetes education alone [31]. However, improved compliance with diabetic treatment and enhanced glycaemic control has been shown to be largely dependent on appropriate intensification of therapy by providers when patients present for their follow-up appointments [98,99]. Thus, attendance at scheduled diabetes appointments (with associated increased intervention by the healthcare team) may be the critical factor in determining whether effective depression treatment improves glycaemic control [100].

Psychopharmacological treatment of depression and diabetes

Since the early 1960s, antidepressant agents have been recognised to affect glucose concentration. Lower plasma glucose concentrations were observed to occur with administration of hydrazine monoamine oxidase inhibitors (MAOIs) such as phenelzine and isocarboxazid [101,102], possibly through increasing extra-hepatic glucose uptake [102]. Despite their potential to cause myriad side effects, tricyclic antidepressants (TCAs) have long been used for the treatment of peripheral neuropathy in diabetic patients. Placebo-controlled double-blind randomised studies have shown that the TCAs desipramine and amitriptyline are more effective than the selective serotonin reuptake inhibitor (SSRI) antidepressant fluoxetine in the treatment of diabetic neuropathy [103,104]. Nevertheless, these benefits must be balanced with the risks of TCA-induced weight gain, hyperglycaemia and orthostatic hypotension [13]. MAOIs and the older atypical antidepressant trazodone are generally free of effects on cardiac conduction. However, like TCAs, MAOIs may cause weight gain and postural hypotension [105]. In addition, the quinidine-like effects of the TCAs and related antidepressants limit their clinical use in patients with diabetes and cardiovascular disease; these agents are contraindicated in patients with left fascicular or bifascular block or a QT corrected (QTc) interval greater than 440 milliseconds [106,107].

The newer SSRIs, the serotonin and noradrenaline reuptake inhibitors (SSNRI) (venlafaxine, paroxetine, duloxetine) and other atypical antidepressants (e.g. bupropion, mirtazapine, nefazodone) offer improved tolerability and safety advantages in depressed patients with diabetes. These newer antidepressants exert less anticholinergic and antiadrenergic effects and lack quinidine-like action and lethality in overdose. Interestingly, some of the SSRIs may also be effective in the treatment of painful diabetic neuropathy [104]. In a double-blind placebo-controlled trial of non-depressed diabetic patients, paroxetine was more tolerable than imipramine, but was somewhat less effective than the TCAs, although better than placebo, in reducing symptoms of peripheral neuropathy. Of note is that all patients with paroxetine plasma concentrations greater than 150–200 nM experienced a therapeutic response, i.e. a 50% decrease in severity of neuropathy symptoms from baseline. Whether paroxetine in plasma concentrations greater than 150–200 nM is as effective as optimal plasma concentrations of imipramine (400–600 nM) for diabetic neuropathy remains to be confirmed [108].

As the SSRIs nefazodone, fluoxetine and fluvoxamine inhibit the cytochrome P450 (CYP) 3A4 isoenzyme, these drugs have the potential to alter the metabolism of certain oral hypoglycaemics, i.e. the thiazolidinedione pioglitazone, meglitinides, repaglinide and nateglinide. Therefore, nefazodone, fluoxetine and fluvoxamine would be expected to confer a risk of hypoglycaemia in patients treated with these hypoglycaemic medications. In addition, the SSRIs fluoxetine, fluvoxamine and sertraline inhibit the CYP 2C9 isoenzyme; thus, these SSRIs could potentially interfere with CYP 2C9 metabolism of the sulfonylureas tolbutamide and glimepiride. However, reports of such potential drug–drug interactions have not been published [109]. In healthy volunteers, high-dose sertraline (200 mg/day) has been shown to decrease tolbutamide clearance by 16% [109,110].

The potential for psychotropic medications, especially antipsychotic and anticonvulsant drugs, to cause weight gain has long been acknowledged. Only relatively recently, however, has the potential of the newer antidepressants to cause weight gain been understood. Of the newer antidepressants, weight gain is often observed with mirtazapine [111,112]. The risk of this side effect must be balanced against the observation that depressed patients with type 2 diabetes are much more likely to fail weight-control interventions in comparison with their non-depressed counterparts [113]. Of note is that the atypical antidepressant bupropion is associated with minimal weight gain, sexual dysfunction [114] and inhibition of CYP enzymes, and is also effective in the treatment of nicotine dependence.

Given the potential changes in glucose regulation with antidepressant administration, especially after augmentation of these psychotropic agents with antipsychotics [115] and/or anticonvulsants [116–119], healthcare providers and patients should be aware of the current American Diabetes Association (ADA) recommendations to monitor HbA1c, fasting blood glucose and lipid levels every three months in patients known to have diabetes or ADA criteria for testing for diabetes and impaired glucose tolerance in undiagnosed individuals (Table 8.5) [120]. Indeed, improvement (or not) of glucoregulatory function after six months or more of antidepressant treatment is largely unstudied [121]. Whether antidepressant treatment can exert direct drug effects, such as increased glycogen synthase activity in skeletal muscle [122], a direct effect on glucose transport mechanisms or improved dietary compliance [123], remains unknown. Fluoxetine at a dose of 60 mg/day for four weeks has been associated with improved insulin sensitivity when administered to obese non-depressed patients with type 2 diabetes, and without reduction in HbA1c or corresponding weight loss [123,124]. After six months

Table 8.5 Criteria for testing diabetes in asymptomatic, undiagnosed individuals [120]

1. Testing for diabetes should be considered in all individuals at age 45 years and above and, if normal, repeated at 3-year intervals.
2. Testing should be considered at a younger age or be carried out more frequently in individuals who:
   - are overweight (BMI $\geq$ 25 kg/m^2)
   - have a first-degree relative with diabetes
   - are members of a high-risk ethnic population (e.g. African American, Pacific Islander)
   - have delivered a baby weighing > 9 lb or have been diagnosed with GDM
   - are hypertensive ($\geq$ 140/90mmHg)
   - have an HDL cholesterol level $\leq$ 35 mg/dl (0.90 mmol/l) and/or a triglyceride level $\geq$ 250 mg/dl (2.82 mmol/l)
   - on previous testing had IGT or IFG*

The OGTT or FPG test may be used to diagnose diabetes. The FPG test is easier to implement, less expensive and more convenient for patients but will miss the diagnosis in many patients who can be recognised with a 2-h OGTT.

*The terms IGT and IFG refer to a metabolic stage intermediate between normal glucose function and diabetes:
- IGT $=$ plasma glucose levels during an OGTT are above normal but below those defined as diabetes: 2-h plasma glucose levels 140–199 mg/dl (7.8–11.1 mmol/l). Plasma glucose < 140 mg/dl (7.8 mmol/l) is the upper limit of normal glucose levels. A 2-h 75g OGTT plasma glucose level $\geq$ 200 mg/dl (11.1 mmol/l) is indicative of diabetes (confirmatory testing must be performed).
- IFG $=$ individuals with fasting glucose levels between 100 mg/dl (5.6 mmol/l) and 125 mg/dl (6.9 mmol/l) but < 140 mg/dl (7/8 mg/dl). A fasting glucose concentration of < 100 mg/dl (5.6 mmol/l) is the upper limit of normal glucose levels. A fasting glucose $\geq$ 126 mg/dl (7 mmol/l) is indicative of diabetes (confirmatory testing must be performed).

FPG, fasting plasma glucose; GDM, gestational diabetes mellitus; HDL, high-density lipoprotein; IFG, impaired fasting glucose; IGT, impaired glucose tolerance; OGTT, oral glucose tolerance test.

of this dosage, fluoxetine has been associated with clinically significant reductions in HbA1c in patients with type 2 diabetes and weight loss [121,122], but not by 12 months [121].

Impact of psychological interventions on glycaemic control

Because successful diabetes management relies heavily on patient self-care, diabetes education has been considered an important part of diabetes treatment since the 1930s [125]. Diabetes education has been presented most often as patient instruction and information regarding diet, medication use, physical activity, foot care and self-monitoring of blood glucose. Diabetes education has been shown to reduce in-patient length-of-stay and hospitalisation rates for hyperglycaemia and diabetic ketoacidosis and to improve out-patient metabolic control. Unfortunately, studies have revealed that 50–80% of people with diabetes have significant knowledge and skill deficits, and less than half of people with diabetes achieve ideal glycaemic control (HbA1c $< 7.0\%$). To ascertain the efficacy of diabetes self-management education in adults with type 2 diabetes, Norris et al. [125] systematically reviewed a series of randomised controlled trials using diabetes education. Their meta-analysis revealed that self-management education does improve HbA1c levels in the short term (i.e. within six months) and that increased contact time with diabetes healthcare providers enhances this beneficial effect. However, glycaemic deterioration reappears one to three months after the intervention ceases. As the course, severity and outcome of diabetes are likely to be influenced heavily by psychological factors, psychological distress is thought to be an important contributor to the lack of long-term healthy diabetes self-management and subsequent glycaemic control [126], perhaps due in part to interference with patient recall of the diabetes information they received.

Psychological distress often can be reduced through the use of CBT. CBT encompasses a wide range of psychological techniques designed to bring about change in thinking patterns and behaviours, i.e. stress-management programmes. In overview, the studies reviewed here implement CBT and/or stress-management/relaxation interventions (Table 8.6). The primary outcome variables have typically included measures of psychological symptoms and glycaemic control, most commonly HbA1c.

Nearly all of the studies administered individual therapies, but Surwit and colleagues' [130] investigation supports the efficacy of out-patient stress-management training administered in a group format for the improvement of glycaemic control in patients with type 2 diabetes. The impact of stress management did not become evident until the 12-month data-collection point. Control and experimental patients both showed decreased HbA1c up to six months. After that point, the average HbA1c of control subjects deteriorated, while that of stress-management subjects continued to improve.

Future randomised, prospective controlled trials of patients with diabetes would benefit from administration of structured diagnostic interviews in order to ascertain the presence of major mental disorders. The promise of psychological treatments is their potential for salutary effects upon neurophysiological mechanisms, e.g. reduction in stress-induced counter-regulatory hormones and alterations of neuropeptides related to appetite and satiety. In this regard, CBT, the most well-known structured manual-driven treatment for depression, may contribute to glycaemic control, although data supporting this conclusion are sparse. In the ten-week controlled study administering weekly CBT for diabetic patients with major depression (see Tables 8.4 and 8.6), both depressive symptoms and HbA1c improved [94]. Compared with patients receiving only diabetic education (the control group), patients receiving CBT and diabetic education exhibited significantly greater clinical improvement on the BDI (-19 vs. -7) at the end of the 10-week intervention;

Table 8.6 Controlled trials of psychological interventions in patients with diabetes

Study	Diabetes patient population	Primary objective	Intervention	Variables	Psychological results	Glycaemic effects	Comments
Lane et al. [127]	Type 2 n = 38 (26 male, 12 female) patients with poorly controlled diabetes	To examine the benefits of biofeedback-assisted relaxation training and to investigate patient characteristics that could predict a positive response to relaxation training	8 weekly 50-minute biofeedback training sessions (with 4 monthly additional session) + diabetes education vs. diabetes education alone	Eysenck Personality Inventory, Nowicki Strickland Locus of Control, STAI, HbA1c, glucose tolerance	By week 48, individuals who responded best to relaxation training with improvements in glucose tolerance were those with higher trait anxiety and more emotional lability	Both groups achieved significant reductions in HbA1c, but there was no difference between the groups	Biofeedback training did not improve heart rate and blood pressure of intervention group; prevalence of major depression unknown in study population
Spiess et al. [128]	Type 2 n = 23 (14 male, 9 female) patients with poorly controlled diabetes	To assess whether a distress-reduction programme improves psychological variables and whether better coping strategies may be associated with improved metabolic control	Distress-reduction programme (25 weekly 90-minute group sessions) + diabetes education vs. diabetes education	DSM-III-R interview, BDI, LES, STAI, HbA1c	By 3 months follow-up, improved depressive and anxiety symptoms in treatment group compared with control group. By 9 months' follow-up, depressive and anxiety symptoms of two groups similar to pretreatment levels	No differences in HbA1c levels between the groups at 3 and 9 months follow-up, but HbA1c of both groups improved significantly from baseline	Elevated depressive symptoms in study subjects (mean BDI > 26), but no study subject fulfilled DSM-III-R criteria for major depression

Study	Population	Aim	Intervention	Measures	Results	Results (cont.)	Comments
Lustman et al. [94]	Type 2 $n = 51$ (26 male, 25 female) with major depression; 41 complete	To assess the efficacy of CBT for depression in patients with diabetes	10 weeks of individual CBT + diabetes education vs. diabetes education alone	DIS, BDI, HbA1c levels, self-monitoring compliance	By 6 months follow-up, more patients in CBT (58%) achieve remission of depressive symptoms vs. control (26%) ($p = 0.03$)	At immediate post-treatment follow-up, no significant difference in HbA1c between treatment and control groups. By 6 months follow-up, HbA1c levels decrease by 0.7% in CBT group and increase by 0.9% in control group ($p = 0.04$)	All subjects fulfilled categorical diagnosis of major depression
Pouwer et al. [129]	Types 1 and 2 $n = 345$ (168 male, 177 female)	To investigate whether monitoring of psychological wellbeing improves mood or glycaemic control	During 12-month period, subjects completed computerised and self-report psychological questionnaires at initial, interim and 12-month visit. Psychological results discussed with patient by diabetes nurse + standard care vs. standard care alone	WBQ-12	Monitored patients reported improved general wellbeing	No differences for HbA1c levels between the two groups	Prevalence of major depression unknown in study population

(cont.)

Table 8.6 (*cont.*)

Study	Diabetes patient population	Primary objective	Intervention	Variables	Psychological results	Glycaemic effects	Comments
Surwit *et al.* [130]	Type 2 $n = 108$ (63 male, 45 female), 72 complete	To determine whether a stress-management programme can improve glucose metabolism	5 sessions of weekly group stress-management therapy + diabetes education vs. diabetes education alone	STAI, Perceived Stress Scale, General Health Questionnaire, HbA1c levels	By 1 year follow-up, no improvement in anxiety even among highly anxious patients at baseline	Difference between groups in HbA1c appeared at 1 year follow-up, i.e. stress-management-trained patients exhibited approximately a 0.5% reduction in HbA1c compared with control patients	Group therapy improves glycaemic control over time, but may take several months to appear, is modest in effect and is not due to changes in exercise, diet or BMI. Prevalence of major depression unknown in study population

| Williams et al. [131] | Type 1 and 2 n = 417 (194 male; 223 female) with major depression or dysthymia; 232 complete | Multicentre study to determine whether depression treatment improves mood and diabetic outcomes in adults with diabetes and depression | Depression care management (educational materials + 6–8 brief sessions of depression psychotherapy) over 12-month period vs. usual care for depression | DSM-IV structured interview, Symptom Checklist-20, HbA1c levels | By 12 month follow-up, treatment group exhibited significantly improved depressive symptoms and overall function | By 12 months follow-up, intervention did not improve glycaemic control | Study sample exhibited relatively good glycaemic control at baseline (HbA1c level: 7.3 +/− 1.4%). Diabetes status based on patient self-report. Intervention group significantly more likely to utilise antidepressant or psychotherapy |

BDI, Beck Depression Inventory [10]; BDQ, Barriers in Diabetes Questionnaire; CBT, cognitive–behavioural therapy; DIS, National Institute of Mental Health (NIMH) Diagnostic Interview Schedule [132]; DSCI, Diabetes Self-care Inventory [132]; DSM-III-R, Diagnostic and Statistical Manual, 3rd edition, revised [133]; HbA1c, haemoglobin A1c; HFS, Fear of Hypoglycemia Survey; LES, Life Events Scale [134]; PAID, Problem Areas in Diabetes; SCL-90, Symptom Checklist 90 [135]; STAI, State-Trait Anxiety Inventory [136]; WBQ-12, Well-Being Questionnaire [8].

more of the CBT-treated patients experienced remission of their depressive symptoms (85% vs. 27%). Although there was not a significant improvement in HbA1c levels by the end of ten weeks of weekly CBT, at six-month follow-up the HbA1c levels of the CBT group had decreased significantly, even after controlling for initial levels. Moreover, CBT-treated patients who failed to achieve full remission of their depression reported poor compliance with self-monitoring of blood glucose, accounting for 25% of the variance in post-treatment levels of depression [94]. The longer-term follow-up (six months after the intervention) of this CBT trial may have been necessary for the decrease in HbA1c to become apparent, as HbA1c reflects the three prior months of glycaemic control). Lastly, most of the studies listed in Table 8.6 did not determine the presence or absence of major mental disorders in their study populations or whether there were specific patient attitudes or behaviours that interfered with patient self-care (e.g. fears of hypoglycaemia, pessimism, needle phobias, avoidance of medical clinics), which CBT techniques such as systematic desensitisation, cognitive restructuring and token economies can alleviate, resulting in improved compliance and glycaemic control [93].

Combination psychotherapy and psychopharmacology interventions

Psychotherapeutic and/or psychopharmacological treatment of the 9–27% of patients with diabetes who experience considerable dysphoria, whether subsyndromal or syndromal major depression, may have a significant effect (positive or negative) on both diabetes-related morbidity and mortality. The fact that psychotherapy and stress-management treatments yield inconclusive results raises the question of the effectiveness and parsimony of introducing psychological treatments to an already complicated treatment regimen. Providing psychological treatments that may not have added benefits will be unnecessarily burdensome to patients, while antidepressant pharmacotherapy is a less effortful intervention. However, the mixed results may be a consequence of not only methodological considerations (e.g. small sample size, design flaws) but also the fact that patients with diabetes may be struggling with complicated severe forms of depression and anxiety that do not respond immediately to intervention. Combined treatment with psychotherapy and psychopharmacology has been found to be significantly more efficacious in the treatment of depression than either treatment alone [137]. Current practice guidelines for primary-care physicians and psychiatrists promote combined psychotherapy with drug treatment as the treatment of choice for depression [138]. Sequential interventions may be even more efficacious than simultaneous drug and therapy treatments. As such, further investigation is necessary regarding the efficacy and relative benefits of combined therapy and drug regimens, both simultaneous and sequential, in the treatment of depression in diabetic patients.

Future directions for research

The principal unanswered questions in this field remain primarily prognostic, aetiologic and treatment-related: By what mechanisms do dysphoria and other symptoms such as hostility [139] affect glucoregulatory systems? Conversely, will treatment of depression prevent or reduce incidence of diabetes and diabetes-associated complications? Investigative strategies should certainly include additional prospective rather than cross-sectional studies of diabetic patients with comorbid depression [140] as well as studies of genetic susceptibilities or neurobiological mechanisms common to both of these debilitating disorders. The disease burden of diabetes increases with time, and prospective studies will allow attention to outcomes of cost, quality of life and control of pain. Certainly the temporal and reciprocal relationship of depression with diabetes can be informed most optimally by prospective examination of whether resolution of hyperglycaemia is consistently associated with improvement in depressive symptoms.

Effective treatment of depression in patients with type 1 or type 2 diabetes may normalise neuroendocrine and immuno-inflammatory hyperactivation, facilitate adherence to diet and exercise, and improve glycaemic control [141]. However, investigative strategies must confirm whether effective depression treatment reduces continuous proximal short-term outcomes such as hyperglycaemia, peripheral neuropathy, impotence and impaired vision versus discrete long-term outcomes, such as onset of dialysis, limb amputation, myocardial infarction and long-term survival. Given the rising number of children with type 2 diabetes and the disparities in health suffered by minority communities, future studies should also focus on these understudied populations [142].

Clearly, important information can be gleaned from animal models of diabetes and the vulnerability of certain brain structures such as the hippocampus to damage in situations of stress [143]. Whether impairments in the insulin signalling pathway in the periphery and brain in patients with depression parallel those observed in Alzheimer's disease, diabetes and ageing [144] remains to be determined. Undoubtedly, further elucidation of specialised metabolic integrative neuronal pathways in the brain that contain glucose-sensing, glucose-responsive neurons will improve our understanding of the complex systems that regulate nutrient intake, calorie storage and energy expenditure [145–147]. Fascinating discoveries will certainly result from future efforts to understand the role of the brain in the integration of mental and metabolic homeostasis [146].

Acknowledgements

This research was supported by grants RR-00039 from the National Institutes of Health, Bethesda, MD, and HS-07922 (Dr Phillips), and MH-069254

(Dr Musselman). We are grateful for the assistance of Ms Erica Bruce, BSA, in the preparation of the manuscript, and the nursing and laboratory staff of the Emory General Clinical Research Center, Emory University Hospital, and the Diabetes Clinic at Grady Memorial Hospital.

REFERENCES

1. World Health Organization. *Diabetes: The Cost of Diabetes* (Geneva: World Health Organization, 2002).
2. Diabetes Control and Complications Trial Research Group. The effect of intensive treatment of diabetes on the development and progression of long-term complications in insulin-dependent diabetes mellitus. *N. Engl. J. Med.* **329** (1993), 977–86.
3. R. Klein, B. E. K. Klein, S. E. Moss, M. D. Davis, D. L. DeMets, The Wisconsin Epidemiologic Study of Diabetes Retinopathy III: prevalence and risk of diabetic retinopathy when age at diagnosis is 30 or more years. *Arch. Opthalmol.* **102** (1984), 527–32.
4. Associated Press. Estimate of Americans with pre-diabetes doubles. *Wall Street Journal*, April 29, 2004.
5. World Health Organization. *Laboratory Diagnosis and Monitoring of Diabetes Mellitus* (Geneva: World Health Organization, 2002).
6. Guidelines Subcommittee of the WHO/ISH Mild Hypertension Liaison Committee. Guidelines for the management of mild hypertension. *Hypertension* **22** (1993), 392–403.
7. J. S. McDaniel, D. L. Musselman, M. R. Porter, D. A. Reed, C. B. Nemeroff, Depression in the cancer patient: a commentary on diagnosis, biology, and treatment. *Arch. Gen. Psychiatry* **52** (1995), 89–99.
8. C. Bradley, The well-being questionnaire. In *Handbook of Psychology and Diabetes*, ed. C. Bradley (chur, Switzerland: Harwood Academic Publishers, 1994), pp. 89–109.
9. P. J. Lustman, H. Amado, R. D. Wetzel, Depression in diabetics: a critical appraisal. *Comp. Psychiatry* **1** (1983), 65–74.
10. A. T. Beck, C. H. Ward, M. Mendelson, J. Mock, J. Erbaugh, An inventory for measuring depression. *Arch. Gen. Psychiatry* **4** (1961), 561–71.
11. P. J. Lustman, L. S. Griffith, J. A. Gavard, R. E. Clouse, Depression in adults with diabetes. *Diabetes Care* **15** (1992), 1631–9.
12. P. J. Lustman, K. E. Freedland, R. M. Carney, B. A. Hong, R. E. Clouse, Similarity of depression in diabetic and psychiatric patients. *Psychosom. Med.* **54** (1992), 602–11.
13. P. J Lustman, L. S. Griffith, R. E. Clouse, *et al.*, Effects of nortriptyline on depression and glucose regulation in diabetes: results of a double-blind, placebo-controlled trial. *Psychosom. Med.* **59** (1997), 241–50.
14. P. Ciechanowski, W. Katon, J. Russo, The relationship of depressive symptoms to symptom reporting, self-care and glucose control in diabetes. *Diabetes Care* **25** (2002), 731–6.
15. L. E. Edge, D. Zheng, K. Simpson, Comorbid depression is associated with increased health care use and expenditures in individuals with diabetes. *Diabetes Care* **25** (2002), 464–70.

16. J. A. Gavard, P. J. Lustman, R. E. Clouse, Prevalence of depression in adults with diabetes: an epidemiological evaluation. *Diabetes Care* **16** (1993), 1167–78.

17. R. J. Anderson, K. E. Freedland, R. E. Clouse, P. J. Lustman, The prevalence of comorbid depression in adults with diabetes: a meta-analysis. *Diabetes Care* **24** (2001), 1069–78.

18. T. L. Gary, R. M. Crum, L. Cooper-Patrick, D. Ford, F. L. Brancati, Depressive symptoms and metabolic control in African-Americans with type 2 diabetes. *Diabetes Care* **23** (2000), 23–9.

19. S. A. Black, J. S. Goodwin, K. S. Markides, The association between chronic diseases and depressive symptomatology in older Mexican Americans. *J. Gerontol. A Biol. Sci. Med. Sci.* **53A** (1998), M188–94.

20. A. Grandinetti, J. K. Kaholokula, K. M. Crabbe, *et al.*, Relationship between depressive symptoms and diabetes among native Hawaiians. *Psychoneuroendocrinology* **25** (2000), 239–46.

21. J. K. Warnock, E. M. Mutzig, Diabetes mellitus and major depression: considerations for treatment of Native Americans. *J. Okla. State Med. Assoc.* **91** (1998), 488–93.

22. K. Ostler, C. Thompson, A. L. Kinmonth, *et al.*, Influence of socio-economic deprivation on the prevalence and outcome of depression in primary care: the Hampshire Depression project. *Br. J. Psychiatry* **178** (2001), 12–17.

23. S. A. Everson, S. C. Saty, J. W. Lynch, G. A. Kaplan, Epidemiologic evidence for the relation between socioeconomic status and depression, obesity, and diabetes. *J. Psychosom. Res.* **53** (2002), 891–5.

24. J. W. Lynch, G. A. Kaplan, S. J. Shema, Cumulative impact of sustained economic hardship on physical, cognitive, psychological, and social functioning. *N. Engl. J. Med.* **337** (1997), 1889–95.

25. C. E. Ross, Neighborhood disadvantage and adult depression. *J. Health Soc. Behav.* **41** (2000), 177–87.

26. C. Saul, N. Payne, How does the prevalence of specific morbidities compare with measures of socio-economic status at small area level? *J. Public Health Med.* **21** (1999), 340–47.

27. L. Fisher, C. A. Chesla, J. T. Mullan, M. M. Skaff, R. A. Kanter, Contributors to depression in Latino and European-American patients with type 2 diabetes. *Diabetes Care* **24** (2001), 1751–7.

28. M. Peyrot, R. R. Rubin, Levels and risk of depression and anxiety symptomatology among diabetic adults. *Diabetes Care* **20** (1997), 585–90.

29. P. J. Lustman, L. S. Griffith, R. E. Clouse, P. E. Cryer, Psychiatric illness in diabetes: relationship to symptoms and glucose control. *J. Nerv. Ment. Dis.* **174** (1986), 736–42.

30. C. E. Lloyd, K. A. Matthews, R. R. Wing, T. J. Orchard, Psychosocial factors and complications of IDDM: the Pittsburgh Epidemiology of Diabetes Complications Study. *Diabetes Care* **15** (1992), 166–72.

31. P. J. Lustman, L. S. Griffith, R. E. Clouse, Depression in adults with diabetes: results of 5-year follow-up study. *Diabetes Care* **11** (1988), 605–12.

32. P. J. Lustman, R. J. Anderson, K. E. Freedland, *et al.*, Depression and poor glycemic control: a meta-analytic review of the literature. *Diabetes Care* **23** (2000), 934–42.

33. D. C. Ziemer, S. F. Ferguson, R. L. Kieltyka, W. Slocum, Barriers to appointment keeping in a municipal hospital diabetes clinic. *Diabetes* **47**, Suppl 1 (1998), A144.

34. M. de Groot, R. Anderson, K. E. Freedland, R. E. Clouse, P. J. Lustman, Association of depression and diabetes complications: a meta-analysis. *Psychosom. Med.* **63** (2001), 619–30.

35. H. Vinnamaki, L. Niskanen, M. Uusitupa, Mental well-being in people with non-insulin dependent diabetes. *Acta Psychiatr. Scand.* **92** (1995), 392–7.

36. R. S. Mazze, D. Lucido, H. Shamoon, Psychological and social correlates of glycemic control. *Diabetes Care* **7** (1984), 360–66.

37. M. A. Testa, D. C. Simonson, Health economic benefits and quality of life during improved glycemic control in patients with type 2 diabetes mellitus. *J. Am. Med. Assoc.* **280** (1998), 1490–96.

38. C. Hayward, Psychiatric illness and cardiovascular disease risk. *Epidemiol. Rev.* **17** (1995), 129–38.

39. W. W. Eaton, H. Armenian, J. Gallo, L. Pratt, E. Ford, Depression and risk for onset of type II diabetes: a prospective population-based study. *Diabetes Care* **22** (1996), 1097–102.

40. L. N. Robins, J. E. Helzer, J. L. Croughan, J. B. W. Williams, R. L. Spitzer, *The NIMH Diagnostic Interview Schedule, Version III* (Washington, DC: Public Health Service [HSS], 1981).

41. W. W. Zung, A self-rating depression scale. *Arch. Gen. Psychiatry* **12** (1965), 63–70.

42. S. A. Everson-Rose, P. M. Meyer, L. H. Powell, *et al.*, Depressive symptoms, insulin resistance, and risk of diabetes in women in midlife. *Diabetes Care* **27** (2004), 2856–62.

43. L. S. Radloff, The CES-D scale: a self-report depression scale for research in the general population. *J. Appl. Psychol. Meas.* **1** (1977), 385–401.

44. N. Kawakami, N. Tkatsuka, H. Shimizu, H. Ishibashi, Depressive symptoms and occurrence of type 2 diabetes among Japanese men. *Diabetes Care* **22** (1999), 1071–6.

45. P. S. Ciechanowski, W. J. Katon, J. E. Russo, Depression and diabetes: impact of depressive symptoms on adherence, function, and costs. *Arch. Intern. Med.* **1160** (2000), 3278–85.

46. W. J. Katon, M. Von Korff, E. Lin, *et al.*, Population-based care of depression: effective disease management strategies to decrease prevalence. *Gen. Hosp. Psychiatry* **19** (1997), 169–78.

47. L. E. Egede, D. Zheng, K. Simpson, Comorbid depression is associated with increased health care use and expenditure in individuals with diabetes. *Diabetes Care* **25** (2002), 464–70.

48. R. E. Clouse, P. J. Lustman, K. E. Freedland, *et al.*, Depression and coronary heart disease in women with diabetes. *Psychosom. Med.* **65** (2003), 376–83.

49. N. Frasure-Smith, F. Lesperance, M. Juneau, M. Talajic, M. G. Bourassa, Gender, depression, and one-year prognosis after myocardial infarction. *Psychosom. Med.* **61** (1999), 26–37.

50. R. M. Sapolsky, L. M. Romero, A. U. Munck, How do glucocorticoids influence stress responses? Integrating permissive, suppressive, stimulator and preparative actions. *Endocrinol. Rev.* **21** (2000), 55–89.

51. D. L. Musselman, C. DeBatista, K. I. Nathan, *et al.*, Biology of mood disorders. In *Textbook of Psychopharmacology*, 2nd edn, ed. A. F. Schatzberg, C. B. Nemeroff (Washington, DC: American Psychiatric Press, 1998), pp. 550–88.

52. A. Munck, A. Naray-Fejes-Toth, Glucocorticoid action: physiology. In *Endocrinology*, ed. L. J. de Groot (Philadelphia: W. B. Saunders, 1995), pp. 1642–56.

53. N. Eigler, L. Sacca, R. S. Sherwin, Synergistic interactions of physiologic increments of glucagon, epinephrine and cortisol in the dog: a model for stress-induced hyperglycemia. *J. Clin. Invest.* **63** (1979), 114–23.

54. R. DeFronzo, R. S. Sherwin, P. Felig, Synergistic interactions of counterregulatory hormones: a mechanism for stress hyperglycemia. *Acta Chir. Scand. Suppl.* **498** (1980), 33–9.

55. D. N. Brindley, Y. Rolland, Possible connections between stress, diabetes, obesity, hypertension and altered lipoprotein metabolism that may result in atherosclerosis. *Clin. Sci.* (Land.) **77** (1989), 453–61.

56. M. F. Dallman, A. M. Strack, S. F. Akana, *et al.*, Feast and famine: critical role of glucocorticoids with insulin in daily energy flow. *Front. Neuroendocrinol.* **14** (1993), 303–47.

57. S. P. Weinstein, T. Paquin, A. Pritsker, R. A. Haber, Glucocorticoid-induced insulin resistance: dexamethsone inhibits the activation of glucose transport in rat skeletal muscle by both insulin- and non-insulin-related stimuli. *Diabetes* **44** (1995), 441–5.

58. P. S. Mueller, G. R. Heninger, R. K. McDonald, Intravenous glucose tolerance test in depression. *Arch. Gen. Psychiatry* **21** (1968), 470–77.

59. J. H. Wright, J. J. Jacisin, N. S. Radin, Glucose metabolism in unipolar depression. *Br. J. Psychiatry* **132** (1978), 386–93.

60. A. Winokur, G. Maislin, J. L. Phillips, J. D. Amsterdam, Insulin resistance after oral glucose tolerance testing in patients with major depression. *Am. J. Psychiatry* **145** (1988), 325–30.

61. E. J. Sachar, J. Finkelstein, L. Hellman, Growth hormone responses in depressive illness: 1. Response to insulin tolerance test. *Arch. Gen. Psychiatry* **25** (1971), 263–9.

62. R. C. Casper, J. M. Davis, G. Pandey, D. Garver, H. Dekirmenjian, Neuroendocrine and amine studies in affective illness. *Psychoneuroendocrinology* **2** (1977), 105–13.

63. R. Duelli, W. Kuschinsky, Brain glucose transporters: relationship to local energy demand. *N. Physiol. Sci.* **16** (2001), 71–6.

64. L. R. Baxter, M. E. Phelps, J. C. Mazziotta, *et al.*, Cerebral metabolic rates for glucose in mood disorders studied with positron emission tomography (PET) and (F-18)-fluro-2-deoxyglucose (FDG). *Arch. Gen. Psychiatry* **42** (1985), 441–7.

65. L. R. Baxter, J. M. Schwartz, M. E. Phelps, *et al.*, Reduction of prefrontal cortex glucose metabolism common to three types of depression. *Arch. Gen. Psychiatry* **46** (1989), 243–50.

66. J. L. Martinot, P. Hardy, A. Feline, *et al.*, Left prefrontal glucose metabolism in the depressed state: a confirmation. *Am. J. Psychiatry* **147** (1990), 1313–17.

67. I. A. Simpson, K. R. Chundru, T. Davies-Hill, W. G. Honer, P. Davies, Decreased concentrations of GLUT1 and GLUT3 glucose transporters in the brains of patients with Alzheimer's disease. *Ann. Neurol.* **35** (1994), 511–12.

68. W. C. Gamberino, W. A. Brennan, Jr, Glucose transporter isoform expression in Huntington's disease brain. *J. Neurochem.* **63** (1994), 1392–7.

69. D. E. Kuhl, M. E. Phelps, C. H. Markham, *et al.*, Cerebral metabolism and atrophy in Huntington's disease. *Ann. Neurol.* **12** (1982), 425–34.

70. D. L. Rothman, I. Magnusson, G. Cline, *et al.*, Decreased muscle glucose transport/phosphorylation is an early defect in the pathogenesis of non-insulin-dependent diabetes mellitus. *Proc. Natl. Acad. Sci. U. S. A.* **92** (1995), 983–7.

71. K. F. Petersen, G. I. Shulman, Pathogenesis of skeletal muscle insulin resistance in type 2 diabetes mellitus. *Am. J. Cardiol.* **90** (2002), 11–18G.

72. G. I. Shulman, D. L. Rothman, T. Jue, *et al.*, Quantitation of muscle glycogen synthesis in normal subjects and subjects with non-insulin dependent diabetes mellitus by ^{13}C nuclear magnetic resonance spectroscopy. *N. Engl. J. Med.* **322** (1990), 223–8.

73. R. Ross, Atherosclerosis: an inflammatory disease. *N. Engl. J. Med.* **340** (1999), 115–26.

74. S. K. Fried, D. A. Bunkin, A. S. Greenburg, Omental and subcutaneous adipose tissue of obese subjects release interleukin-6: depot difference and regulation by glucocorticoid. *J. Clin. Endocrinol. Metab.* **83** (1998), 847–50.

75. J. M. Fernandez-Real, M. Vayred, C. Richart, *et al.*, Circulating interleukin 6 levels, blood pressure, and insulin insensitivity in apparently healthy men and women. *J. Clin. Endocrinol. Metab.* **86** (2001), 1154–9.

76. G. Paolisso, M. R. Rizzo, G. Mazziotti, *et al.*, Advancing age and insulin resistance: role of plasma tumor necrosis factor-alpha. *Am. J. Physiol.* **275** (1998), E294–9.

77. G. S. Hotamisligil, N. S. Shargill, B. M. Spiegelman, Adipose expression of tumor necrosis factor-alpha: direct role in obesity-linked insulin resistance. *Science* **259** (1993), 87–91.

78. G. S. Hotamisligil, A. Budavari, D. Murray, B. M. Spiegelman, Reduced tyrosine kinase activity of the insulin receptor in obesity-diabetes. *J. Clin. Invest.* **94** (1994), 1543–9.

79. G. S. Hotamisligil, B. M. Spiegelman, Tumor necrosis factor a: a key component of the obesity-diabetes link. *Diabetes* **43** (1994), 1271–8.

80. G. S. Hotamisligil, P. Arner, J. F. Caro, R. L. Atkinson, B. M. Spiegelman, Increased adipose tissue expression of tumor necrosis factor-a in human obesity and insulin resistance. *J. Clin. Invest.* **95** (1995), 2409–15.

81. P. A. Kern, M. Szaghizadah, J. M. Ong, *et al.*, The expression of tumor necrosis factor in human adipose tissue: regulation by obesity, weight loss, and relationship to lipoprotein lipase. *J. Clin. Invest.* **95** (1995), 2111–19.

82. G. S. Hotamisligil, P. Peraldi, A. Budavari, *et al.*, IRS-1-mediated inhibition of insulin receptor tyrosine kinase activity in TNF-alpha- and obesity-induced insulin resistance. *Science* **271** (1996), 665–8.

83. M. Saghizadeh, J. M. Ong, W. T. Garvey, R. R. Henry, P. A. Kern, The expression of TNFa by human muscle: relationship to insulin resistance. *J. Clin. Invest.* **97** (1996), 1111–16.

84. S. Kent, R. M. Bluthe, K. W. Kelley, R. Dantzer, Sickness behavior as a new target for drug development. *Trends Pharmacol. Sci.* **13** (1992), 24–8.

85. R. Yirmiya, Endotoxin produces a depressive-like episode in rats. *Brain Res.* **711** (1996), 163–74.

86. M. Maes, S. Scharpe, H. Y. Meltzer, *et al.*, Increased neopterin and interferon-gamma secretion and lower availability of L-tryptophan in major depression: further evidence for an immune response. *Psychiatr. Res.* **54** (1994), 143–60.

87. M. Maes, E. Vendoolaeghe, R. Ranjan, *et al.*, Increased serum interleukin-1-receptor-antagonist concentrations in major depression. *J. Affect. Dis.* **36** (1995), 2–36.

88. M. Maes, R. Smith, A. Christophe, *et al.*, Fatty acid composition in major depression: decreased omega 3 fractions in cholesteryl esters and increased C20:4 omega-6/C20:5 omega-3 ratio in cholesteryl esters and phospholipids. *J. Affect. Dis.* **38** (1996), 35–46.

89. M. Berk, A. A. Wadee, R. H. Kuschke, A. O'Neill-Kerr, Acute-phase proteins in major depression. *J. Psychosom. Res.* **43** (1997), 529–34.

90. U. H. Frommberger, J. Bauer, P. Haselbauer, *et al.*, Interleukin-6-(IL-6) plasma levels in depression and schizophrenia: comparison between the acute state and after remission. *Eur. Arch. Psychiatry Clin. Neurosci.* **247** (1997), 228–33.

91. G. E. Miller, C. A. Stetler, R. M. Carney, K. E. Freedland, W. A. Banks, Clinical depression and inflammatory risk markers for coronary heart disease. *Am. J. Cardiol.* **90** (2002), 1279–83.

92. D. L. Musselman, A. H. Miller, M. R. Porter, *et al.*, Higher than normal plasma interleukin-6 concentrations in cancer patients with depression: preliminary findings. *Am. J. Psychiatry* **158** (2001), 1252–7.

93. F. J. Snoek, T. C. Skinner, Psychological counselling in problematic diabetes: does it help? *Diabetes Med.* **19** (2002), 265–73.

94. P. J. Lustman, L. S. Griffith, K. E. Freedland, S. S. Kissel, R. E. Clouse, Cognitive behavior therapy for depression in type 2 diabetes mellitus: a randomized, controlled trial. *Ann. Intern. Med.* **129** (1998), 613–21.

95. Diabetes Control and Complications Trial Research Group. The effect of intensive treatment of diabetes on the development and progression of long-term complications in insulin-dependent diabetes mellitus. *N. Engl. J. Med.* **329** (1993), 977–86.

96. L. M. Thaler, D. C. Ziemer, D. L. Gallina, *et al.*, Availability of rapid HbA1c measurements enhances clinical decision-making. *Diabetes Care* **22** (1999), 1415–21.

97. P. J. Lustman, G. W. Harper, Nonpsychiatric physicians' identification and treatment of depression in patients with diabetes. *Comp. Psychiatry* **28** (1987), 22–7.

98. C. B. Cook, L. S. Phillips, I. M. El-Kebbi, *et al.*, Diabetes in urban African-Americans: XVII. Improved diabetes management over five years with nurse provider-led care at a large municipal hospital. *Diabetes Care* **22** (1999), 1494–500.

99. C. D. Miller, L. S. Phillips, D. C. Ziemer, *et al.*, Hypoglycemia in patients with type 2 diabetes. *Arch. Intern. Med.* **161** (2001), 1653–9.

100. W. Slocum, D. C. Ziemer, S. D. Culler, C. Cook, S. Y. Ferguson, Poor appointment keeping behavior worsens glycemic control. *Diabetes* **48**: Suppl 1 (1999), A197.

101. P. J. Goodnick, J. H. Henry, V. M. V. Buki, Treatment of depression in patients with diabetes mellitus. *J. Clin. Psychiatry* **56** (1995), 128–36.

102. H. M. van Praag, B. Leijnse, Depression, glucose tolerance, peripheral glucose uptake and their alterations under the influence of anti-depressive drugs of the hydrazine type. *Psychopharmacologia* **8** (1965), 67–78.

103. M. B. Max, R. Kishore-Kumar, S. C. Schafer, *et al.*, Efficacy of desipramine in painful diabetic neuropathy: a placebo-controlled trial. *Pain* **45** (1991), 3–9.

104. M. B. Max, S. A. Lynch, J. Muir, *et al.*, Effects of desipramine, amitriptyline, and fluoxetine in diabetic neuropathy. *N. Engl. J. Med.* **326** (1992), 1250–56.

105. J. Rabkin, F. Quitkin, W. Harrison, P. McGrath, E. Tricamo, Adverse reactions to monoamine oxidase inhibitors: I. A comparative study. *J. Clin. Psychopharmacol.* **4** (1984), 270–78.

106. P. R. Muskin, A. H. Glassman, The use of tricyclic antidepressants in a medical setting. In *Consultation-liaison Psychiatry: Current Trends and Future Perspectives*, ed. J. B. Finkel (New York: Grune & Stratton, 1983), pp. 137–58.

107. S. P. Roose, G. W. Dalack, Treating the depressed patient with cardiovascular problems. *J. Clin. Psychiatry* **53** (1992), 25–31.

108. S. H. Sindrup, L. F. Gram, K. Brosen, O. Eshoj, E. F. Mogensen, The selective serotonin reuptake inhibitor paroxetine is effective in the treatment of diabetic neuropathy symptoms. *Pain* **42** (1990), 135–44.

109. C. L. DeVane, J. S. Markowitz, Psychoactive drug interactions with pharmacotherapy for diabetes. *Psychopharmacol. Bull.* **36** (2002), 40–52.

110. L. M. Tremaine, K. D. Wilner, S. H. Preskorn, A study of the potential effect of sertraline on the pharmacokinetics and protein binding of tolbutamide. *Clin. Pharmacokinet.* **32**: Suppl 1 (1992), 31–6.

111. N. Sussman, D. L. Ginsberg, J. Bikoff, Effects of nefazodone on body weight: a pooled analysis of selective serotonin reuptake inhibitor-and imipramine-controlled trials. *J. Clin. Psychiatry* **62** (2001), 256–60.

112. M. Fava, Weight gain and antidepressants. *J. Clin. Psychiatry* **61**: Suppl 11 (2000), 37–41.

113. M. D. Marcus, R. R. Wing, J. Guare, E. H. Blaire, A. Jawad, Lifetime prevalence of major depression and its effect on treatment outcome in obese type II diabetic patients. *Diabetes Care* **15** (1992), 253–5.

114. D. L. Rowland, L. Myers, A. Culver, J. M. Davidson, Bupropion and sexual function: a placebo-controlled prospective study on diabetic men with erectile dysfunction. *J. Clin. Psychopharmacol.* **17** (1997), 350–57.

115. C. E. Koro, D. O. Fedder, G. J. L'Italien, *et al.*, Assessment of independent effect of olanzapine and risperidone on risk of diabetes among patients with schizophrenia: population based nested case–control study. *Br. Med. J.* **325** (2002), 243–7.

116. P. S. Masand, Atypical antipsychotics and DKA: issues and controversies. *Thomson Professional Postgraduate Services* **2** (2002), 1–3.

117. M. J. Serynak, D. L. Leslie, R. D. Alarcon, M. F. Losonczy, R. Rosenheck, Association of diabetes mellitus with use of atypical neuroleptics in the treatment of schizophrenia. *Am. J. Psychiatry* **159** (2002), 561–6.

118. J. I. Isojarvi, J. Rattya, V. V. Myllyla, *et al.*, Valproate, lamotrigine, and insulin-mediated risks in women with epilepsy. *Ann. Neurol.* **43** (1998), 446–51.

119. H. Jin, J. M. Meyer, D. V. Jeste, Phenomenology of and risk factors for new-onset diabetes mellitus and diabetic ketoacidosis associated with atypical antipsychotics: an analysis of 45 published cases. *Ann. Clin. Psychiatry* **14** (2002), 59–64.

120. Report of the expert committee on the diagnosis and classification of diabetes mellitus. *Diabetes Care* **26**: Suppl 1 (2003), 5–20.

121. M. O'Kane, P. G. Wiles, J. K. Wales, Fluoxetine in the treatment of obese type 2 diabetic patients. *Diabetes Med.* **11** (1994), 105–10.

122. L. Breum, U. Bjerre, J. F. Bak, S. Jacobsen, A. Astrup, Long-term effects of fluoxetine on glycemic control in obese patients with non-insulin-dependent diabetes mellitus or glucose intolerance: influence on muscle glycogen synthase and insulin receptor kinase activity. *Metabolism* **44** (1995), 1570–76.

123. P. Mahuex, F. Ducros, J. Bourque, J. Garon, J.-L. Chiasson, Fluoxetine improves insulin sensitivity in obese patients with non-insulin-dependent diabetes mellitus independently of weight loss. *Int. J. Obes.* **21** (1997), 97–102.

124. B. J. P. van Loon, J. K. Radder, M. Frolich, Fluoxetine increases insulin action in obese nondiabetic and in obese noninsulin-dependent diabetic individuals. *Int. J. Obes.* **16** (1992), 79–85.

125. S. L. Norris, J. Lau, S. J. Smith, C. H. Schmid, M. M. Engelgau, Self-management education for adults with type 2 diabetes: a meta-analysis of the effect on glycemic control. *Diabetes Care* **25** (2002), 1159–71.

126. B. A. Hamburg, G. E. Inoff, Coping with predictable crises of diabetes. *Diabetes Care* **6** (1983), 409–16.

127. J. D. Lane, C. C. McCaskill, S. L. Ross, M. N. Feinglos, R. S. Surwit, Relaxation training for NIDDM: predicting who may benefit. *Diabetes Care* **16** (1993), 1087–94.

128. K. Spiess, G. Sachs, P. Pietschmann, R. Prager, A program to reduce onset distress in unselected type I diabetic patients: effects on psychological variables and metabolic control. *Eur. J. Endocrinol.* **132** (1995), 580–86.

129. F. Pouwer, F. J. Snoek, H. M. van der Ploeg, H. J. Ader, R. J. Heine, Monitoring of psychological well-being in outpatients with diabetes: effects on mood, HbA(1c), and the patient's evaluation of the quality of diabetes care: a randomized controlled trial. *Diabetes Care* **24** (2001), 1929–35.

130. R. S. Surwit, M. A. L. Van Tilburg, N. Zucker, *et al.*, Stress management improves long-term glycemic control in type 2 diabetes. *Diabetes Care* **25** (2002), 30–34.

131. J. W. Williams, Jr, W. Katon, E. H. Lin, *et al.*, The effectiveness of depression care management on diabetes-related outcomes in older patients. *Ann. Intern. Med.* **140** (2004), 1015–24.

132. L. N. Robins, J. E. Helzer, J. Croughnan, J. B. W. Williams, R. L. Spitzer, *NIMH Diagnostic Interview Schedule: Version III-R* (Rockville, MD: National Institutes of Mental Health, 1987).

133. American Psychiatric Association *Diagnostic and Statistical Manual of Mental Disorders*, 4th edn. (Washington, DC: American Psychiatric Association, 1994).

134. E. S. Paykel, Methodology of live events research. *Adv. Psychosom. Med.* **17** (1987), 13–29.

135. W. A. Arrundell, *SCL-90: Manual for a Multi-dimensional Indicator of Psychopathology* (Lisse: Swets and Zeitinger, 1986).

136. C. D. Spielberger, R. L. Gorsuch, R. Luschene, *Test Manual for the State-Trait Anxiety Inventory* (Palo Alto, CA: Consulting Psychologists Press, 1970).

137. M. B. Keller, J. P. McCullough, D. N. Klein, *et al.*, A comparison of nefazodone, the cognitive behavioral-analysis system of psychotherapy, and their combination for the treatment of chronic depression. *N. Engl. J. Med.* **342** (2000), 1462–70.

138. H. C. Schulberg, W. Katon, G. E. Simon, J. Rush, Treating major depression in primary care practice: an update of the Agency for Health Care Policy and Research Practice Guidelines. *Arch. Gen. Psychiatry* **55** (1998), 1121–7.

139. R. S. Surwit, R. B. Williams, I. C. Siegler, J. D. Lane, M. Helms, Hostility, race, and glucose metabolism in nondiabetic individuals. *Diabetes Care* **25** (2002), 835–9.

140. V. W. Persky, J. Kempthorne-Rawson, R. B. Shekelle, Personality and risk of cancer: 20-year follow-up of the Western Electric study. *Psychosom. Med.* **49** (1987), 435–49.

141. P. J. Lustman, L. S. Griffith, R. E. Clouse, *et al.*, Improvement in depression is associated with improvement in glycemic control. *Diabetes* **4**: Suppl 1 (1995), 27A.

142. R. Sinha, G. Fisch, B. Teague, *et al.*, Prevalence of impaired glucose tolerance among children and adolescents with marked obesity. *N. Engl. J. Med.* **346** (2002), 802–10.

143. B. S. McEwen, A. M. Magarinos, L. P. Reagan, Studies of hormone action in the hippocampal formation: possible relevance to depression and diabetes. *J. Psychosom. Res.* **53** (2002), 883–90.

144. W. H. Gispen, G.-J. Biessels, Cognition and synaptic plasticity in diabetes mellitus. *Trends Neurosci.* **23** (2000), 542–9.

145. B. E. Levin, A. A. Dunn-Meynell, V. H. Routh, Brain glucose sensing and body energy homeostasis: role in obesity and diabetes. *Am. J. Physiol. Endocrinol. Metab.* **276** (1999), R1223–31.

146. B. E. Levin, Glucosensing neurons do more than just sense glucose. *Int. J. Obes.* **25**: Suppl 5 (2001), 68–72.

147. A. A. Dunn-Meyell, N. E. Rawson, B. E. Levin, Distribution and phenotype of neurons containing the ATP-sensitive K^+ channel. *Brain Res.* **814** (1998), 41–54.

148. P. J. Lustman, K. E. Freedland, L. S. Griffith, R. E. Clouse, Fluoxetine for depression in diabetes: a randomized double-blind placebo-controlled trial. *Diabetes Care* **23** (2000), 618–23.

9

Depression and chronic fatigue

Peter D. White

Introduction

This chapter reviews fatigue as a symptom and some of its syndromes, including chronic fatigue syndrome and vital exhaustion. The chapter also reviews the similarities and differences between fatigue and depression. The links include common symptoms, sleep disturbance, physical inactivity and common treatments with both cognitive – behavioural therapy (CBT) and graded exercise therapy. The differences involve aetiology, pathophysiology, nosology and response to antidepressants. Depression and fatigue should be considered as separate phenomena with common presentations and associations.

Epidemiology of fatigue

Fatigue is a common symptom in both the community and primary care. Between 10% and 20% of people in the community, if asked, will admit to feeling abnormally tired at any one time [1]. At the same time, fatigue is distributed continuously within the community, with no point of rarity [2]. Therefore, any cut-off is arbitrary, and the prevalence will vary by definition of fatigue, how the question is asked or the symptom volunteered, and its context; for instance, fewer people volunteer fatigue to their general practitioner (GP). Studies of fatigue reporting to primary-care doctors from Ireland and Holland calculated annual incidences of 6.5 and 5.3 reports per 100 patients, respectively [3,4]. One study showed that the incidence of the complaint of fatigue and its synonyms (e.g. tired, worn out, exhausted) recorded by GPs in the UK did not change in the 12 years between 1990 and 2001, being reported by 1.5% of GP attenders per annum [5]. The differences in incidence were probably due to different denominator populations, particularly in age ranges, with the later study involving patients of all ages rather than only adults.

Depression and Physical Illness, ed. A. Steptoe.
Published by Cambridge University Press. © Cambridge University Press 2006.

Women report fatigue more commonly than men. Fatigue is uncommon before puberty [5]. The commonest aetiological associations with the complaint of fatigue are depression, anxiety and reported 'stress' [6]. Physical diseases or states are uncommon causes, but thyroid disease, pregnancy, breastfeeding and certain infections, such as infectious mononucleosis, are well described causes of both acute and persistent fatigue [1,7].

Chronic fatigue syndrome

About a third of patients presenting with six months of fatigue will meet criteria for a chronic fatigue syndrome [8]. Prolonged or chronic fatigue is significantly less common than the symptom of fatigue, and there has been uncertainty about the existence of a chronic fatigue syndrome (CFS), also called myalgic encephalomyelitis (ME) [9,10]. CFS is now accepted as a valid diagnosis by medical authorities in the UK [9], in the USA and internationally [11]. Its primary symptom is physical fatigue, which particularly follows exertion [1,12]. Other symptoms agreed in consensual guidelines include poor concentration and memory, sleep disturbance, headache, sore throat, tender lymph glands and muscle and joint pain [11]. There are several criterion-based definitions of CFS [13–15]. These definitions were derived by consensus, have not been supported consistently by empirical studies and continue to be refined [11].

The aetiology of the syndrome is unknown, but there is evidence that different risk markers are associated with predisposition, triggering and maintenance of the illness [1]. Predisposing risk markers may include mood disorders (especially depressive disorders), other 'functional' syndromes (such as irritable bowel syndrome), female sex [1] and possibly genetic factors [16,17]. These risk markers are similar to those of depressive illness, with the possible exception of independent genetic factors.

Triggering risk markers are less established, but there is sufficient evidence to support certain infections as aetiological triggering factors not only for fatigue but also CFS (see below). This contrasts with depressive illness.

Maintaining or perpetuating risk markers are most important in determining treatment programmes, since reversing maintaining factors should lead to improvement. Reasonably well-established factors include mood disorders such as dysthymia, illness beliefs such as believing the whole condition is physical, pervasive inactivity, avoidant coping, membership of a patient-support group, and being in receipt of or dispute about financial benefits [18–22].

Membership of a patient support group is an interesting risk marker. This may be confounded by ascertainment, in that those patients who have not been helped by treatment may join such groups for support since the healthcare system has failed to help them. The other possibility is that the process of being a member and, for example, hearing stories of non-recovery reduces motivation and hope for recovery. This may particularly be the case if one of the aims of the support group is public advocacy to legitimise the illness as a real and chronic disabling disease that cannot be cured [23–25].

The role of abnormal illness behaviour in predisposing to or maintaining CFS is uncertain. Patients with CFS have higher scores on measures of hypochondriasis and disease conviction when compared with general practice controls [26] but not when compared with chronically ill controls suffering from multiple sclerosis [27]. Hall and colleagues [28] reported a case – control study of the pre-claim medical reports of 133 claimants of income protection, diagnosed as suffering from CFS. They compared these CFS claimants with multiple sclerosis claimants and non-claimants, controlling for age but not for gender. They found that CFS claimants had reported significantly more illnesses at the time of proposal for insurance compared with the two comparison groups. The illnesses were many and various, but lethargy and infections (glandular fever, upper-respiratory-tract infections, chest infections) were reported most commonly. This group also made significantly more claims between their accepted proposal and the diagnosis of CFS. There were several methodological weaknesses in this study: There was a significantly greater proportion of women in the CFS group. It is well known that women report more symptoms in general [29], and fatigue in particular [30], than men. Without a comparison group of sufferers with another 'functional' disorder, we cannot know whether the differences were specific to CFS or to a more general problem. The same group went on to study GP attenders with CFS or ME, and replicated their findings of excess consultations for those with CFS/ME up to 15 years before diagnosis compared with patients with multiple sclerosis [31].

Fatigue as part of depressive illness

Tiredness and lack of energy are common symptoms of depressive illness [32,33]. When this occurs, the patient normally complains of feeling 'tired all the time'. Such fatigue is often both mental and physical and can be relieved by physical activity and exercise. This contrasts with the features of fatigue in chronic fatigue syndrome, whereby physical exertion normally exacerbates the condition. The mental fatigue of depression is often reported as a problem with concentration and memory.

Sleep disturbance is common to both depressive illness and CFS [34,35], and it is likely that the sleep disturbance of depressive illness at least exacerbates fatigue reported by such patients. Sleep disturbance has been reported to be a trait marker for recurrent depressive illness [34], but this has not been studied in CFS.

Is chronic fatigue syndrome a subclinical depressive illness?

Many studies demonstrate the close association between mood disorders, especially depressive illness, and CFS [1,36]. The point prevalence of depressive disorder in patients with CFS is significantly higher that of medical conditions that are disabling and equally chronic [1]. This suggests that the higher rates of depressive illness are not simply an understandable reaction to having a chronic disabling medical condition. Something more must explain these findings.

There are several possibilities. One explanation is that the high rates may be due to the uncertainty of suffering from a medically unexplained condition, but rates are still higher than those related to conditions such as irritable bowel syndrome, even though no study has directly compared rates. Another possible explanation is that the high rates may be due to the stigma attached to the label of CFS [25]. Some qualitative evidence supports this, and one comparative study has been published [37]. Patients with CFS felt more stigmatised than not only patients with established medical diseases such as multiple sclerosis, rheumatoid arthritis and inflammatory bowel disease but also patients with other functional disorders, such as fibromyalgia and irritable bowel syndrome. The authors suggested that this was due to the particular ambiguity of the status of CFS as a medical condition.

An equally convincing and simpler explanation is that some of the symptoms of the two conditions are identical, e.g. poor concentration and memory, fatigue and unrefreshing sleep. So, the threshold of having both disorders is lowered, since all that is needed is persistent low mood or anhedonia in order for the criteria for both disorders to be met [11,32]. Therefore, the mutual presence of both conditions is artificially raised by these means.

This leaves the issue as to which is the primary diagnosis in these comorbid states. As might be expected, longitudinal studies suggest that mood disorders may follow and precede CFS, as well as occur at the same time, so each may be primary in different patients [38–41].

This brings us to the issue of how CFS is classified. CFS is an uncertain diagnosis that does not fit neatly into taxonomic classifications of diseases [1,36]. Some authors classify CFS as a neurological disease – 'myalgic encephalomyelitis' – others as the psychiatric disorder neurasthenia and others as a non-specific somatoform disorder [32,33] or even as part of a general functional somatic syndrome [42]. These classifications have been questioned by many authors, with the most significant criticisms being made of trying to force CFS into either a medical or a psychiatric grouping, with its attendant dualistic connotations [43,44]. This categorisation is meaningless, in any case, since psychiatric disorders are, of necessity, disorders of the brain and thus neurological at least at one level of understanding.

CFS is thus an 'orphan' illness, belonging entirely to neither neurological nor psychiatric classifications [43].

Of relevance to this, multivariate analytical approaches to symptoms and other clinical features support the apparent independence of CFS from mood disorders. Hickie and colleagues [45] showed that both the individuals and clinical presentations of attenders at a chronic fatigue clinic could be divided into two main groups: three-quarters of patients had symptoms similar to descriptions of neurasthenia, with mainly fatigue-related symptoms; a quarter of patients had a larger number of symptoms, with greater chronicity, whom the authors thought had presentations more consistent with a somatoform disorder. The authors replicated this work with patients from an international cross-section of mainly fatigue clinics [46]. Other studies have supported the independence and reliability over time of a chronic or persistent fatigue syndrome in primary care or the community using similar methodologies [38,39,41,47]. These studies all suggest that the nosology of fatigue syndromes is different from that of depressive illness.

Another approach to testing the independence of CFS from mood disorders is to study the development of CFS in high-risk populations. The next section describes such an approach.

Fatigue and depression following infections

The viral aetiology for fatigue is better established than for depressive illness. White and colleagues [7] found a five-fold risk for fatigue six months after infectious mononucleosis (IM) compared with ordinary upper-respiratory-tract infections, a finding that Petersen *et al.* [48] have replicated. But does such fatigue amount to CFS?

Retrospective studies have identified fatigue syndromes after various infections, including viral hepatitis [49], viral meningitis [50], Q fever [51], and infectious mononucleosis (IM) [52]. Cohort studies have concentrated on fatigue following IM (glandular fever). White and colleagues [53] studied 250 patients attending primary care in the UK with glandular fever/IM or an ordinary upper-respiratory-tract infection (most commonly, streptococcal sore throat). They used principal components analyses of physical and psychological symptoms to define an acute fatigue syndrome after IM [53], which evolved into CFS in 9% of those infected [7]. The syndrome was found to be essentially independent of psychiatric disorders and consisted of physical and mental fatigue (especially after physical exertion), excessive sleep, poor concentration, anhedonia, retardation, social withdrawal, emotional lability, transient sore throat and lymph-gland pain and enlargement [54]. The syndrome was shown to have face validity and was a more reliable diagnosis than depressive disorder [53,54]. Symptoms were consistent with acute sickness behaviour [55], suggesting that cytokines might be involved.

Most importantly, in differentiating CFS from depressive disorder, the authors showed that an empirically derived fatigue syndrome was predicted by different risk factors than depressive illness [56]. The fatigue syndrome was predicted most consistently by the immune response close to onset and afterwards by objective evidence of physical deconditioning, the latter finding being replicated by others [57]. In contrast, depressive illness was predicted by life events and difficulties, a past psychiatric history and an emotional personality [56].

Buchwald and colleagues have reported a US cohort of 150 patients studied after acute IM also in primary care [58]. They found that 12% had not recovered by six months [59,60]. Fatigue and excessive sleep were also the most prominent convalescent symptoms. Buchwald and colleagues went on to examine the symptoms associated with fatigue in the same sample, followed up to four years after onset [61]. They used principal components analyses to separate the symptoms into factors and latent class analyses to separate out the patients. They found that patients with IM went on to have two fatigue syndromes – one with hypersomnia and no pain, the other with insomnia and pain. The latter was still discernable and independent four years after onset. Both the syndromes were independent of mood disorder.

Depressive illnesses are reported following infections, but much less commonly than fatigue, and they are usually transient [7,60] and not as clearly related to the infection [48]. It is clear that although infections are aetiological agents in fatigue, this is unlikely to be the case for depression.

Vital exhaustion and ischaemic heart disease

Appels [62] explored the link between 'vital exhaustion' and ischaemic heart disease (IHD) for a quarter of a century. Vital exhaustion comprises unusual fatigue, loss of energy, increased irritability and feelings of demoralisation. The first issue is whether this is any different from either chronic fatigue syndrome or depressive illness. Second, if it is different, then does vital exhaustion independently predict IHD events? Third, if there is a causative link, then how is it mediated?

Appels' research group found a close correlation between vital exhaustion and depression [63]. However, they went on to find that vital exhaustion has an independent effect on IHD outcomes [64]. In contrast, Wojciechowski and colleagues [65] used the same Maastricht questionnaire to measure vital exhaustion and found strong correlations between this scale and two validated self-rated measures of depression (Zung depression scale, and Symptom Checklist 90 [SCL-90] depression subscale) in patients studied up to a year after myocardial infarction. They also found a one-factor solution to a principal components analysis of all three scales combined. This methodologically robust method showed that vital exhaustion and depression were not independent in patients with heart disease.

This finding has been replicated more recently. McGowan and colleagues [66] examined 305 consecutive inpatients about four days after their first myocardial infarction. They confirmed that vital exhaustion, measured by the Maastricht questionnaire, was correlated highly with the Hospital Anxiety and Depression Scale (HADS) depression subscale. A factor analysis of the Maastricht questionnaire showed four independent factors: fatigue, depression, poor concentration and sleep difficulties. The fatigue factor was still correlated highly with the HADS depression subscale score. The authors recommended that future studies should study fatigue separately from vital exhaustion and depression. Prescott and colleagues [67] found that both exhaustion and depression items of a vital exhaustion measure were related to later deaths from IHD in a large community sample.

The influence of depression on IHD is reviewed in Chapters 3 and 4. Relevant and shared pathophysiological mechanisms, found to be associated with vital exhaustion, may include altered haemostasis and cytokine expression [68–70].

The independence of vital exhaustion and CFS has not been examined directly, but the close correlation between vital exhaustion and depression, fatigue as an independent factor subsumed in vital exhaustion, and demoralisation being a central feature of vital exhaustion all suggest some separation between CFS and vital exhaustion, even though they share features of both fatigue and sleep disturbance [71].

Pathophysiology discriminates fatigue and depression

Apart from the stronger evidence for the importance of infections in the aetiology of fatigue more than depression, there are important pathophysiological differences as well. The hypothalamic–pituitary–adrenal (HPA) axis is down-regulated in CFS [72,73] and up-regulated in melancholic depressive illness [74]. This apparent difference is less convincing when one remembers that atypical depressive illness, with hypersomnia and prominent fatigue, has no associated HPA axis up-regulation and may even be down-regulated [74]. The reasons become clear when one considers that the abnormalities in HPA axis regulation in both depressive illness and CFS may be a consequence of changes in activity, sleep and feeding, since reduced eating and sleep deprivation up-regulate the HPA axis [75], and vice versa [76,77]. These abnormalities may therefore be secondary to the behavioural consequences of the illness rather than primary [77,78].

Depressive illness is associated with reduced rapid-eye-movement (REM) latency, and this may even be a trait marker for depression [79]. REM latency is the period between sleep onset and the start of dreaming sleep. Reduced REM latency does not occur in CFS [35]. Sleep in CFS is consistent with psychophysiological disturbance, rather than any specific sleep architecture [35], which may also occur in less severe depressive illness. Hypersomnia is particularly associated with post-infectious fatigue [52,53] but also occurs in atypical depression [80].

The role of the immune system in both CFS and depressive illness is being studied more now than previously [81,82]. Immunological abnormalities are being found in both disorders, particularly in the innate and cell-mediated immune systems [81,83]. Cytokines can induce both depression and fatigue [84,85]. However, no researchers have demonstrated that these immunological abnormalities are functionally important, with regard to more infections or abnormal responses to antigens, or that they are associated with features of either illness [86]. These immune changes may be caused by the sleep disturbance and inactivity, themselves caused by depression and CFS [82,87].

Treatment similarities and differences between fatigue and depression

CBT and graded exercise therapy are useful treatments of both mood disorders and CFS [88–95]. CBT and graded exercise therapy have in common a return to physical activity, which enhances energy in both CFS and depressive illness. Intriguingly, therapeutic exercise does not seem to work in CFS simply by improving fitness, although it does do this. Fulcher and White [90,91] found a significant association between increased fitness and good functional outcome, but there was no association between increased fitness and feeling better. It seems that mere exposure to increased physical activity through exercise is sufficient for feeling better, something also found in depressive illness [94] and the related condition of fibromyalgia [95].

One explanation for this apparent paradox is that exercise is acting as an exposure programme for the previously conditioned avoidance response to activity. Another explanation advanced to explain this finding in individuals with depressive illness is that exercise involves socialisation, and it is this process that determines success. A final explanation is in the effect of aerobic exercise on the brain, since non-aerobic exercise does not seem to relieve depression [95]. No researchers have compared the effects of aerobic versus non-aerobic exercise in CFS.

The other positive results of exercise include positive effects on brain activity and repair [96] and the mood-enhancing effects of endorphins, although these are related more to acute intensive exercise than to a graded exercise programme [97]. A useful clinical diagnostic tip is that acute exercise lifts mood in depressive illness but causes fatigue in CFS.

In marked contrast to depressive illness, several randomised controlled trials (RCTs) of antidepressants for chronic fatigue syndrome have shown little evidence of efficacy [88,89]. One large RCT found that fluoxetine did not even help the depression associated with CFS [98]. Certain antidepressants may be useful in CFS when there is associated insomnia or pain to the extent of also meeting criteria for fibromyalgia [99].

Secondary fatigue

Fatigue is commonly associated with chronic medical disorders, but it should be differentiated from fatiguability. Fatiguability is the onset of a physical sensation of fatigue and weakness after exertion and is commonly reported with neurological diseases such as multiple sclerosis and myopathies. Particularly when fatiguability is associated with post-exertional weakness, neurological diseases are important differential diagnoses.

The diseases with high risks for fatigue (found in the majority of patients) are hormonal (hypothyroidism), metabolic (diabetes mellitus), neoplastic (haematological malignancies), infectious (human immunodeficiency virus [HIV]) and inflammatory (systemic lupus erythematosus). There have been a considerable number of studies of the associations of 'secondary' fatigue [100–105]. Apart from measures of disease activity, other associations repeatedly found include sleep disturbance, mood disorders, inactivity and physical deconditioning [100–102,106].

Studies of fatigue associated with multiple sclerosis are instructive and exemplary. As in all studies of secondary fatigue, measures of the severity or pathophysiology of the disease itself are associated with fatigue [107]. Some cytokines are associated, but others are not [108]. Associations vary depending on the fatigue measure, confirming the multidimensional nature of fatigue, but all measures were associated with depression [109]. Fatigue is associated independently with both depression and disability [110]. Objectively confirmed sleep disturbance is associated with fatigue [111].

There have been a number of studies of various treatments aimed at reversing the associations of secondary fatigue in general, in the hope they would help fatigue directly, with variable results. The most consistent evidence of efficacy has been with graded exercise programmes and CBT. As is the case with CFS, antidepressants seem to help depression but not fatigue [112], with the one possible exception of fatigue associated with multiple sclerosis [113].

Conclusions

This chapter has reviewed the similarities and differences between fatigue and depression. Our current lack of understanding of these symptoms or conditions is exacerbated by the likelihood that both are heterogeneous in either form or causes.

Setting that aside, we can conclude that fatigue and depression can be differentiated from each other in several ways. The syndromes of fatigue and depression share symptoms, which leads to easy misdiagnosis and inflated comorbidity. The concept of vital exhaustion represents aspects of both depression and fatigue, which should be measured separately.

The practical implications are important. Clinicians should assess their patients carefully and differentiate those with one or other condition as their sole problem, while remembering that there will be those who seem to have both at the same time. Treatments will be both different and similar, but should be tailored to the individual needs of the patient.

REFERENCES

1. S. C. Wessely, M. Hotopf, M. Sharpe., *Chronic Fatigue and its Syndromes* (Oxford: Oxford University Press, 1998).

2. T. Pawlikowska, T. Chalder, S. R. Hirsch, *et al.*, Population based study of fatigue and psychological distress. *Br. Med. J.* **308** (1994), 763–6.

3. W. Cullen, Y. Kearney, G. Bury, Prevalence of fatigue in general practice. *Ir. J. Med. Sci.* **171** (2002), 10–12.

4. E. Kenter, I. Okkes, S. Oskam, H. Lamberts, Tiredness in Dutch family practice: data on patients complaining of and/or diagnosed with 'tiredness'. *Fam. Pract.* **20** (2003), 434–40.

5. A. M. Gallagher, J. M. Thomas, W. T. Hamilton, P. D. White, The incidence of fatigue symptoms and diagnoses presenting in UK primary care from 1990 to 2001. *J. R. Soc. Med.* **97** (2004), 571–5.

6. M. K. Chen, The epidemiology of self-perceived fatigue among adults. *Prev. Med.* **15** (1986), 74–81.

7. P. D. White, J. M. Thomas, J. Amess, *et al.*, Incidence, risk and prognosis of acute and chronic fatigue syndromes and psychiatric disorders after glandular fever. *Br. J. Psychiatry* **173** (1998), 475–81.

8. L. Darbishire, L. Ridsdale, P. T. Seed, Distinguishing patients with chronic fatigue from those with chronic fatigue syndrome: a diagnostic study in UK primary care. *Br. J. Gen. Pract.* **53** (2003), 441–5.

9. Royal College of Psychiatrists. Royal College of Physicians and Royal College of General Practitioners, *Chronic Fatigue Syndrome: Report of a Joint Working Group of the Royal Colleges of Physicians, Psychiatrists and General Practitioners* (London, Royal College of Physicians, 1996)

10. CFS/ME working group. Report of the CFS/ME Working Group to the Chief Medical Officer, 2001. www.dh.gov.uk/assetroot/04/05/95/06/04059506.pdf

11. W. C. Reeves, A. Lloyd, S. D. Vernon, *et al.*, Identification of ambiguities in the 1994 chronic fatigue syndrome research case definition and recommendations for resolution. *BMC Health Serv Res* **3** (2003), 25.

12. L. A. Jason, S. R. Torres-Harding, A. W. Carrico, R. R. Taylor, Symptom occurrence in persons with chronic fatigue syndrome. *Biol. Psychol.* **59** (2002), 15–27.

13. A. Lloyd, D. Wakefield, J. Dwyer, C. Boughton, What is myalgic encephalomyelitis? *Lancet* **1** (1988), 1286–7.

14. M. C. Sharpe, L. C. Archard, J. E. Banatvala, *et al.*, A report: chronic fatigue syndrome – guidelines for research. *J. R. Soc. Med.* **84** (1991), 118–21.

15. K. Fukuda, S. E. Straus, I. Hickie, *et al.*, The chronic fatigue syndrome: a comprehensive approach to its definition and study: International Chronic Fatigue Syndrome Study Group. *Ann. Intern. Med.* **21** (1994), 953–9.

16. I. Hickie, K. Kirk, N. Martin, Unique genetic and environmental determinants of prolonged fatigue: a twin study. *Psychol. Med.* **29** (1999), 259–68.

17. R. Powell, J. Ren, G. Lewith, *et al.*, Identification of novel expressed sequences, up-regulated in the leucocytes of chronic fatigue syndrome patients. *Clin. Exper. Allergy* **33** (2003), 1450–56.

18. A. Wilson, I. Hickie, A. Lloyd, *et al.*, Longitudinal study of the outcome of chronic fatigue syndrome. *Br. Med. J.* **308** (1994), 756–60.

19. M. Clark, W. Katon, J. Russo, *et al.*, Chronic fatigue: risk factors for symptom persistence in a 2.5-year follow up study. *Am. J. Med.* **98** (1995), 187–95.

20. J. Vercoulen, C. Swanink, J. Fennis, *et al.*, Prognosis in chronic fatigue syndrome: a prospective study on the natural course. *J. Neurol. Neurosurg. Psychiatry* **60** (1996), 489–94.

21. R. P. Bentall, P. Powell, F. J. Nye, R. H. Edwards, Predictors of response to treatment for chronic fatigue syndrome. *Br. J. Psychiatry* **181** (2002), 248–52.

22. J. B. Prins, E. Bazelmans, S. Van der Werf, J. W. M. Van der Meer, G. Bleijenberg, Cognitive behaviour therapy for chronic fatigue syndrome: predictors of treatment outcome. In *Psycho-neuro-endocrinology: A Common Language for the Whole Human Body*, ed. T. Sivik, D. Byrne, D. R. Lipsitt, *et al.* (Amsterdam: Elsevier, 2002), pp. 131–5.

23. N. M. Hadler, If you have to prove you are ill, you can't get well: the object lesson of fibromyalgia. *Spine* **21** (1996), 2397–400.

24. S. Peters, I. Stanley, M. Rose, P. Salmon, Patients with medically unexplained symptoms: sources of patients' authority and implication for demands on medical care. *Soc. Sci. Med.* **46** (1998), 559–65.

25. L. Page, S. Wessely, Medically unexplained symptoms: exacerbating factors in the doctor–patient encounter. *J. R. Soc. Med.* **96** (2003), 223–7.

26. R. Schweitzer, D. I. Robertson, B. Kelly, J. Whiting, Illness behaviour of patients with chronic fatigue syndrome. *J. Psychosom. Res.* **38** (1994), 41–9.

27. P. Trigwell, S. Hatcher, M. Johnson, P. Stanley, A. House, 'Abnormal' illness behaviour in chronic fatigue syndrome and multiple sclerosis. *Br. Med. J.* **311** (1995), 15–18.

28. G. H. Hall, W. T. Hamilton, A. P. Round, Increased illness experience preceding chronic fatigue syndrome: a case control study. *J. R. Coll. Physicians Lond.* **32** (1998), 44–8.

29. C. M. T. van Wijk, A. T. Kolk, Sex differences in physical symptoms: the contribution of symptom perception theory. *Soc. Sci. Med.* **45** (1997), 231–46.

30. J. Joyce, M. Hotopf, S. Wessely, The prognosis of chronic fatigue and chronic fatigue syndrome: a systematic review. *Q. J. Med.* **90** (1997), 223–33.

31. W. T. Hamilton, G. H. Hall, A. P. Round, Frequency of attendance in general practice and symptoms before development of chronic fatigue syndrome: a case–control study. *Br. J. Gen. Pract.* **51** (2001), 553–8.

32. World Health Organization. *The ICD-10 Classification of Mental and Behavioural Disorders: Clinical Descriptions and Diagnostic Guidelines* (Geneva: World Health Organization, 1992).

33. American Psychiatric Association, *Diagnostic and Statistical Manual of Mental Disorders*, 4th edn (Washington, DC: American Psychiatric Association, 1994).

34. R. H. Jindal, M. E. Thase, A. L. Fasiczka, *et al.*, Electroencephalographic sleep profiles in single-episode and recurrent unipolar forms of major depression II. Comparison during remission. *Biol. Psychiatry* **51** (2002), 230–36.

35. N. F. Watson, V. Kapur, L. M. Arguelles *et al.*, Comparison of subjective and objective measures of insomnia in monozygotic twins discordant for chronic fatigue syndrome. *Sleep* **26**, (2003), 324–8.

36. A. R. Lloyd, Chronic fatigue and chronic fatigue syndrome: shifting boundaries and attributions. *Am. J. Med.* **105** (1998), S7–10.

37. K. J. Looper, L. J. Kirmayer, Perceived stigma in functional somatic syndromes and comparable medical conditions. *J. Psychosom. Res.* **57** (2004), 373–8.

38. G. Van der Linden, T. Chalder, I. Hickie, *et al.*, Fatigue and psychiatric disorder: different or the same? *Psychol. Med.* **29** (1999), 863–8.

39. I. Hickie, A. Koschera, D. Hadzi-Pavlovic, B. Bennett, A. Lloyd, The temporal stability and co-morbidity of prolonged fatigue: a longitudinal study in primary care. *Psychol. Med.* **29** (1999), 855–61.

40. L. A. Aaron, R. Herrell, S. Ashton, *et al.*, Comorbid clinical conditions in chronic fatigue: a co-twin control study. *J. Gen. Intern. Med.* **16** (2001), 24–31.

41. P. Skapinakis, G. Lewis, V. Mavreas, Temporal relations between unexplained fatigue and depression: longitudinal data from an international study in primary care. *Psychosom. Med.* **66** (2004), 330–35.

42. S. Wessely, C. Nimnuan, M. Sharpe, Functional somatic syndromes: one or many? *Lancet* **354** (1999), 936–9.

43. P. D. White, Physical or mental? A perspective on chronic fatigue syndrome. *Adv. Psychiatr. Treat.* **8** (2002), 363–5.

44. S. Wessely, P. D. White, In debate: there is only one functional somatic syndrome. *Br. J. Psychiatry* **185** (2004), 95–6.

45. I. Hickie, A. Lloyd, D. Hadzi-Pavlovic, *et al.*, Can the chronic fatigue syndrome be defined by distinct clinical features? *Psychol. Med.* **25** (1995), 925–35.

46. A. Wilson, I. Hickie, D. Hadzi-Pavlovic, *et al.*, What is chronic fatigue syndrome? Heterogeneity within an international multicentre study. *Aust. N. Z. J. Psychiatry* **35** (2001), 520–27.

47. R. R. Taylor, L. A. Jason, M. E. Schoeny, Evaluating latent variable models of functional somatic distress in a community sample. *J. Ment. Health* **10** (2001), 335–49.

48. I. Petersen, J. M. Thomas, W. T. Hamilton, P. D. White, Risk and predictors of fatigue after infectious mononucleosis in a large primary-care cohort. *Q. J. Red.* **99** (2006), 49–55.

49. G. J. Berelowitz, A. P. Burgess, T. Thanabalasingham, I. M. Murray-Lyon, D. J. Wright, Post-hepatitis syndrome revisited. *J. Viral Hepatol.* **2** (1995), 133–8.

50. M. Hotopf, N. Noah, S. Wessely, Chronic fatigue and psychiatric morbidity following viral meningitis: a controlled study. *J. Neurol. Neurosurg. Psychiatry* **60** (1996), 495–503.

51. J. G. Ayres, N. Flint, E. G. Smith, *et al.*, Post-infection fatigue syndrome following Q fever. *Q. J. Med.* **91** (1998), 105–23.

52. S. Lambore, J. McSherry, A. S. Kraus, Acute and chronic symptoms of mononucleosis. *J. Fam. Pract.* **33** (1991), 33–7.

53. P. D. White, J. M. Thomas, J. Amess, *et al.*, The existence of a fatigue syndrome after glandular fever. *Psychol. Med.* **25** (1995), 907–16.

54. P. D. White, S. A. Grover, H. O. Kangro, *et al.*, The validity and reliability of the fatigue syndrome that follows glandular fever. *Psychol. Med.* **25** (1995), 917–24.

55. R. Dantzer, Cytokine-induced sickness behavior: where do we stand? *Brain Behav. Immun.* **15** (2001), 7–24.

56. P. D. White, J. M. Thomas, H. O. Kangro, *et al.*, Predictions and associations of fatigue syndromes and mood disorders that occur after infectious mononucleosis. *Lancet* **358** (2001), 1946–54.

57. B. Candy, T. Chalder, A. J. Cleare, *et al.*, Predictors of fatigue following the onset of infectious mononucleosis. *Psychol. Med.* **33** (2003), 847–55.

58. T. D. Rea, J. E. Russo, W. Katon, R. L. Ashley, D. S. Buchwald, Prospective study of the natural history of infectious mononucleosis caused by Epstein–Barr virus. *J. Am. Board Fam. Pract.* **14** (2001), 234–42.

59. D. S. Buchwald, T. D. Rea, W. J. Katon, J. E. Russo, R. L. Ashley, Acute infectious mononucleosis: characteristics of patients who report failure to recover. *Am. J. Med.* **109** (2000), 531–7.

60. W. Katon, J. Russo, R. L. Ashley, D. Buchwald, Infectious mononucleosis: psychological symptoms during acute and subacute phases of illness. *Gen. Hosp. Psychiatry* **21** (2000), 21–9.

61. P. D. White, J. M. Thomas, P. F. Sullivan, D. Buchwald, The nosology of sub-acute and chronic fatigue syndromes that follow infectious mononucleosis. *Psychol. Med.* **34** (2004), 499–507.

62. A. Appels, Exhaustion and coronary heart disease the history of a scientific quest. *Patient Educ. Couns.* **55** (2004), 223–9.

63. M. S. Kopp, P. R. Falger, A. Appels, S. Szedmák, Depressive symptomatology and vital exhaustion are differentially related to behavioral risk factors for coronary artery disease. *Psychosom. Med.* **60** (1998), 752–8.

64. A. Appels, W. J. Kop, E. Schouten, The nature of the depressive symptomatology preceding myocardial infarction. *Behav. Med.* **26** (2000), 86–9.

65. F. L. Wojciechowski, J. J. Strik, P. Falger, R. Lousberg, A. Honig, The relationship between depressive and vital exhaustion symptomatology post-myocardial infarction. *Acta Psychiatr. Scand.* **102** (2000), 359–65.

66. L. McGowan, C. Dickens, C. Percival, *et al.*, The relationship between vital exhaustion, depression and comorbid illnesses in patients following first myocardial infarction. *J. Psychosom. Res.* **57** (2004), 183–8.

67. E. Prescott, C. Holst, M. Grønbaek, *et al.*, Vital exhaustion as a risk factor for ischaemic heart disease and all-cause mortality in a community sample: a prospective study of 4084 men and 5479 women in the Copenhagen City Heart Study. *Int. J. Epidemiol.* **32** (2003), 990–97.

68. W. J. Kop, K. Hamulyák, C. Pernot, A. Appels, Relationship of blood coagulation and fibrinolysis to vital exhaustion. *Psychosom. Med.* **60** (1998), 352–8.

69. A. Van der Ven, R. van Diest, K. Hamulyák, *et al.*, Herpes viruses, cytokines, and altered hemostasis in vital exhaustion. *Psychosom. Med.* **65** (2003), 194–200.

70. P. Jeanmonod, R. von Känel, F. E. Maly, J. E. Fischer, Elevated plasma C-reactive protein in chronically distressed subjects who carry the A allele of the TNF-alpha-308 G/A polymorphism. *Psychosom. Med.* **66** (2004), 501–6.

71. R. Van Diest, W. P. Appels, Sleep physiological characteristics of exhausted men. *Psychosom. Med.* **56** (1994), 28–35.

72. A. J. Cleare, D. Blair, S. Chambers, S. Wessely, Urinary free cortisol in chronic fatigue syndrome. *Am. J. Psychiatry* **158** (2001), 641–3.

73. A. J. Cleare, The neuroendocrinology of chronic fatigue syndrome. *Endocr. Rev.* **24** (2003), 236–52.

74. J. W. Kasckow, D. Baker, T. D. Geracioti, Jr, Corticotropin-releasing hormone in depression and post-traumatic stress disorder. *Peptides* **22** (2001), 845–51.

75. P. E. Mullen, C. R. Linsell, D. Parker, Influence of sleep disruption and calorie restriction on biological markers for depression. *Lancet* **2** (1986), 1051–5.

76. G. Leese, P. Chattington, W. Fraser, *et al.*, Short-term night-shift working mimics the pituitary-adrenocortical dysfunction in chronic fatigue syndrome. *J. Clin. Endocrinol. Metabol.* **81** (1996), 1867–70.

77. A. J. Cleare, The HPA axis and the genesis of chronic fatigue syndrome. *Trends Endocrinol. Metabol.* **15** (2004), 55–9.

78. J. Gaab, V. Engert, V. Heitz, *et al.*, Associations between neuroendocrine responses to the insulin tolerance test and patient characteristics in chronic fatigue syndrome. *J. Psychosom. Res.* **56** (2004), 419–24.

79. D. E. Giles, D. J. Kupfer, A. J. Rush, H. P. Roffwarg, Controlled comparison of electrophysiological sleep in families of probands with unipolar depression. *Am. J. Psychiatry* **155** (1998), 192–9.

80. A. Korszun, V. Moskvina, S. Brewster, *et al.*, Familiality of symptom dimensions in depression. *Arch. Gen. Psychiatry* **61** (2004), 468–74.

81. M. Irwin, Psychoneuroimmunology of depression: clinical implications. *Brain Behav. Immun.* **16** (2002), 1–16.

82. M. Lyall, M. Peakman, S. Wessely, A systematic review and critical evaluation of the immunology of chronic fatigue syndrome. *J. Psychosom. Res.* **55** (2003), 79–90.

83. A. Skowera, A. Cleare, D. Blair, *et al.*, High levels of type 2 cytokine-producing cells in chronic fatigue syndrome. *Clin. Exp. Immunol.* **135** (2004), 294–302.

84. M. Wichers, M. Maes, The psychoneuroimmuno-pathophysiology of cytokine-induced depression in humans. *Int. J. Neuropsychopharmacol.* **5** (2002), 375–88.

85. K. W. Kelley, R. M. Bluthe, R. Dantzer, *et al.*, Cytokine-induced sickness behavior. *Brain Behav. Immun.* **17**: Suppl 1 (2003), 112–18.

86. M. Peakman, A. Deale, R. Field, M. Mahalingam, S. Wessely, Clinical improvement in chronic fatigue syndrome is not associated with lymphocyte subsets of function or activation. *Clin. Immunol. Immunopathol.* **82** (1997), 83–91.

87. M. Irwin, Effects of sleep and sleep loss on immunity and cytokines. *Brain Behav. Immun.* **16** (2002), 503–12.

88. P. Whiting, A. M. Bagnall, A. J. Sowden, *et al.*, Interventions for the treatment and management of chronic fatigue syndrome: a systematic review. *J. Am. Med. Assoc.* **286** (2001), 1360–68.

89. D. A. Lawlor, S. W. Hopker, The effectiveness of exercise as an intervention in the management of depression: systematic review and meta-regression analysis of randomised controlled trials. *Br. Med. J.* **322** (2001), 763–7.

90. K. Y. Fulcher, P. D. White, Randomised controlled trial of graded exercise in patients with the chronic fatigue syndrome. *Br. Med. J.* **314** (1997), 1647–52.

91. K. Y. Fulcher, P. D. White, Strength and physiological response to exercise in patients with the chronic fatigue syndrome. *J. Neurol. Neurosurg. Psychiatry* **69** (2000), 302–7.

92. B. W. Penninx, W. J. Rejeski, J. Pandya, *et al.*, Exercise and depressive symptoms: a comparison of aerobic and resistance exercise effects on emotional and physical function in older persons with high and low depressive symptomatology. *J. Gerontol. B Psychol. Sci. Soc. Sci.* **57** (2002), 124–32.

93. R. Raine, A. Haines, T. Sensky *et al.*, Systematic review of mental health interventions for patients with common somatic: can research evidence from secondary care be extrapolated to primary care? *Br. Med. J.* **325** (2002), 1082–5.

94. D. Veale, K. Le Fevre, C. Pantelis, *et al.*, Aerobic exercise in the adjunctive treatment of depression: a randomized controlled trial. *J. R. Soc. Med.* **85** (1992), 541–4.

95. V. Valim, L. Oliveira, A. Suda, *et al.*, Aerobic fitness effects in fibromyalgia. *J. Rheumatol.* **30** (2003), 1060–69.

96. G. Kempermann, H. van Praag, F. H. Gage, Activity-dependent regulation of neuronal plasticity and self repair. *Progr. Brain Res.* **127** (2000), 35–48.

97. C. Ekdahl, R. Ekman, S. I. Andersson, A. Melander, B. Svensson, Dynamic training and circulating levels of corticotropin-releasing factor, beta-lipotropin and beta-endorphin in rheumatoid arthritis. *Pain* **40** (1990), 35–42.

98. J. Vercoulen, C. M. A. Swanink, F. G. Zitman, *et al.*, Randomised, double-blind, placebo-controlled study of fluoxetine in chronic fatigue syndrome. *Lancet* **347** (1996), 858–61.

99. L. M. Arnold, P. E. Keck, J. A. Welge, Antidepressant treatment of fibromyalgia: a meta-analysis and review. *Psychosomatics* **41** (2000), 104–13.

100. J. H. Vercoulen, C. M. Swanink, J. M. Galama, *et al.*, The persistence of fatigue in chronic fatigue syndrome and multiple sclerosis: development of a model. *J. Psychosom. Res.* **45** (1998), 507–17.

101. C. M. Tench, I. McCurdie, P. D. White, D. P. D'Cruz, The prevalence and associations of fatigue in systemic lupus erythematosus. *Rheumatology (Oxford)* **39** (2000), 1249–54.

102. C. Tench, D. Bentley, V. Vleck, *et al.*, Aerobic fitness, fatigue, and physical disability in systemic lupus erythematosus. *J. Rheumatol.* **29** (2002), 474–81.

103. P. Servaes, J. Prins, C. Verhagen, G. Bleijenberg, Fatigue after breast cancer and in chronic fatigue syndrome, similarities and differences. *J. Psychosom. Res.* **52** (2002), 453–9.

104. F. Dimeo, A. Schmittel, T. Fietz, *et al.*, Physical performance, depression, immune status and fatigue in patients with hematological malignancies after treatment. *Ann. Oncol.* **15** (2004), 1237–42.

105. A. Romani, R. Bergamaschi, E. Candeloro, *et al.*, Fatigue in multiple sclerosis: multidimensional assessment and response to symptomatic treatment. *Mult. Scler.* **10** (2004), 462–8.

106. K. Reuter, M. Harter, The concepts of fatigue and depression in cancer. *Eur. J. Cancer Care* **13** (2004), 127–34.

107. M. C. Tartaglia, S. Narayanan, S. J. Francis, *et al.*, The relationship between diffuse axonal damage and fatigue in multiple sclerosis. *Arch. Neurol.* **61** (2004), 201–7.

108. P. Flachenecker, T. Kümpfel, B. Kallmann, *et al.*, Fatigue in multiple sclerosis: a comparison of different rating scales and correlation to clinical parameters. *Mult. Scler.* **8** (2002), 523–6.

109. P. Flachenecker, I. Bihler, F. Weber, *et al.*, Cytokine mRNA expression in patients with multiple sclerosis and fatigue. *Mult. Scler.* **10** (2004), 165–9.

110. D. C. Kroencke, S. G. Lynch, D. R. Denney, Fatigue in multiple sclerosis: relationship to depression, disability, and disease pattern. *Mult. Scler.* **6** (2000), 131–6.

111. H. P. Attarian, K. M. Brown, S. P. Duntley, J. D. Carter, A. H. Cross, The relationship of sleep disturbances and fatigue in multiple sclerosis. *Arch. Neurol.* **61** (2004), 525–8.

112. G. R. Morrow, J. T. Hickok, J. A. Roscoe, *et al.*, Differential effects of paroxetine on fatigue and depression: a randomized, double-blind trial. *J. Clin. Oncol.* **21** (2003), 4635–41.

113. D. C. Mohr, S. L. Hart, A. Goldberg, Effects of treatment for depression on fatigue in multiple sclerosis. *Psychosom. Med.* **65** (2003), 542–7.

10

Cancer and depression

Alice E. Simon, Steven C. Palmer and James C. Coyne

Introduction

Recent advances in the detection [1] and treatment [2] of cancer have led to longer survival times [3]; for example, the five-year survival rate of localised breast cancer is now 97% [4]. As a result of this lengthened life expectancy, greater attention is being paid to quality of life and psychosocial care for cancer patients. In the short term, this means ensuring that patients maintain their quality of life during diagnostic and treatment phases. In the longer term, the aim is to ensure that psychological problems are prevented or ameliorated so that cancer patients can rehabilitate and resume functioning at the level they maintained before their cancer.

Cancer remains a life-threatening illness linked by many authors with fears about incapacity, disfigurement and death [5,6]. Unsurprisingly, many individuals diagnosed with cancer experience at least transient psychological distress. This recognition, however, can lead to a dismissal of depression as a normative response to cancer and missed opportunities to address a highly impairing, but readily treatable, psychiatric disorder when depression does occur. On the other hand, overestimation of the extent to which cancer results in depression can misguide allocation of resources, leading to an emphasis on strategies for aggressively detecting psychiatric disorders at the expense of follow-up care for patients who have already been identified, as well as attention to more common problems and basic supportive needs that affect quality of life among cancer patients more generally.

In addition to concern about depression as an added disease burden, there is considerable speculation about depression as a cause of cancer and predictor of disease progression and survival [7]. If depression can be shown to affect progression and survival, then ensuring that it is detected and treated effectively becomes all the more important. Yet, tying the value of treatment of depression to its effect on disease course and an extension of life can lead to a discrediting of quality of life as

Depression and Physical Illness, ed. A. Steptoe.
Published by Cambridge University Press. © Cambridge University Press 2006.

a valuable outcome for mental health and psychosocial interventions, particularly if stronger claims about effects on progression and survival are not substantiated.

The relationship between cancer and depression is the focus of a large and growing literature. One review identifies more than 3000 published abstracts in the period 1966–2001 [8]. In this chapter, we discuss three main areas: (i) the prevalence of depression among cancer patients, (ii) the identification and treatment of depression among cancer patients and (iii) the relationship between depression and cancer incidence, progression and survival. We propose that although the diagnosis and treatment of cancer are associated with depression for some people, the prevalence of depression in patients with cancer has been overestimated. Inaccurate estimates of the prevalence of depression impede the design of effective services and the rational allocation of clinical resources. A number of treatments for depression have been shown to be efficacious, but there remains a lack of demonstrated effectiveness in the delivery of these interventions in the routine care of cancer patients, in part because the competing demands of managing a life-threatening illness interfere with the delivery of quality care for depression. We argue that the greatest challenge in the management of depression in cancer patients is ensuring the adequacy of the delivery of treatment within the confines of these competing demands, rather than the lack of efficacious treatments. Finally, available data suggest a lack of support for speculations that depression causes cancer or directly accelerates its progression, but depression remains an additional disease burden and threat to quality of life.

Prevalence of depression among cancer patients

Depression is widely believed to be a highly prevalent condition among cancer patients, but estimates of its prevalence vary greatly. Massie's [9] review of papers published up to 2002 cites a range of 0–38% for major depression and 0–58% for depression spectrum disorders (including more mild and moderate symptom reporting of depression), but both estimates are too imprecise to provide a guide to the need for services. In studies published since 2002, this variability is still common. At the lower end, one study of a breast-cancer waiting-room sample found that 29% of patients were in the distressed range. Follow-up interviews found that approximately 9% met criteria for major depression, 7% met criteria for minor depression and 6% met criteria for generalised anxiety disorder [10], quite consistent with other recent estimates [11–13]. One of the recent higher-end estimates is Burgess and colleagues' [14] report that 48% of patients with breast cancer experienced 'clinically significant' depression or anxiety in the first year after diagnosis. However, this figure grouped individuals meeting full diagnostic criteria for major depressive disorder (MDD) and generalised anxiety disorders with 'borderline' cases of depression and anxiety, for which the efficacy of intervention has not been established. Burgess and colleagues note that a year after diagnosis, the prevalence of 'clinically significant' depression and anxiety was only 15%, and thereafter the risk of anxiety and depression was no greater than in the general population, suggesting that the depression and anxiety being discussed are largely self-limiting and not enduring clinical disorders.

There are a number of factors that contribute to the wide variation in reporting of depression in cancer patients. As mentioned already, levels of depression are likely to vary according to the length of time that has elapsed since diagnosis of cancer, and this may be particularly true where subclinical cases are concerned, e.g. [14]. Higher estimates may also reflect use of self-report questionnaires of 'depressive symptoms' rather than diagnostic interviews to ascertain formal clinical diagnoses [15] or the sampling of in-patients with more severe somatic disturbance or advanced stage of disease [16,17].

In older adults (age 60–74 years) in the UK, the group most likely to experience a diagnosis of cancer, the one-month prevalence is 7% for mixed anxiety and depressive disorder, 3% for general anxiety disorder and 1% for depressive episodes [18]. Using an index of depressive symptoms and a wider age range (16–74 years), the one-month prevalence is 10% for all adults in the UK [19]. In the USA, Kessler *et al.* [20] found a 16.6% lifetime prevalence of depression and a 6.6% 12-month prevalence. Some studies of the prevalence of depression among cancer patients report levels comparable to or lower than these, suggesting that cancer itself may provide no additional risk for depression. This hypothesis was tested systematically in a meta-analysis of 58 studies comparing levels of anxiety and depression in cancer patients with the general population. This showed that levels of depression were higher in cancer patients than in the general population, but levels of anxiety and general psychological distress were not [21]. Other reviews also conclude that depression is more common in cancer patients than among the general population [8,15,22]. However, differences in sampling and assessment strategies, definitions of depression and diagnostic criteria, and handling of overlap between somatic symptoms of disease/treatment and depression make it difficult to draw definitive conclusions.

Another useful comparison is between levels of depression in cancer patients and other patient groups. Rates in patients with neurological disorders appear to be more consistently higher (30–50%) than in those with cancer or other medical illnesses [9]. Analyses of a longitudinal study of depressive symptoms in a sample of 8387 adults (aged 51–61 years) suggested that cancer patients have more depressive symptoms than those with hypertension, arthritis, heart disease, diabetes or stroke in the first two years after diagnosis. Levels of depressive symptoms in cancer patients were comparable to levels found in patients with chronic lung disease [23].

However, the age range for this study is lower than the mean age of diagnosis of most cancers, and among cancer patients lower age is associated with greater distress. More generally, estimates of the prevalence of major depressive disorder among cancer patients based on semi-structured diagnostic interviews with representative samples overlap with the 5–13% range found in primary-care patients [24–28].

The best estimates of the prevalence of depression in cancer patients suggest that the disorder is more common than in the general population, but perhaps only as common as or a little more common than in general medical patients, including primary-care patients. Even accepting the higher estimates of prevalence in cancer patients, the majority of individuals with cancer will not develop major depression. As Raison and Miller's [22] review concludes, 'cancer is a risk factor, rather than a mandate, for depression' (p. 283). This raises an interesting but overlooked issue. If cancer does not raise the level of current depression as once thought, then what effect does it have on lifetime rates of depression? Depression is a recurrent episodic condition with a mean first onset in the early twenties, long before the mean age at which most cancers are diagnosed. If most cases of depression during cancer treatment are recurrences, then this would have important implications for efforts to detect and treat this depression, and perhaps even prevent it among cancer patients vulnerable on the basis of past history.

Dilemmas in the diagnosis and assessment of depression in cancer patients

Cancer poses many of the same challenges as other medical conditions in terms of accurate diagnosis of depression and the suitability of various strategies for detection and assessment. Symptoms that discriminate well between psychiatric and non-medical patients may prove less efficient in cancer patients, necessitating adjustment in diagnostic criteria. The overlap between depressive symptoms and the symptoms of cancer and side effects of treatment may pose problems in the interpretation of self-report and interview measures of depression

Controversy in the diagnosis of depression

Many cancer patients report symptoms of fatigue, loss of appetite and cognitive impairment, which could be attributed to the illness itself, side effects of treatment, or depression. It has been particularly difficult to resolve the overlap between the fatigue that accompanies treatment for cancer and depression [29]. Confusion about the overlap between the symptoms of MDD and those of cancer and its treatment could result in invalid diagnoses, leading to inappropriate treatment of non-depressed individuals with antidepressants in lieu of more appropriate supportive services or empirically supported interventions for other forms of symptom distress [30]. The philosophy of the *Diagnostic and Statistical Manual of Mental Disorders*, fourth edition (DSM-IV) [31] definition of MDD is inclusive and non-aetiological, and although the criteria for attributing a symptom to a medical illness are strict (i.e. the symptom must be the *direct* physiological consequence of a medical condition), the validity of this approach remains unsettled.

Studies provide contradictory suggestions as to whether overlapping symptoms should be given equal [28,32] or lesser [33–35] weight. Various strategies have been proposed for diagnosing MDD among cancer patients [36–38]. Inclusive strategies count all symptoms, regardless of their aetiology, and offer high sensitivity for MDD at the expense of low specificity and overdiagnosis, e.g. [39]. Exclusive strategies allow only symptoms clearly unrelated to the diagnosis and treatment of cancer to count towards an MDD diagnosis. However, this approach may require the diagnostician to possess more knowledge than is readily available in the literature [38]. The substitutive approach [40] replaces somatic symptoms with additional cognitive symptoms. However, there are currently no clear, agreed guidelines as to which symptoms to replace, the symptoms that should replace these, or whether and how to weigh various symptoms to arrive at an accurate diagnosis. Aetiological approaches count symptoms only if they are clearly not a result of physical illness, and thus these can be the most restrictive of the classification schemes. Indeed, prevalence rates for depression among medical patients can vary as much as 210% when comparing inclusive and aetiological strategies [41]. The confusion over which strategy is most 'accurate' in the sense of clinically useful remains unresolved; existing data [39], although sparse, indicate that small changes in diagnostic strategies can substantially affect the nature and prevalence of MDD identified.

In the absence of conclusive data, the most prudent strategy may be to apply what is known about depression among other patient groups. Most cases of MDD in adults are recurrences. Among primary-care patients, individuals with current depression are eight times more likely to have a history of depression than non-depressed individuals; after taking history into account, the risk of depression proffered by other putative factors is substantially lowered, e.g. [42]. Given this, it may be most reasonable for clinicians to have a variable threshold for counting symptoms, taking an inclusive approach among individuals with a history of depressive disorder and a more aetiological approach among those without such a history, but being prepared to revise a provisional diagnosis based on course or response to treatment. This resolution, although less than ideal, may allow for identification of those most likely to benefit from intervention while reducing the chance of introducing new treatment to individuals unlikely to benefit. Whether such a resolution can be readily implemented is unclear. It is somewhat reassuring that mental health professionals can be trained to discriminate between symptoms of depression and symptoms of physical illness and side effects of treatment when using structured interview protocols and formal diagnostic criteria [43]. On the other hand, lay interviewers required to accept patient reports at face value without probing, e.g. as in [44], produce dubious diagnoses, rendering the conclusions of some research studies suspect [45].

Prevalence of depression by cancer type, stage and treatment

Disease site

Patients with cancer are not, of course, a homogeneous group in terms of the cancers they have. For this reason alone, differences exist in the levels of distress experienced by patients with cancer. Zabora *et al.* [46] studied 5000 cancer patients, of whom 58% had received a diagnosis within the past 90 days. The highest prevalence of distress was found in those with lung cancer, where 43.4% of the sample showed high levels of distress. Similarly high levels of distress were experienced by patients with brain, liver, pancreatic and head and neck cancers. Significantly lower levels of distress were experienced in patients with gynaecological, breast, colon and prostate cancers. This may be because of the better prognosis for the latter cancer sites. Other studies report similar findings; for example, Stommel *et al.* [47] found higher levels of depression in patients with lung cancer compared with those with breast, colon or prostate cancers in their sample of 860 older (≥ 65 years) patients.

Disease stage

Stage of disease at diagnosis is another factor that affects reporting of psychological adjustment. Being diagnosed with more advanced disease implies a poorer prognosis and, understandably, can be expected to pose a greater threat to psychological wellbeing. A number of studies show that more advanced disease is associated with increased psychological distress, e.g. [48–50], although other studies find little or no relationship between stage and psychological outcomes [51–53]. Studies that fail to find an effect often do not include patients with the most advanced disease stages [14,52], or make a comparison between early- and advanced-stage patients in widely different timeframes since diagnosis, e.g. [51]. These varied responses may also reflect the fact that patients are notoriously poor at understanding the precise implication of their diagnoses [54–57].

Treatments of cancer

Some cancer treatments are also associated with increased levels of depression. Immunotherapeutic agents, such as interferon alfa and interleukin, used to treat some cancers (e.g. kidney, melanoma) induce depressed mood as a direct side effect [58–60]. Other more extreme treatments such as bone-marrow and stem-cell transplants appear to result in higher levels of distress than cancers with other treatment modalities indirectly because of the more severe trauma to the body and isolation of the patient [61–63]. More widespread treatments such as chemotherapy, radiotherapy and surgery commonly cause symptoms of illness, including fatigue, pain and sickness (see Chapter 12). These symptoms experienced at chronic levels are debilitating and are connected to psychological distress [47,64–66]. The studies cited here find that different treatments can increase levels of distress. Patients undergoing treatment may differ in terms of distress compared with those who have completed or who are still awaiting treatment.

There are also studies that conclude that type of treatment is not associated with distress, e.g. [14,47,53]. Burgess *et al.*'s [14] study of depression and anxiety in 222 women with breast cancer concludes that risk factors such as younger age, past history of depression and lack of social support are more important risk factors for depression than cancer-related variables. This possibility cannot be discussed within the parameters of this chapter. These variables are risk factors for depression in general population samples.

Detection and treatment of depression in cancer patients

Regardless of the prevalence of depression, its occurrence represents a burden to the patient. Nonetheless, the clinical significance of distress remains unclear. Zabora *et al.* [46] suggest that two-thirds of distressed patients improve without intervention, but the authors provide no supporting data. Others suggest that most patients experience a reduction in initial distress within weeks of diagnosis and considerable improvement within three to four months [14,67–69]. At least one effort to monitor intensively the emergence of any distress and to intervene quickly failed to demonstrate an effect, apparently because of the high rate of resolution without any intervention beyond routine care [70]. Yet, there is a consensus that not all distress among cancer patients resolves so readily and that appropriately identifying and treating distressed patients is imperative. A more useful approach may be to identify groups of people who are most at risk for developing psychological problems and to direct available services towards them. Unfortunately, there has not been much progress in identifying such patients.

It is well documented that depression is frequently overlooked by healthcare professionals and that depression that goes undetected in routine medical care is not likely to be addressed elsewhere [71]. Cancer care professionals are often not well equipped to deal with depression in their patients, lacking the time, communication skills, diagnostic skills and treatment and referral resources that are needed. Fallowfield and colleagues [72] assessed 143 cancer physicians' ability to detect distress in their patients. Over 70% (595/827) of patients with probable psychiatric morbidity (measured by the General Health Questionnaire [GHQ-12]) were missed by their physicians. Physicians and nurses are able to recognise obvious signs of distress such as crying but miss symptoms such as suicidal thoughts and hopelessness, which would require more involved interviewing or direct enquiry to elicit [73,74]. Undetected depression in cancer patients represents a missed opportunity to reduce suffering and impairment. This has led to a growing chorus of calls for routine screening of cancer patients for psychological distress and depression [75–77].

Screening for depression in cancer patients

Screening for depression involves patients completing self-report questionnaires or computer touch-screen measures, with the results being passed on to doctors or allied health professionals for follow-up evaluation and, if appropriate, treatment or referral. Screening instruments that have been proposed range from a simple distress thermometer, e.g. [78], to the full range of standardised measures developed in other populations, such as the Center for Epidemiologic Studies Depression Scale (CES-D) [79], Brief Symptom Inventory [80], Hospital Anxiety and Depression Scale (HADS) [81] and two- and nine-item versions of the Patient Health Questionnaire (PHQ) [82,83].

With appropriate cut-off points, as few as two screening items may prove as valid and efficient as longer instruments [84], reducing patient and staff burden. Yet, regardless of the length or other details of a screening instrument, a clinical interview is necessary to confirm a diagnosis. Conceptually, empirically and clinically, there is a distinction between a score on a self-report measure and a clinical diagnosis of depression sufficient for decision-making [25]. The imperfect fit between scores on a screening instrument and diagnosis dictates that efficient cut-off points for a screening instrument inevitably involve a balance between sensitivity in identifying the disorder and specificity for ruling out individuals without diagnosis. Lower cut-off points ensure that fewer depressed patients are missed, but at the expense of requiring more follow-up interviews of patients who turn out to be not depressed. Resolution of these false-positive cases is costly and likely diverts resources from improving the treatment of individuals with known depression. In one large-scale study of depression screening in primary-care settings, Spitzer *et al.* [85] estimated that an additional 8.4 minutes for resolution of a positive screen had to be added to what would have otherwise have been a 6- to 12-minute encounter. This observation was in the context of a research study with enriched resources and training for staff, which are unlikely to be available in routine oncology settings. Other research has demonstrated that such resolution of positive screens can cost an additional US$60 per patient [86].

A study conducted by two of the authors of this chapter [10] raised some issues about the efficiency of screening. Almost a third of a sample of women recruited from the waiting room of a specialty breast cancer treatment setting screened positive for depression, despite many of them being long-term survivors report-ing for a follow-up visit. This figure could be cited as evidence of the enduring distress associated with breast cancer, but it is actually almost identical to what would be obtained in a primary-care waiting room [87]. Furthermore, only 8% of the waiting-room sample was subsequently found to have MDD, and the odds of an individual screening positively having MDD were only 21%. Many of the depressed women had a recent or current prescription for an antidepressant, and so the probability that an interview with a woman who screened positive would yield an untreated case of MDD was only 7%. In short, two-stage screening and interviewing in this sample could provide little in terms of improved detection of untreated depression for a lot of effort.

There is some evidence that the introduction of screening with adequate feedback to medical staff can increase the number of cases of MDD that are identified [13] and the number of patients who are referred for psychiatric care [88]. This should, presumably, result in a reduction in the overall level of depression in the screened sample [89]. However, there has been no demonstration that routine screening for depression reduces the rate of the disorder or level of depressive symptoms among cancer patients on a clinic or population basis. The consistent finding in the general medical literature is that screening does not improve patient outcomes without the introduction of considerable resources, and it is exceedingly difficult to identify any enduring benefits after the enriched resources of a demonstration project are withdrawn [90]. We know of no demonstration that screening by itself reduces depression on a population basis, despite an extensive review of the literature [90]. The result of one pilot study with patients with prostate cancer raises some issues that deserve more attention. Roth and colleagues [91] were able to get 77% (93/121) of a waiting-room sample to complete questionnaires; 29 scored above a cut-off point on one or both screening instruments. These 29 patients were referred for further evaluation, but 12 missed or refused an appointment. One recurrent issue in dealing with these patients was the difficulty of getting such an evaluation without requiring a return visit by the patient. Of the 17 evaluated, three patients not currently receiving treatment were given a psychiatric diagnosis. A re-evaluation was recommended to them, but there is no report of how many patients completed this. Consistent with some of the difficulties that Roth and colleagues encountered, Shimizu and colleagues [88] found that only 28% (19/67) of cancer patients who scored positive on a screening test for depression accepted a referral to a psychiatrist.

Screening is clearly not a panacea in the improvement of the outcome of depres-sion on a cancer setting or population basis. We would urge caution before any commitment to screening as the sole or primary means to address depression in a cancer-care setting and would urge careful consideration of its likely costs, benefits and alternatives. Maguire [92] apparently shares our concerns and recommends training cancer-care professionals in better detecting distress and depression in conversations with patients. We would also recommend strategies such as greater surveillance of cancer patients with histories of depression, given the importance of this background as a predictor of depression during cancer care [93–95]; monitoring of the adequacy of existing treatment of patients identified as depressed; and lowering the barriers for cancer patients who are motivated to seek specialty mental health care.

Treatment for depression in cancer patients

In light of conventional assumptions that cancer is a strong risk factor for depression, it might seem ironic that there is a paucity of clinical trials examining treatment for depression in cancer patients. An expert scientific review and consensus conference commissioned by the Depression and Bipolar Support Alliance (DBSA) [96] concluded: 'Available evidence strongly suggests that depression in the patient with cancer responds to tricyclic antidepressants (TCAs), selective serotonin reuptake inhibitors (SSRIs), mirtazapine, and mianserin' (p. 16). This statement is based on seven studies: two were double-blind randomised placebo-controlled trials supporting the efficacy of mianserin, a heterocyclic antidepressant that is not commonly prescribed. Apart from these, none of the other studies was a double-blind randomised placebo-controlled trial in which an antidepressant was shown to be superior to placebo. Although one randomised placebo-controlled trial obtained null effects for fluoxetine [97], the lack of evidence is mainly a matter of the paucity of research with adequate statistical power and other minimal methodological rigour. Pirl [8] cites nine relevant studies, but his additions do not change our conclusion. Thus, currently the strength of the recommendation of treatment of depression in cancer patients with antidepressants must come from studies of the treatment of depression with antidepressants in the presence of comorbid physical illness more generally. However, the evidence is that depressed patients with comorbid physical illness have worse treatment outcomes than those without physical comorbidity [98].

Evidence that psychotherapy is efficacious for depression in cancer patients is similarly limited. Sheard and Maguire [99] have provided what is becoming a widely cited meta-analysis of the effects of psychological interventions on depression in cancer patients. They initially identified 20 intervention trials in which depression was measured as an outcome, but only ten allowed assessment of an effect size. Sheard and Maguire found an effect size of 0.36, but the data were found to be highly heterogeneous, and elimination of three positive outliers with small sample sizes and other serious design flaws reduced the effect size by a half to 0.19. Although these results can hardly be seen as demonstrating the efficacy of psychotherapy for depressed cancer patients, neither can they be taken as decisive evidence against the efficacy of treatment; particularly in this instance, absence of evidence of an effect is not evidence of an absence of effect. Sheard and Maguire [99] note that most of these studies did not involve recruitment of patients on the basis of them being depressed, and those that did so relied on self-reported distress as the criterion. What Sheard and Maguire do conclude for the studies in which patients were recruited without regard to level of depression is that there is no evidence that providing psychotherapy to non-depressed patients prevents depression.

In the midst of what may seem a discouraging assessment of the literature, it would be useful to point to a promising recent study. Nezu and colleagues [100] randomised 132 cancer patients to individual problem-solving therapy, or problem-solving therapy with the involvement of a significant other, or waiting-list control. Patients were not recruited on the basis of a diagnosis of depression, but the requirement that they were experiencing a significant level of distress yielded a sample that had depressive symptoms of a mean severity typically seen in clinical trials with depressed out-patients. Both of the problem-solving therapy conditions resulted in significant reductions in distress on most of a set of outcome measures, whereas baseline levels of distress were maintained in the waiting-list control groups. The patients who had the involvement of their significant others experienced greater gain than those receiving individual problem-solving therapy. Improvements in the patients receiving active treatment were still evident at one-year follow-up.

Another promising, but preliminary, study supports patients' use of antidepressant medication before receiving treatment with interferon alfa in order to prevent the development of depression, a side effect serious enough to require discontinuation of interferon in the treatment of melanoma. Musselman *et al.* [59] conducted a double-blind study using paroxetine in patients with malignant melanoma ($n = 40$) before the start of interferon alfa treatment. Only 2 of 18 patients receiving paroxetine developed depression compared with 9 of 20 in the placebo group. Furthermore, only one patient in the paroxetine group, compared with seven in the placebo group, discontinued interferon treatment because of severe depression. This suggests that there may be a role for antidepressants as a preventive measure in patients receiving this type of treatment. These results need to be replicated, and long-term effects are still unknown.

A third innovative study is more troubling in its implications, particularly given the investigators' interpretation of their results. Fisch and colleagues [101] randomised cancer patients in the community to receive by mail either fluoxetine or placebo, with the instructions that patients contact their oncologist if they experienced vomiting or nausea after taking the drug. Participants in this study had been screened for depression, but screening served as a basis for excluding patients who did not have at least some symptoms, rather than to ensure clinically significant levels of symptoms. The authors concluded from their results: 'Our data may broaden the comfort zone of oncologists for prescribing antidepressants for some patients' (p. 1942). There were numerous methodological problems with this study, starting with difficulties accruing patients despite a US statewide recruitment effort. Moreover, the differences between their intervention and placebo groups were greater at baseline than at follow-up, and in the follow-up assessment on which they base their claim of effectiveness data were available for only 14 of the 81 intervention patients and 19 of the 78 placebo patients. Our major concerns with this study are three-fold (see also [102,103]): first, there is more generally a lack of evidence that antidepressants are effective for individuals who have subthreshold depression, and the investigators' encouragement of such use is counter to available evidence. Second, it is already difficult to get non-psychiatric physicians such as oncologists to adhere to diagnostic criteria and provide adequate patient education and follow-up; Fisch and colleagues imply that neither is needed. Finally, from the point of view of policy, it would be unfortunate if inaccurate claims about the effectiveness of mailing antidepressants to patients who are not even depressed were used to argue against the provision of appropriate psychosocial services. Substantial rates of prescription of antidepressants to cancer patients who are not depressed is already an important issue in quality and economics of mental healthcare for cancer patients [102].

In summary, the case for the efficacy of intervention for depression among cancer patients depends mainly on evidence derived from other populations. Demonstrations that such claims can be validly extended to cancer patients are sorely overdue. However, our earlier review of the prevalence of depression among cancer patients suggests a challenge in the mounting of methodologically adequate studies: if only 9% of patients with breast cancer suffer from major depression and a substantial proportion are already receiving treatment, then a multisite trial with massive amounts of screening may be necessary to accrue a sufficient sample.

Effectiveness of delivery versus efficacy of treatment of depression in cancer

Even if we provisionally accept that what is efficacious in the treatment of depression more generally should work for cancer patients as well, there is the question of the effectiveness with which care for depression can be delivered to cancer patients. Aside from the urgent and competing demands of treating a life-threatening illness, there are formidable issues concerning patient acceptance and access to quality care. A high proportion of patients reject psychological intervention [88,104,105]. Moynihan et al. [104] reported that only 40% (73/184) of their sample of patients with testicular cancer accepted psychological therapy. 'We make a plea for caution with regard to the blind faith that counselling will be gratefully received and will be effective despite a dearth of sound evidence' (p. 128). Sharpe and colleagues [105] report that 53% of patients rejected their problem-solving intervention, but 37% also rejected the control condition where there was simply monitoring of depression and 'usual care'. Sollner and colleagues [106] found that only 42% of patients with breast cancer who screened positive on a measure of distress endorsed an interest in counselling, a proportion no greater than for non-distressed patients with breast cancer. In the study by Roth and colleagues [91], one of the patients with prostate cancer refusing screening outright stated: 'This is a psychiatric evaluation? Right now I have my own problems and I don't want to get involved.'

The data are mixed as to the extent to whether cancer-care professionals influence patient uptake of mental health and psychosocial treatment. Although most (68%) of a sample of patients with prostate cancer reported that they would prefer not to take medication for depression, 75% indicated that they would do so if advised by their physician [107]. However, Eakin and Strycker [108] found that although clinicians reported referring 70% of cancer patients to support services, only 24% of these patients recalled having discussed the issue.

The problems of low uptake and patient resistance to mental health and psychosocial services is often framed in terms of stigma, with the requisite solution being a destigmatisation of help-seeking [109]. However, there is consistent evidence that offered a choice, patients with cancer prefer more support and communication from oncologists and oncological nurses than interactions with mental health professionals, and interventions designed to increase their access to quality, understandable information about their condition and its treatment to counselling and psychotherapy [107,110–113]. Perhaps, not unreasonably, patients prefer to deal directly with the perceived source of their distress and depression [106]. It remains an important but unaddressed question as to whether improved access to care specialists and medical information is a more acceptable and effective means of preventing and ameliorating depression than formal mental health services, or, if not, whether such improved access and information might function as an effective first-stage response, such that patients who do not benefit sufficiently are particularly appropriate for specialty mental health interventions.

Even when depressed cancer patients are interested in empirically supported treatments, they may have difficulty accessing such services. Cancer care tends to be provided in tertiary-care settings to which patients travel many miles [10,107]. It may be logistically difficult or undesirable to coordinate mental healthcare with visits for chemotherapy or radiation and unrealistic to expect that patients will make regular return visits expressly for care for depression.

Then there is the issue of the availability in cancer-care settings of professionals trained in the effective treatment of depression. It has been argued that quality mental health and psychosocial care is an essential component of comprehensive cancer care, but psycho-oncology units, if present at all in routine cancer care, tend to be understaffed [76]. Pamphlets for the Memorial Sloane Kettering Cancer Center, which has been instrumental in the development of psycho-oncology, state flatly that specialty psychosocial services are not available in their affiliated cancer-care settings. Furthermore, the patient base needed for interventions targeting focused groups of cancer patients, such as those with early breast cancer or metastatic breast cancer, has not usually been appreciated. Goodwin *et al.*'s [114] presentation of lessons learned in a randomised trial of supportive expressive therapy for patients with metastatic breast cancer deserves careful consideration.

The unfortunate state of affairs for treatment of depression in routine care for cancer is that if depression is addressed at all, then it is likely to be with peer- or professionally led support groups with patients of varying cancer sites, stages of cancer and time since diagnosis; non-specific individual counselling and psychotherapy; or, more predominately, prescription of antidepressants by non-psychiatric physicians and nurses that is both non-specific and followed up poorly. The gap in outcome is likely to be great between what occurs with these treatments and what is obtained with empirically supported treatments in the context of a clinical trial.

Relevance of primary medical care

In closing our discussion of care for depression in cancer patients, there are three reasons for giving attention to primary medical care. First, the de facto mental health system for the treatment of depression in North America and the UK is centred on primary medical care [115]. Cancer patients who are suspected of being depressed are likely to be started by their oncology clinicians on antidepressants with expectations of follow-up in primary care or to be referred directly to their primary-care physicians for further evaluation for treatment with medication [116]. The quality of care for depression in primary care is thus likely to be the quality of care available to depressed cancer patients.

Second, over 15 years of research on treatment of outcome of depression in primary care document well the difficulties in ensuring quality of care in non-psychiatric medical settings [71,117]. This large body of literature indicates that in routine primary care, treatments with established efficacy are delivered with effectiveness that is no greater than that observed for placebo in clinical trials in specialty mental health settings, apparently due to the low quality of routine care. It is estimated that only 20% of depressed primary-care patients receive adequate care, and there are notable deficiencies in patient education, scheduling of follow-up visits and a failure to adjust medications in the face of unacceptable side effects or lack of improvement [71,118]. Approximately 40–50% of depressed patients will need such adjustments [119], but in the absence of adequate monitoring and follow-up problems with medication and non-adherence are not likely to be detected.

It has become clear that simply identifying more depressed primary-care patients will not improve patient outcomes on a practice or population basis, that physician education alone is insufficient to improve these outcomes [117,120], and that more fundamental changes in the structure of practice are needed. In a comprehensive review, Brody [121] (p. 21) has identified some components that contribute to the effectiveness of multi-component strategies to improve the outcome of depression in primary care:

We have learned that improving the care and outcomes of depression in primary care requires some or all of the following: a systematic approach to the recognition and assessment of depression; evidence-based decision support; patient education and activation; ongoing monitoring and feedback regarding patient adherence and outcomes; integration of mental health specialists for patients who are not improving as expected; and physician education.

Brody [121] notes, however, that serious difficulties have been encountered in attempting to sustain these innovations beyond well-funded demonstration projects.

Depression-management specialists, who are usually Master's level nurses or social workers who take responsibility for assessment and follow-up, are becoming a basic component of cost-effective strategies for improving the outcome of depression in general medical care [122,123]. These managers can be trained to meet patient preferences by offering either medication management or brief structured psychotherapies. One promising extension of this work is the utilisation of centralised systems of telephone management of depressed patients, with regular direct contact of depression-management specialists with patients and support and feedback to treating professionals [124,125].

The challenges of improving the effectiveness with which depression is managed in cancer care are undoubtedly even more overwhelming than what has been encountered in primary medical care. Yet, innovations developed in primary care are now being disseminated into cancer care, at least on a pilot and demonstration project basis. Strong *et al.* [126] delivered a nurse-led intervention to cancer patients with a diagnosis of major depression in which a cancer nurse was trained to deliver a problem-solving therapy and encourage the patient to consult with a primary-care physician concerning antidepressants. Patients receiving the intervention showed significant reductions in depression compared with the control group. Strong *et al.* [126] noted a number of difficulties associated with patient rejection of participation in the programme and primary-care physicians rejecting the advice of the depression specialists, but this pilot project nonetheless shows the promise of depression-management specialists in the context of cancer care. In a study in which the depression-management specialist had responsibility for promoting adherence to antidepressants, Dwight-Johnson *et al.* [127] randomised 55 low-income Hispanic American patients from a public-sector hospital with breast or cervical cancer and comorbid depression to either collaborative care delivered by a depression-management specialist or usual care. The usual-care arm of the study involved informing the patient of her diagnosis of depression and encouraging her to seek treatment. The patients receiving the intervention experienced significantly greater reduction in depressive symptoms, which the investigators attributed to both the effectiveness of the intervention and the difficulties the control women experienced in obtaining care for their depression.

Depression and cancer incidence, progression and survival: death is not everything

The established rationale for improving the detection and treatment of depression in cancer care is that the toll of depression on the wellbeing and quality of life of cancer patients is unnecessary in terms of the availability of efficacious treatments. However, considerable attention has been given to controversial claims that depression is implicated in the incidence and progression of cancer and that, as demonstrated in the effects of group psychotherapy on survival, treating depression can extend the lives of cancer patients [7,96]. Indeed, the view that mood and morale affect the progression and outcome of cancer has become prevalent among the lay public and even some oncology professionals [128,129]. However, even the mechanism by which depression might influence development of cancer is highly speculative and controversial. The effect of depression on immune functioning is commonly cited as a plausible mechanism [7], but there is a limited range of cancers for which immune functioning is conceivably relevant, and research has consistently failed to find effects of psychosocial interventions on the immune functioning of cancer patients [130].

Spiegel and Giese-Davis [7] noted that the literature concerning depressed mood predicting cancer incidence is at best mixed, 'although there is support in the literature for an association between lingering depression and faster cancer progression, the field has yet to sort out the overlapping symptoms of increased tumour burden and vegetative depression' (p. 273). Currently, there is considerable scepticism in the literature concerning whether a causal role for depression or emotional wellbeing in cancer progression can be demonstrated when appropriate controls are introduced for known biological prognostic indicators, physical symptoms and side effects of treatment [131]. Large-scale observational studies have failed to find that emotional wellbeing predicts survival in patients with metastatic [132] or early [133,134] breast cancer. In a review of prospective studies, Garssen [135] characterised depression as 'an influence that cannot be totally dismissed' (p. 315), rather than being among the pool of the most promising psychosocial variables.

Some of the research interest in this topic stemmed from Greer and colleagues' [136] study of survival in patients with breast cancer, which found an association between denial, helplessness/hopelessness, fighting spirit and survival in a group of early-stage breast cancer patients. This group was followed for 15 years and the effect persisted over that time. However, the sample size was relatively small ($n = 69$). Watson *et al.*'s ongoing study of survival in breast cancer patients ($n = 578$) also shows that helplessness/hopelessness is related to decreased survival at both five [137] and ten [138] years' follow-up. Watson *et al.*'s study fails to replicate the findings for fighting spirit found in the study by Greer *et al.* [136]. Watson *et al.* reported a very limited effect for depression at the five-year follow-up, but this was no longer present at the ten-year follow-up [137,138].

With regard to the possibility that psychological interventions can improve survival, Spiegel's group [7,139,140] have argued that there is evidence to support this possibility. They cite [7,140] five studies that support this hypothesis [139,141–144] and five studies that do not [133,145–148]. Since Spiegel and colleagues' reviews, an additional negative finding has been obtained [51]. Palmer and Coyne [149] note that three of the studies cited by Spiegel and colleagues ([142–144]) involved a confounding of improved medical surveillance and more intensive medical care with psychological intervention, so that any improvement in survival cannot be attributed unambiguously to psychological intervention. The remaining two studies ([139,141]) have serious statistical problems. Survival data for cancer patients is highly skewed, with a small number of patients typically living much longer than the rest, making medians better summary statistics than means. When the Spiegel *et al.* [139] data are summarised in terms of median survival time, the advantage for the patients receiving the intervention is non-significant, being only a few months. Fawzy *et al.* [141] dropped a number of patients from their analyses, including one patient because he was clinically depressed and so did not provide the intention-to-treat analyses that are standard in evaluating medical interventions. Not only do the available studies not support an effect of psychological intervention on survival, but also their relevance to the question of a role for depression in cancer progression is unclear. Spiegel and Giese-Davis's [7] question 'What are the aspects of psychosocial intervention that seem to be most effective in reducing depression . . . ?' (p. 275) seemed quite unanswerable. As noted, Fawzy *et al.* [141] dropped the one depressed patient in their study; other studies do not target depression or assess it as an outcome, and in general these studies have recruited patients that are not notably depressed, even when suffering metastatic disease.

In summary, the evidence that depression causes cancer or accelerates its progression or that intervention for depression improves survival is largely absent or negative. This stands in sharp contrast to the robust prognostic value for depression in cardiovascular disease [150]. In the absence of credible evidence, continued claims for a role for depression in cancer and claims that psychological interventions promote survival can prove damaging to the field. Lesperance and Frasure-Smith [151] stated: 'Although the prevention of death is a powerful tool to influence many of our medical colleagues who use it to justify the allocation of resources, death is not everything' (p. 19). When strong claims about the role of depression in cancer ultimately need to be abandoned, it will seem to be an undignified retreat to claim that the usefulness of detecting and treating depression based on the 'mere' benefits for wellbeing or quality of life. An unwarranted strong claim thus could rob the credibility of what had always been a reasonable claim.

Conclusions

Depression is unlikely to cause or accelerate cancer progression. This is in contrast to the apparent role of depression in other diseases, such as cardiac morbidity and mortality discussed in Chapters 3 and 4 of this book. The prevalence of depression in cancer patients is relatively low but is an additional, and often unrecognised, problem for some patients. Difficulties assessing prevalence and identifying cases of depression in cancer patients have hampered efforts to provide appropriate clinical services. There are a number of effective treatments for depression, but there is often limited availability of trained staff to deliver them, and many cancer patients continue to reject interventions for psychological problems. Depression could be reduced in cancer patients by providing more effective symptom-management or behavioural interventions. These forms of treatment could be more acceptable to patients and delivered more easily by existing oncology staff, but data concerning the potential of these methods are still limited.

Acknowledgements

Preparation of this chapter was supported in part by National Cancer Center (NCI) grant 5R01MH063172 and by Cancer Research, UK.

REFERENCES

1. D. Stockton, T. Davies, N. Day, J. McCann, Retrospective study of reasons for improved survival in patients with breast cancer in East Anglia: earlier diagnosis or better treatment. *Br. Med. J.* **314** (1997), 472–5.

2. C. S. McArdle, D. J. Hole, Outcome following surgery for colorectal cancer. *Br. Med. Bull.* **64** (2002), 119–25.

3. M. Coleman, P. Babb, P. Damiecki, *et al.*, *Cancer Survival Trends in England and Wales, 1971–1995* (London: The Stationary Office, 1999).

4. American Cancer Society. *Cancer Facts and Figures.* (Atlanta, GA: American Cancer Society, 2005).

5. M. McMenamin, H. Barry, A. M. Lennon, *et al.*, A survey of breast cancer awareness and knowledge in a Western population: lots of light but little illumination. *Eur. J. Cancer* **41** (2005), 393–7.

6. K. McCaffery, J. Wardle, J. Waller, Knowledge, attitudes, and behavioral intentions in relation to the early detection of colorectal cancer in the United Kingdom. *Prev. Med.* **36** (2003), 525–35.

7. D. Spiegel, J. Giese-Davis, Depression and cancer: mechanisms and disease progression. *Biol. Psychiatry* **54** (2003), 269–82.

8. W. F. Pirl, Evidence report on the occurrence, assessment, and treatment of depression in cancer patients. *J. Natl. Cancer Inst. Monogr.* (2004), 32–9.

9. M. J. Massie, Prevalence of depression in patients with cancer. *J. Natl. Cancer Inst. Monogr.* (2004), 57–71.

10. J. C. Coyne, S. C. Palmer, P. J. Shapiro, R. Thompson, A. DeMichele, Distress, psychiatric morbidity, and prescriptions for psychotropic medication in a breast cancer waiting room sample. *Gen. Hosp. Psychiatry* **26** (2004), 121–8.

11. M. Harter, K. Reuter, A. Aschenbrenner, *et al.*, Psychiatric disorders and associated factors in cancer: results of an interview study with patients in inpatient, rehabilitation and outpatient treatment. *Eur. J. Cancer* **37** (2001), 1385–93.

12. D. W. Kissane, D. M. Clarke, J. Ikin, *et al.*, Psychological morbidity and quality of life in Australian women with early-stage breast cancer: a cross-sectional survey. *Med. J. Aust.* **169** (1998), 192–6.

13. M. Sharpe, V. Strong, K. Allen, *et al.*, Major depression in outpatients attending a regional cancer centre: screening and unmet treatment needs. *Br. J. Cancer* **90** (2004), 314–20.

14. C. Burgess, V. Cornelius, S. Love, *et al.*, Depression and anxiety in women with early breast cancer: five year observational cohort study. *Br. Med. J.* **330** (2005), 702.

15. M. Hotopf, J. Chidgey, J. J. Addington-Hall, K. L. Ly. Depression in advanced disease: a systematic review. Part 1. Prevalence and case finding. *Palliat. Med.* **16** (2002), 81–97.

16. C. Classen, L. D. Butler, C. Koopman, *et al.*, Supportive-expressive group therapy and distress in patients with metastatic breast cancer: a randomized clinical intervention trial. *Arch. Gen. Psychiatry* **58** (2001), 494–501.

17. M. E. Lynch. The assessment and prevalence of affective disorders in advanced cancer. *J. Palliat. Care* **11** (1995), 10–18.

18. O. Evans, N. Singleton, H. Meltzer, R. Stewart, M. Prince. *The Mental Health of Older People* (London: The Stationery Office, 2003).

19. N. Singleton, R. Bumpstead, M. O'Brien, A. Lee, H. Meltzer *Psychiatric Morbidity among Adults Living in Private Households 2000* (London: The Stationery Office, 2001).

20. R. C. Kessler, P. Berglund, O. Demler, *et al.*, The epidemiology of major depressive disorder: results from the National Comorbidity Survey Replication (NCS-R). *J. Am. Med. Assoc.* **289** (2003), 3095–105.

21. A. van't Spijker, R. W. Trijsburg, H. J. Duivenvoorden, Psychological sequelae of cancer diagnosis: a meta-analytical review of 58 studies after 1980. *Psychosom. Med.* **59** (1997), 280–93.

22. C. L. Raison, A. H. Miller, Depression in cancer: new developments regarding diagnosis and treatment. *Biol. Psychiatry* **54** (2003), 283–94.

23. D. Polsky, J. A. Doshi, S. Marcus, *et al.*, Long-term risk for depressive symptoms after a medical diagnosis. *Arch. Intern. Med.* **165** (2005), 1260–66.

24. J. E. Barrett, J. A. Barrett, T. E. Oxman, P. D. Gerber, The prevalence of psychiatric disorders in a primary care practice. *Arch. Gen. Psychiatry* **45** (1988), 1100–106.

25. J. C. Coyne. Self-reported distress: analog or Ersatz depression? *Psychol. Bull.* **116** (1994), 29–45.

26. L. G. Kessler, P. D. Cleary, J. D. Burke, Jr, Psychiatric disorders in primary care. Results of a follow-up study. *Arch. Gen. Psychiatry* **42** (1985), 583–7.

27. H. C. Schulberg, M. McClelland, B. J. Burns, Depression and physical illness: the prevalence, causation and diagnosis of co-morbidity. *Clin. Psychol. Rev.* **7** (1987), 145–67.

28. W. Katon, The epidemiology of depression in medical care. *Int. J. Psychiatry Med.* **17** (1987), 93–112.

29. K. Reuter, M. Harter, The concepts of fatigue and depression in cancer. *Eur. J. Cancer Care* **13** (2004), 127–34.

30. J. C. Coyne, S. C. Palmer, P. A. Sullivan, Screening for depression in adults. *Ann. Intern. Med.* **138** (2003), 767–8.

31. American Psychiatric Association. *Diagnostic and Statistical Manual of Mental Disorders*, 4th edn (Washington, DC: American Psychiatric Association, 1994).

32. W. Katon, Depression: somatic symptoms and medical disorders in primary care. *Compr. Psychiatry* **23** (1982), 274–87.

33. S. Cavanaugh, D. C. Clark, R. D. Gibbons, Diagnosing depression in the hospitalized medically ill. *Psychosomatics* **24** (1983), 809–15.

34. D. A. Clark, A. Cook, D. Snow, Depressive symptom differences in hospitalized, medically ill, depressed psychiatric inpatients and nonmedical controls. *J. Abnorm. Psychol.* **107** (1998), 38–48.

35. D. C. Clark, C. S. vonAmmon, R. D. Gibbons, The core symptoms of depression in medical and psychiatric patients. *J. Nerv. Ment. Dis.* **171** (1983), 705–13.

36. S. A. Cohen-Cole, A. Stoudemire, Major depression and physical illness. Special considerations in diagnosis and biologic treatment. *Psychiatr. Clin. North Am.* **10** (1987), 1–17.

37. M. K. Popkin, A. L. Callies, E. A. Colon, A framework for the study of medical depression. *Psychosomatics* **28** (1987), 27–33.

38. P. C. Trask, Assessment of depression in cancer patients. *J. Natl. Cancer Inst. Monogr.* (2004), 80–92.

39. R. G. Kathol, A. Mutgi, J. Williams, G. Clamon, R. Noyes, Jr, Diagnosis of major depression in cancer patients according to four sets of criteria. *Am. J. Psychiatry* **147** (1990), 1021–4.

40. J. Endicott, Measurement of depression in patients with cancer. *Cancer* **53** (1984), 2243–9.

41. H. G. Koenig, L. K. George, B. L. Peterson, C. F. Pieper, Depression in medically ill hospitalized older adults: prevalence, characteristics, and course of symptoms according to six diagnostic schemes. *Am. J. Psychiatry* **154** (1997), 1376–83.

42. J. C. Coyne, C. M. Pepper, H. Flynn, Significance of prior episodes of depression in two patient populations. *J. Consult. Clin. Psychol.* **67** (1999), 76–81.

43. H. G. Koenig, P. Pappas, T. Holsinger, J. R. Bachar, Assessing diagnostic approaches to depression in medically ill older adults: how reliably can mental health professionals make judgments about the cause of symptoms? *J. Am. Geriatr. Soc.* **43** (1995), 472–8.

44. K. Honda, R. D. Goodwin, Cancer and mental disorders in a national community sample: findings from the national comorbidity survey. *Psychother. Psychosom.* **73** (2004), 235–42.

45. J. C. Coyne, S. C. Palmer, National Comorbidity Survey data concerning cancer and depression lack credibility. *Psychother. Psychosom.* **74** (2005), 260–61.

46. J. Zabora, K. BrintzenhofeSzoc, B. Curbow, C. Hooker, The prevalence of psychological distress by cancer site. *Psychooncology* **10** (2001), 19–28.

47. M. Stommel, M. E. Kurtz, J. C. Kurtz, C. W. Given, B. A. Given, A longitudinal analysis of the course of depressive symptomatology in geriatric patients with cancer of the breast, colon, lung, or prostate. *Health Psychol.* **23** (2004), 564–73.

48. R. H. Osborne, G. R. Elsworth, J. L. Hopper, Age-specific norms and determinants of anxiety and depression in 731 women with breast cancer recruited through a population-based cancer registry. *Eur. J. Cancer* **39** (2003), 755–62.

49. J. Gallagher, M. Parle, D. Cairns, Appraisal and psychological distress six months after diagnosis of breast cancer. *Br. J. Health Psychol.* **7** (2002), 365–76.

50. K. Shimozuma, P. A. Ganz, L. Petersen, K. Hirji, Quality of life in the first year after breast cancer surgery rehabilitation needs and patterns of recovery. *Breast Cancer Res. Treat.* **56** (1999), 45–57.

51. D. W. Kissane, B. Grabsch, A. Love, *et al.*, Psychiatric disorder in women with early stage and advanced breast cancer a comparative analysis. *Aust. N. Z. J. Psychiatry* **38** (2004), 320–26.

52. E. M. Bleiker, F. Pouwer, H. M. van der Ploeg, J. W. Leer, H. J. Ader, Psychological distress two years after diagnosis of breast cancer: frequency and prediction. *Patient. Educ. Couns.* **40** (2000), 209–17.

53. J. Norum, Adjuvant chemotherapy in Dukes' B and C colorectal cancer has only a minor influence on psychological distress. *Support. Care Cancer* **5** (1997), 318–21.

54. J. C. Weeks, E. F. Cook, S. J. O'Day, *et al.*, Relationship between cancer patients' predictions of prognosis and their treatment preferences. *J. Am. Med. Assoc.* **279** (1998), 1709–14.

55. C. F. Quirt, W. J. Mackillop, A. D. Ginsburg, *et al.*, Do doctors know when their patients don't? A survey of doctor–patient communication in lung cancer. *Lung Cancer* **18** (1997), 1–20.

56. E. Chow, L. Andersson, R. Wong, *et al.*, Patients with advanced cancer: a survey of the understanding of their illness and expectations from palliative radiotherapy for symptomatic metastases. *Clin. Oncol. (R. Coll. Radiol.)* **13** (2001), 204–8.

57. M. Gattellari, P. N. Butow, M. H. Tattersall, S. M. Dunn, C. A. MacLeod, Misunderstanding in cancer patients: why shoot the messenger? *Ann. Oncol.* **10** (1999), 39–46.

58. L. Capuron, A. Ravaud, N. Gualde, *et al.*, Association between immune activation and early depressive symptoms in cancer patients treated with interleukin-2-based therapy. *Psychoneuroendocrinology* **26** (2001), 797–808.

59. D. L. Musselman, D. H. Lawson, J. F. Gumnick *et al.*, Paroxetine for the prevention of depression induced by high-dose interferon alfa. *N. Engl. J. Med.* **344** (2001), 961–6.

60. A. G. Paterson, P. C. Trask, L. I. Wagner, P. Esper, B. Redman, Validation of the FACT-BRM with interferon-alpha treated melanoma patients. *Qual. Life Res.* **14** (2005), 133–9.

61. B. Holzner, G. Kemmler, D. Cella, *et al.*, Normative data for functional assessment of cancer therapy: general scale and its use for the interpretation of quality of life scores in cancer survivors. *Acta Oncol.* **43** (2004), 153–60.

62. C. S. Neitzert, P. Ritvo, J. Dancey, *et al.*, The psychosocial impact of bone marrow transplantation a review of the literature. *Bone Marrow Transplant.* **22** (1998), 409–22.

63. R. Illescas-Rico, F. Amaya-Ayala, J. L. Jimenez-Lopez, M. E. Caballero-Mendez, J. Gonzalez-Llaven, Increased incidence of anxiety and depression during bone marrow transplantation. *Arch. Med. Res.* **33** (2002), 144–7.

64. R. K. Portenoy, H. T. Thaler, A. B. Kornblith, *et al.*, Symptom prevalence, characteristics and distress in a cancer population. *Qual. Life Res.* **3** (1994), 183–9.

65. P. Hopwood, R. J. Stephens, Depression in patients with lung cancer: prevalence and risk factors derived from quality-of-life data. *J. Clin. Oncol.* **18** (2000), 893–903.

66. B. Bennett, D. Goldstein, A. Lloyd, T. Davenport, I. Hickie, Fatigue and psychological distress: exploring the relationship in women treated for breast cancer. *Eur. J. Cancer* **40** (2004), 1689–95.

67. B. L. Andersen, Psychological interventions for cancer patients to enhance the quality of life. *J. Consult Clin. Psychol.* **60** (1992), 552–68.

68. E. Maunsell, J. Brisson, L. Deschenes, Psychological distress after initial treatment of breast cancer: assessment of potential risk factors. *Cancer* **70** (1992), 120–25.

69. A. J. Ramirez, M. A. Richards, S. R. Jarrett, I. S. Fentiman, Can mood disorder in women with breast cancer be identified preoperatively? *Br. J. Cancer* **72** (1995), 1509–12.

70. E. Maunsell, J. Brisson, L. Deschenes, N. Frasure-Smith, Randomized trial of a psychologic distress screening program after breast cancer: effects on quality of life. *J. Clin. Oncol.* **14** (1996), 2747–55.

71. J. C. Coyne, R. Thompson, M. S. Klinkman, D. E. Nease, Jr, Emotional disorders in primary care. *J. Consult. Clin. Psychol.* **70** (2002), 798–809.

72. L. Fallowfield, D. Ratcliffe, V. Jenkins, J. Saul, Psychiatric morbidity and its recognition by doctors in patients with cancer. *Br. J. Cancer* **84** (2001), 1011–15.

73. S. D. Passik, W. Dugan, M. V. McDonald, *et al.*, Oncologists' recognition of depression in their patients with cancer. *J. Clin. Oncol.* **16** (1998), 1594–600.

74. M. V. McDonald, S. D. Passik, W. Dugan, *et al.*, Nurses' recognition of depression in their patients with cancer. *Oncol. Nurs. Forum* **26** (1999), 593–9.

75. B. M. Hoffman, M. A. Zevon, M. C. D'Arrigo, T. B. Cecchini, Screening for distress in cancer patients: the NCCN rapid-screening measure. *Psychooncology* **13** (2004), 792–9.

76. L. E. Carlson, B. D. Bultz, Efficacy and medical cost offset of psychosocial interventions in cancer care: making the case for economic analyses. *Psychooncology* **13** (2004), 837–49.

77. N. Akizuki, T. Akechi, T. Nakanishi, *et al.*, Development of a brief screening interview for adjustment disorders and major depression in patients with cancer. *Cancer* **97** (2003), 2605–13.

78. P. B. Jacobsen, K. A. Donovan, P. C. Trask, *et al.*, Screening for psychologic distress in ambulatory cancer patients. *Cancer* **103** (2005), 1494–502.

79. L. S. Radloff, The CES-D scale: a self-report depression scale for research in the general population. *Appl. Psychol. Meas.* **1** (1977), 385–401.

80. L. R. Derogatis, N. Melisaratos, The Brief Symptom Inventory: an introductory report. *Psychol. Med.* **13** (1983), 595–605.

81. A. Zigmond, R. Snaith, The Hospital Anxiety and Depression Scale. *Acta Psychiatr. Scand.* **67** (1983), 361–70.

82. B. Lowe, K. Kroenke, K. Grafe, Detecting and monitoring depression with a two-item questionnaire (PHQ-2). *J. Psychosom. Res.* **58** (2005), 163–71.

83. B. Lowe, J. Unutzer, C. M. Callahan, A. J. Perkins, K. Kroenke, Monitoring depression treatment outcomes with the patient health questionnaire-9. *Med. Care* **42** (2004), 1194–201.

84. V. Henkel, R. Mergl, J. C. Coyne, *et al.*, Screening for depression in primary care: will one or two items suffice? *Eur. Arch. Psychiatry Clin. Neurosci.* **254** (2004), 215–23.

85. R. L. Spitzer, J. B. Williams, K. Kroenke, *et al.*, Utility of a new procedure for diagnosing mental disorders in primary care: the PRIME-MD 1000 study. *J. Am. Med. Assoc.* **272** (1994), 1749–56.

86. A. C. Leon, J. E. Kelsey, A. Pleil, *et al.*, An evaluation of a computer assisted telephone interview for screening for mental disorders among primary care patients. *J. Nerv. Ment. Dis.* **187** (1999), 308–11.

87. S. Fechner-Bates, J. C. Coyne, T. L. Schwenk, The relationship of self-reported distress to depressive disorders and other psychopathology. *J. Consult. Clin. Psychol.* **62** (1994), 550–9.

88. K. Shimizu, T. Akechi, M. Okamura, *et al.*, Usefulness of the nurse-assisted screening and psychiatric referral program. *Cancer* **103** (2005), 1949–56.

89. S. A. McLachlan, A. Allenby, J. Matthews, *et al.*, Randomized trial of coordinated psychosocial interventions based on patient self-assessments versus standard care to improve the psychosocial functioning of patients with cancer. *J. Clin. Oncol.* **19** (2001), 4117–25.

90. S. C. Palmer, J. C. Coyne, Screening for depression in medical care: pitfalls, alternatives, and revised priorities. *J. Psychosom. Res.* **54** (2003), 279–87.

91. A. J. Roth, A. B. Kornblith, L. Batel-Copel, *et al.*, Rapid screening for psychologic distress in men with prostate carcinoma: a pilot study. *Cancer* **82** (1998), 1904–8.

92. P. Maguire, Improving communication with cancer patients. *Eur. J. Cancer* **35** (1999), 1415–22.

93. C. Dean, Psychiatric morbidity following mastectomy: preoperative predictors and types of illness. *J. Psychosom. Res.* **31** (1987), 385–92.

94. J. Harrison, P. Maguire, Predictors of psychiatric morbidity in cancer patients. *Br. J. Psychiatry* **165** (1994), 593–8.

95. J. S. McDaniel, D. L. Musselman, C. B. Nemerof, Cancer and depression: Theory and treatment. *Psychiatr. Ann.* **27** (1997), 360–64.

96. D. L. Evans, D. S. Charney, L. Lewis, *et al.*, Mood disorders in the medically ill: scientific review and recommendations. *Biol. Psychiaty* **58** (2005), 175–89.

97. D. Razavi, J. F. Allilaire, M. Smith, *et al.*, The effect of fluoxetine on anxiety and depression symptoms in cancer patients. *Acta Psychiatr. Scand.* **94** (1996), 205–10.

98. A. K. Koike, J. Unutzer, K. B. Wells, Improving the care for depression in patients with comorbid medical illness. *Am. J. Psychiatry* **159** (2002), 1738–45.

99. T. Sheard, P. Maguire, The effect of psychological interventions on anxiety and depression in cancer patients results of two meta-analyses. *Br. J. Cancer* **80** (1999), 1770–80.

100. A. M. Nezu, C. M. Nezu, S. H. Felgoise, K. S. McClure, P. S. Houts, Project Genesis: assessing the efficacy of problem-solving therapy for distressed adult cancer patients. *J. Consult. Clin. Psychol.* **71** (2003), 1036–48.

101. M. J. Fisch, P. J. Loehrer, J. Kristeller, *et al.*, Fluoxetine versus placebo in advanced cancer outpatients: a double-blinded trial of the Hoosier Oncology Group. *J. Clin. Oncol.* **21** (2003), 1937–43.

102. J. C. Coyne, S. C. Palmer, P. J. Shapiro, Prescribing antidepressants to advanced cancer patients with mild depressive symptoms is not justified. *J. Clin. Oncol.* **22** (2004), 205–6.

103. B. A. Erwin, P. A. Sullivan, T. R. ten Have, Trial of antidepressants for mildly depressed cancer patients should have been reported in a manner allowing independent evaluation of investigators' claims. *J. Clin. Oncol.* **22** (2004), 753–4.

104. C. Moynihan, J. M. Bliss, J. Davidson, L. Burchell, A. Horwich, Evaluation of adjuvant psychological therapy in patients with testicular cancer: randomised controlled trial. *Br. Med. J.* **316** (1998), 429–35.

105. M. Sharpe, V. Strong, K. Allen, *et al.*, Management of major depression in outpatients attending a cancer centre: a preliminary evaluation of a multicomponent cancer nurse-delivered intervention. *Br. J. Cancer* **90** (2004), 310–13.

106. W. Sollner, S. Maislinger, A. Konig, A. Devries, P. Lukas, Providing psychosocial support for breast cancer patients based on screening for distress within a consultation-liaison service. *Psychooncology.* **13** (2004), 893–7.

107. P. J. Shapiro, J. C. Coyne, L. K. Kruus, *et al.*, Interest in services among prostate cancer patients receiving androgen deprivation therapy. *Psychooncology* **13** (2004), 512–25.

108. E. G. Eakin, L. A. Strycker, Awareness and barriers to use of cancer support and information resources by HMO patients with breast, prostate, or colon cancer: patient and provider perspectives. *Psychooncology* **10** (2001), 103–13.

109. J. C. Holland, History of psycho-oncology overcoming attitudinal and conceptual barriers. *Psychosom. Med.* **64** (2002), 206–21.

110. M. Beutel, G. Henrich, A. Sellschopp, M. Keller, W. Adermayer, Needs and utilization of ambulatory psychosocial services by cancer patients – exemplified by the oncologic day clinic. *Psychother. Psychosom. Med. Psychol.* **46** (1996), 304–11.

111. R. E. Gray, M. Fitch, C. Davis, C. Phillips, Interviews with men with prostate cancer about their self-help group experience. *J. Palliat. Care* **13** (1997), 15–21.

112. K. N. Moore, A. Estey, The early post-operative concerns of men after radical prostatectomy. *J. Adv. Nurs.* **29** (1999), 1121–9.

113. F. Wong, D. E. Stewart, J. Dancey, *et al.*, Men with prostate cancer: influence of psychological factors on informational needs and decision making. *J. Psychosom. Res.* **49** (2000), 13–9.

114. P. J. Goodwin, M. Leszcz, G. Quirt, *et al.*, Lessons learned from enrollment in the BEST study: a multicenter, randomized trial of group psychosocial support in metastatic breast cancer. *J. Clin. Epidemiol.* **53** (2000), 47–55.

115. D. A. Regier, W. E. Narrow, D. S. Rae, *et al.*, The de facto US mental and addictive disorders service system: Epidemiologic Catchment Area prospective 1-year prevalence rates of disorders and services. *Arch. Gen. Psychiatry* **50** (1993), 85–94.

116. P. A. Sullivan, J. C. Coyne, S. C. Palmer, J. M. Metz, Antidepressant use in breast cancer patients: an Oncolink study. Presented at the 27th annual meeting of the American Society of Preventive Oncology, Philadelphia, PA, 3 March 2003.

117. W. J. Katon, J. Unutzer, G. Simon, Treatment of depression in primary care: where we are, where we can go. *Med. Care* **42** (2004), 1153–7.

118. J. W. Williams, Jr, C. D. Mulrow, E. Chiquette, *et al.*, A systematic review of newer pharmacotherapies for depression in adults: evidence report summary. *Ann. Intern. Med.* **132** (2000), 743–56.

119. W. Katon, K. M. Von, E. Lin, *et al.*, Collaborative management to achieve treatment guidelines: impact on depression in primary care. *J. Am. Med. Assoc.* **273** (1995), 1026–31.

120. J. C. Coyne, S. C. Palmer, P. A. Sullivan, Is case-finding an inefficient way of addressing depression as a public health problem? *Pharmacoepidemiol. Drug Saf.* **11** (2002), 545–7.

121. D. S. Brody, Improving the management of depression in primary care: recent accomplishments and ongoing challenges. *Dis. Manage Health Outcomes* **11** (2003), 21–31.

122. T. E. Oxman, A. J. Dietrich, H. C. Schulberg, The depression care manager and mental health specialist as collaborators within primary care. *Am. J. Geriatr. Psychiatry* **11** (2003), 507–16.

123. H. C. Schulberg, C. Bryce, K. Chism, *et al.*, Managing late-life depression in primary care practice: a case study of the health specialist's role. *Int. J. Geriatr. Psychiatry* **16** (2001), 577–84.

124. E. M. Hunkeler, J. F. Meresman, W. A. Hargreaves, *et al.*, Efficacy of nurse telehealth care and peer support in augmenting treatment of depression in primary care. *Arch. Fam. Med.* **9** (2000), 700–708.

125. G. E. Simon, M. VonKorff, C. Rutter, E. Wagner, Randomised trial of monitoring, feedback, and management of care by telephone to improve treatment of depression in primary care. *Br. Med. J.* **320** (2000), 550–54.

126. V. Strong, M. Sharpe, A. Cull, *et al.*, Can oncology nurses treat depression? A pilot project. *J. Adv. Nurs.* **46** (2004), 542–8.

127. M. Dwight-Johnson, K. Ell, P. J. Lee, Can collaborative care address the needs of low-income Latinas with comorbid depression and cancer? Results from a randomized pilot study. *Psychosomatics* **46** (2005), 224–32.

128. J. Lemon, S. Edelman, Perceptions of the 'mind-cancer' relationship among the public, cancer patients, and oncologists. *J. Psychosoc. Oncol.* **21** (2004), 43–58.

129. B. D. Doan, R. E. Gray, C. S. Davis, Belief in psychological effects on cancer. *Psychooncology* **2** (1993), 139–50.

130. B. L. Andersen, W. B. Farrar, D. M. Golden-Kreutz, *et al.*, Psychological, behavioral, and immune changes after a psychological intervention: a clinical trial. *J. Clin. Oncol.* **22** (2004), 3570–80.

131. H. Faller, M. Schmidt, Prognostic value of depressive coping and depression in survival of lung cancer patients. *Psychooncology* **13** (2004), 359–63.

132. F. Efficace, L. Biganzoli, M. Piccart, *et al.*, Baseline health-related quality-of-life data as prognostic factors in a phase III multicentre study of women with metastatic breast cancer. *Eur. J. Cancer* **40** (2004), 1021–30.

133. P. J. Goodwin, M. Leszcz, M. Ennis, *et al.*, The effect of group psychosocial support on survival in metastatic breast cancer. *N. Engl. J. Med.* **345** (2001), 1719–26.

134. F. Efficace, P. Therasse, M. J. Piccart, *et al.*, Health-related quality of life parameters as prognostic factors in a nonmetastatic breast cancer population an international multicenter study. *J. Clin. Oncol.* **22** (2004), 3381–8.

135. B. Garssen, Psychological factors and cancer development: evidence after 30 years of research. *Clin. Psychol. Rev.* **24** (2004), 315–38.

136. S. Greer, T. Morris, K. W. Pettingale, Psychological response to breast cancer: effect on outcome. *Lancet* **2** (1979), 785–7.

137. M. Watson, J. S. Haviland, S. Greer, J. Davidson, J. M. Bliss, Influence of psychological response on survival in breast cancer: a population-based cohort study. *Lancet* **354** (1999), 1331–6.

138. M. Watson, J. Homewood, J. Haviland, J. M. Bliss, Influence of psychological response on breast cancer survival: 10-year follow-up of a population-based cohort. *Eur. J. Cancer* **41** (2005), 1665–6.

139. D. Spiegel, J. R. Bloom, H. C. Kraemer, E. Gottheil, Effect of psychosocial treatment on survival of patients with metastatic breast cancer. *Lancet* **2** (1989), 888–91.

140. D. Spiegel, Effects of psychotherapy on cancer survival. *Nat. Rev. Cancer* **2** (2002), 383–9.

141. F. I. Fawzy, N. W. Fawzy, C. S. Hyun, *et al.*, Malignant melanoma: effects of an early structured psychiatric intervention, coping, and affective state on recurrence and survival 6 years later. *Arch. Gen. Psychiatry* **50** (1993), 681–9.

142. J. L. Richardson, D. R. Shelton, M. Krailo, A. M. Levine, The effect of compliance with treatment on survival among patients with hematologic malignancies. *J. Clin. Oncol.* **8** (1990), 356–64.

143. T. Kuchler, D. Henne-Bruns, S. Rappat, *et al.*, Impact of psychotherapeutic support on gastrointestinal cancer patients undergoing surgery: survival results of a trial. *Hepatogastroenterology* **46** (1999), 322–35.

144. R. McCorkle, N. E. Strumpf, I. F. Nuamah, *et al.*, A specialized home care intervention improves survival among older post-surgical cancer patients. *J. Am. Geriatr. Soc.* **48** (2000), 1707–13.

145. M. W. Linn, B. S. Linn, R. Harris, Effects of counseling for late stage cancer patients. *Cancer* **49** (1982), 1048–55.

146. A. Ilnyckyj, J. Farber, M. Cheang, B. Weinerman, A randomized controlled trial of psychotherapeutic intervention in cancer patients. *Ann. R. Coll. Physicians Surg. Can.* **27** (1994), 93–6.

147. A. J. Cunningham, C. V. Edmonds, G. P. Jenkins, *et al.*, A randomized controlled trial of the effects of group psychological therapy on survival in women with metastatic breast cancer. *Psychooncology* **7** (1998), 508–17.

148. S. Edelman, J. Lemon, D. R. Bell, A. D. Kidman, Effects of group CBT on the survival time of patients with metastatic breast cancer. *Psychooncology* **8** (1999), 474–81.

149. S. C. Palmer, J. C. Coyne, Examining the evidence that psychotherapy improves the survival of cancer patients. *Biol. Psychiatry* **56** (2004), 61–2.

150. N. Frasure-Smith, F. Lesperance, Reflections on depression as a cardiac risk factor. *Psychosom. Med.* **67**: Suppl 1 (2005), 19–25.

151. F. Lesperance, N. Frasure-Smith, The seduction of death. *Psychosom. Med.* **61** (1999), 18–20.

11

Depression and obesity

Lucy Cooke and Jane Wardle

Introduction

It is estimated that at least 300 million people worldwide are obese and two to three times more are overweight [1]. Rates vary enormously from country to country, but the situation in the USA is particularly alarming: current figures suggest that over 65% of US adults are overweight, of whom over 30% are obese (body mass index [BMI] $\geq$ 30) and almost 5% are severely obese (BMI $\geq$ 40) [2]. Although associations between obesity and physical health consequences such as diabetes, heart disease and cancer, as well as all-cause mortality, are well documented [3–6], the psychological impact of obesity remains poorly characterised.

In the heyday of psychosomatics, obesity was believed to be a consequence of either misinterpreting emotional arousal as hunger or using food as a form of self-medication in order to cope with distress [7]. Obese people were assumed to have extensive psychopathology, and the treatment of choice was psychotherapy. However, when larger-scale epidemiological studies were carried out, it became clear that there were no systematic differences in either personality or rates of psychiatric illness between obese and normal-weight adults [8]. With time, the psychosomatic theory lost ground as a basis for management of obesity, but interest in the link with depression has lived on. Recent years have seen evidence that stress is associated with adiposity [9,10], and both cortisol and leptin have been implicated in linking the hypothalamic-pituitary-adrenocortical (HPA) axis and adipose tissue [11,12]. Along with new ideas on the role of 'comfort foods' as moderators of HPA function [13], interest has revived in the idea that distress could contribute to overeating and overweight.

The major emphasis in contemporary research is on the emotional consequences of obesity, reflecting the range of difficulties faced by obese people living in Western countries, where fatness is widely regarded as abhorrent. Negative attitudes towards

Depression and Physical Illness, ed. A. Steptoe.
Published by Cambridge University Press. © Cambridge University Press 2006.

obesity are compounded by it being stereotyped as self-inflicted: the result of laziness, greed and other failures of self-control [14]. Hostile social attitudes towards obesity have resulted in discrimination, social exclusion and bullying, which have been documented across a variety of educational, occupational and social settings [15]. The psychosocial adversities come on top of the functional limitations imposed by adiposity itself or its comorbidities. This heavy burden of social, psychological and physical difficulties is understandably assumed to greatly increase the risk of depression.

In 1995, Friedman and Brownell published a seminal review examining the psychological correlates of obesity [16]. Since that time, there have been three more reviews of the adult literature [17–19]. This chapter summarises the findings of earlier reviews and presents a more detailed examination of recent research into associations between obesity and depression in both community-based and clinical samples. We also include tables covering the principal studies in the field since the publication of Friedman and Brownell's review.

Community-based cross-sectional studies

In their review of the literature, Friedman and Brownell [16] included a meta-analysis of four community-based studies. This revealed a very small and non-significant association between obesity and depression (Pearson's $r = -0.06$), although there was significant variation between studies, with positive results reported by Istvan and colleagues [20] in women but not in men and negative results reported by Wadden *et al.* [21], Stewart and Brook [22] and Seegers and Mertens [23]. More recently, Faith *et al.* [17] updated the literature review and concluded similarly that the majority of community studies find no significant association, but they also noted that some individual studies have reported positive associations, e.g. [24,25]. Both reviews raised the possibility that heterogeneity in sample selection and measures of depression, and inaccurate assessments of adiposity in some studies, could disguise stronger associations between obesity and depression in some population groups. Table 11.1 gives details of some important community-based cross-sectional studies published since 1995.

One of the largest studies of recent years [26] looked at relationships between weight and suicidal ideation, suicide attempts, and past-year major depressive disorder in over 40 000 national survey respondents who were interviewed face to face. Unadjusted analyses using a categorical indicator of weight status showed that although the obese group had increased odds of suicide ideation relative to all other respondents, there were no differences in suicide attempts or depression. However, the associations between weight status and psychiatric outcomes differed for men and women. Relative to men with a BMI less than 30, obese men (BMI $\geq$ 30) had

Table 11.1 Large-scale community-based cross-sectional studies, 1995–2004

Ref.	Sample details	Measure of obesity	Measure of depression	Association between obesity and depression	Gender differences	Comments
Bin Li et al. [34]	n = 56 167 Over 65 years old (Chinese)	BMI (measured) Obese = BMI ≥ 25	Geriatric Depression Scale (interview)	Obesity related to lower risk of depression	Not tested	Significant linear trend with depressive symptoms decreasing with increasing BMI
Carpenter et al. [26]	n = 40 086 Mean age 44 years (African American and white)	BMI (self-report) Obese = BMI ≥ 30	AUDADIS (interview)	No significant effect on depression overall	Significant gender by weight status interaction – lower risk of depression in obese men and higher risk in obese women	No significant interaction with race
Dong et al. [29]	n = 482 families (n = 2103 individuals) (African and European Americans)	BMI (measured) Obese = BMI ≥ 30	Structured questionnaire on depression, anxiety and suicide (interview)	Significant association between obesity and depression	Not tested	Effect still significant after controlling for chronic disease and other potential confounders, although measure of chronic illness was somewhat basic Stronger effect in BMI > 40
Jorm et al. [30]	n = 2280 age 20–24 years n = 1334 age 40–44 years n = 2305 age 60–64 years (Australian)	BMI (self-report) Obese = BMI ≥ 30	Goldberg Depression Scale (Questionnaire)	Significant association between obesity and depression	Interaction not tested Effects seen in men and women	After controlling for confounders the effect was reversed – underweight women were most depressed; overweight and obese women were least depressed

Study	Sample	BMI (obesity definition)	Measure	Results	Gender interaction	Comments
Johnston et al. [27]	n = 2482 adults (Canadian)	BMI (measured) Obese = BMI ≥ 30	CES-D (questionnaire)	More obese participants met the clinical cut-off point for depression	Not tested	Tables giving CES-D mean scores by age, gender and weight status show a somewhat variable effect
Kaplan et al. [33]	n = 12 823 Over 65 years old (Canadian)	BMI (self-report) Obese = BMI ≥ 30	Psychological Distress (6 items) (telephone interview)	Significant association between psychological distress and obesity	Psychological distress and obesity significantly associated in women; in men the same association was not quite significant	Unadjusted analyses would probably have shown stronger effects but are not presented here
Onyike et al. [28]	N = 84 1015 39 years old (North American)	BMI (measured) Obese = BMI ≥ 30	DIS (interview)	Significant association with past month depression	No evidence of interaction between gender and obesity Significant effect in women; same effect size was not quite significant in men	Adjusted odds ratios for obesity (BMI > 30) were rendered non-significant, but effect in severely obese people (BMI > 40) remained strong and significant
* Roberts et al. [45]	N = 2298 Alameda County Study participants Over 50 years old	BMI (self-report) Obese = > 85th percentile	DSM-12D (questionnaire)	Significant association between obesity and depression	Not tested in cross-sectional analyses	Effect still significant in adjusted analyses Using BMI > 30 as definition of obese, effect was significant in unadjusted but non-significant after adjusting for confounders

*This study included a one-year follow-up. AUDADIS, Alcohol Use Disorders and Associated Disabilities Schedule; BMI, body mass index; CES-D, Center for Epidemiologic Studies Depression Scale; DIS, Diagnostic Interview Schedule; DSM-12D, Diagnostic and Statistical Manual 12-Item Depression Scale.

decreased odds of a major depressive disorder and of suicide attempts, whereas obese women had increased odds of past-year major depression compared with other women. This was a much more striking gender difference than had been found previously [20] and renewed interest in the role of gender as a moderating variable. It also had implications for mechanisms, suggesting that social attitudes to obesity – assumed to be more severe for women – may play an important part.

Researchers in Canada, using data from the Nova Scotia Health Survey [27] found that a significantly higher proportion of obese than normal-weight respondents had Center for Epidemiologic Study Depression Scale (CES-D) scores within the clinical range. Onyike and colleagues [28] used data on young adults (aged 15–39 years) from the third National Health and Nutrition Examination Survey (NHANES III) to examine the relationship between obesity and past-month, past-year, lifetime and recurrent major depression. Odds ratios (OR) for the association between weight status and past-month depression were significantly increased for obese people, especially severely obese (BMI > 40) individuals. The relationship between severe obesity and past-month depression remained strong and significant in adjusted analyses. Significant effects were found for both men and women, although neither of these studies specifically tested the gender by weight-status interactions. Onyike *et al.*'s finding of stronger effects in participants with a BMI over 40 highlights the fact that most older studies did not examine *severity* of obesity as a moderating variable. In many Western countries, a BMI over 30 is so common in some gender/race/age groups that the adverse social effects may come into play only at higher levels of obesity. In fact, this remains a neglected area, although an exception is a family-based study [29] that examined the relationship between depression and obesity and found a stronger association in severely obese individuals that held across race and gender.

Jorm and colleagues [30] investigated the association between weight status and emotional wellbeing in a sample of over 2000 people in each of three age groups (20–24 years, 40–44 years, 60–64 years) and also addressed issues of possible confounding by demographic factors and health status. Overall and for both sexes separately, a significant association between obesity and depression was observed. However, when physical ill-health, lack of physical activity, low social support, low education and financial problems were controlled for, a different picture emerged, with the underweight women being more depressed and obese women having relatively better mental health than the normal-weight group. Physical health alone accounted for all of the association between obesity and depression in women.

Several studies over the years have specifically examined middle-aged or older populations, where obesity levels are higher. Two studies that have examined the link between depression and abdominal adiposity in middle-aged women [25] and men [31] reported positive associations between depression and abdominal obesity that were stronger than associations with BMI and that remained significant after adjusting for BMI. Cross-sectional analyses of data from the Alameda County Study revealed that obese participants (BMI ≥ 30) aged 50 years or older were more than twice as likely to be depressed than their non-obese counterparts [32]. Kaplan *et al.* [33] examined data from 12 823 Canadian community dwellers aged 65 and over. Obesity was related to high psychological distress overall, although in men the association did not reach significance. The presence of comorbid physical conditions, as well as a number of other potential confounds, was controlled for in these analyses, and it is likely therefore that unadjusted odds ratios would have been considerably higher. In contrast, a study of 56 167 elderly Chinese men and women enrolled as members of 'elderly health centres' reported data showing that obese individuals of both sexes were approximately 20% less likely to suffer from depressive symptoms than those of normal weight [34]. The authors explain that in Chinese culture, there is an association between happiness or good fortune and body fat, and this may be protective against depressive symptoms.

Taken together, these studies suggest that at least in Western countries, obesity, particularly severe obesity, is associated with depression, especially among women. Overall, the size of the association is modest. In Onyike and colleagues' [28] data, for example, past-month depression rates were increased from 2.8% to 5.1%. This is important in public health terms but highlights the fact that the majority of obese people in community samples are not depressed. The few studies that have examined physical health consequences have raised the possibility that poor physical health might play an important role in explaining why some obese people are depressed, but results have been mixed [30,33] and more research is needed.

Community-based prospective studies

Cross-sectional studies can identify associations between obesity and depression but are unable to address the direction of causation: does depression raise the risk of obesity, or does obesity raise the risk of depression? Prospective data can provide a temporal perspective that is informative but not definitive, but to date very few studies have been published (see Table 11.2 for details of community-based prospective studies published since 1995). An early study [35] reported that the most severely depressed of a sample of 800 middle-aged women were at greatest risk of subsequent weight gain, and the effect was independent of the use of psychotropic drugs. However, these results were not confirmed by DiPietro *et al.* [36], who reported an extremely complex association by which depressed older adults (> 55 years old) lost more weight than their non-depressed peers, whereas depressed younger men gained more weight and depressed younger women gained less weight; neither have studies of depressed samples found higher rates of obesity [37].

Table 11.2 Community-based prospective studies, 1995–2004

Ref.	Sample details	Measure of obesity	Measure of depression	Baseline obesity associated with depression at follow-up?	Baseline depression associated with obesity at follow-up?	Gender differences	Controlled for	Comments
Bardone et al. [38]	$n = 459$ girls Age 15 years at baseline (New Zealanders)	BMI (measured)	DISC-C (interview)	Not tested	Adolescent depression did not predict BMI at follow-up at age 21 years	Not tested	SES, age at menarche, absence of father figure, parental smoking, childhood health, maternal health and maternal BMI	
Barefoot et al. [42]	$n = 3560$ (mostly men) <25 years old at baseline (North American)	BMI (measured at baseline, self-report at follow-up)	MMPI (OBD subscale) at baseline; NEOPI (depression subscale) at follow-up (questionnaires)	Not tested	No main effect of depression, but those with high baseline depression gained less weight than non-depressed if they were initially lean but more if they were initially heavy; trend strongest in those who were more depressed at baseline and follow-up	Gender by depression interaction was not significant	Gender, baseline BMI, gender by BMI interaction, exercise, smoking	Lack of gender effects might have been due to small number of women in this sample
Hasler et al. [43]	$n = 591$ Age 19–40 years (Swiss)	BMI (self-report) Overweight = BMI ≥ 25	SPIKE (interview)	Being overweight and increased weight gain associated with atypical depression in men and women but not with major, recurrent brief, or minor depression	Not tested	No	Substance use, levels of physical activity, demographic variables, family history of weight problems	Association not stronger if higher thresholds for defining overweight (BMI > 27.5 or BMI > 30.0) used

Study	Sample	BMI/obesity measure	Depression measure		Findings	Gender interaction	Confounders adjusted for	Comments
Pine et al. [39]	n = 644 Aged 9–18 years at baseline (North American)	BMI (self-report) Obese = BMI > 80th percentile	DIS-C (interview)	Not tested.	Obesity in young adulthood related to adolescent depression in the whole sample	Yes: obesity associated with adult depression in both genders, but negative association in males and positive in females	Age, gender, ethnicity, parental social class, parental sociopathy, physical health status, childhood IQ, smoking and alcohol	Associations persisted after controlling for potential confounding variables
Pine et al. [40]	n = 90 with major depression n = 87 with no psychiatric disorder Aged 6–17 years at baseline (USA)	BMI (measured at baseline, self-report at follow-up)	Schedule for Affective Disorders (interview)	Not tested	Depression in childhood associated positively with BMI in adulthood; duration of depression also emerged as predictor of adult BMI	No gender by depression interaction	Age, gender social class, ethnicity, physical health status, number of pregnancies, smoking, alcohol/medication use	
Richardson et al. [41]	n = 1037 Aged 11 years at baseline (New Zealanders)	BMI (measured) Obese = BMI ≥ 30	DIS-C (interview)	Not tested	Adjusted for baseline BMI, depressed late adolescent girls were more than twice as likely to be obese at 26 years than non-depressed	Yes: girls only; no relationship among boys, nor in either gender for depression in early adolescence	Childhood BMI, gender, parental obesity, SES, maternal depression	Dose–response relationship observed with number of episodes of depression (N.B. same cohort as Bardone et al. [38])
Roberts et al. [32, 44]	Participants in the Alameda County Study n = 1739 (2002) n = 2123 (2003) Mean age 63 years (waves of data 1994–95 and 1999)	BMI (self-report) Obese = BMI ≥ 30 (2002 and 2003)	DSM-12D (questionnaire)	Greater relative risk for depression at 5-year follow-up among those who were obese at baseline	Relationship did not operate in reverse direction – depression at baseline did not predict obesity at follow-up (2003)	No significant obesity–gender interaction	Age, gender, education, marital status, mental health problems at baseline, social isolation, social support, chronic medical problems, functional impairment, life events, financial strain, physical activity	

BMI, body mass index; DIS-C, Diagnostic Interview Schedule for Children; DISC-C, Diagnostic Interview Schedule for Children; DSM-12D, Diagnostic and Statistical Manual 12-Item Depression Scale; MMPI, Minnesota Multiphasic Personality Inventory; NEOPI, NEO Personality Inventory; OBD, Obvious Depression Scale; SES, socioeconomic status; SPIKE, Structured Psychopathological Interview and Rating of the Social Consequences for Epidemiology.

The possibility that depression in early life might have even more adverse consequences on future weight trajectories has been addressed in several studies looking at adolescent depression as a predictor of adult obesity, with mixed results. The Dunedin Multidisciplinary Health and Development study failed to find a greater risk of early adult obesity among depressed adolescents in New Zealand [38]. Similarly, a study of over 700 North American adolescents found that an association between depression in childhood and adult BMI was rendered non-significant when conduct disorder symptoms were controlled for [39]. However, two more recent studies have reported positive results. In the first of these, a small sample ($n = 90$) of children aged between 6 and 17 years with major depression were followed up after 10–15 years [40]. At baseline, depressed children did not differ in BMI from healthy controls, but at follow-up they were on average almost two BMI points above the healthy controls (26.1 vs. 24.2), a difference that appeared not to be explained by a number of confounding factors, including medication history. In addition, duration of depression emerged as a predictor of adult BMI.

The second study assessed whether major depression in early or late-adolescence increased risk of obesity at 26 years of age in the Dunedin cohort [41]. After adjusting for baseline BMI, depressed late-adolescent girls were more than twice as likely to be obese as adults compared with their non-depressed peers, with a dose–response relationship with number of episodes of depression, although there was no relationship in boys, or in either sex in relation to depression in early adolescence.

One possibility, rarely explored in the epidemiological literature, is that depression may exacerbate pre-existing weight-change tendencies. In their sample of college students, Barefoot and colleagues [42] found no main effect of depression but found a significant interaction between depression status and baseline BMI, such that individuals with high baseline depression scores gained less weight than their non-depressed peers if they were lean at baseline, but gained more weight if they were overweight at baseline.

The alternative direction of causation is that obesity is a risk factor for development of depression. In a community sample of young adults, Hasler *et al.* [43] found that being consistently overweight in early adulthood was associated with atypical but not typical depression, but the fact that overeating is part of the clinical diagnosis of atypical depression suggests that the mechanism is unlikely to be a true effect of weight on depression. Again using data from the Alameda County Study, Roberts and colleagues [44,45] found that obese older adults (> 50 years of age at baseline) were at increased risk of subsequent depression. In an attempt to clarify the temporal relation between the two factors, the researchers looked at two waves of data collected five years apart [32]. Individuals who were obese at baseline were at increased risk of depression five years later, but no evidence was found to support the reverse hypothesis.

Uncertainty remains as to the temporal relationship, if any, between depression and obesity, partly because so few prospective studies have been attempted to date. There is evidence to support both causal pathways, although effects are not always large. As with cross-sectional studies, some findings suggest an increased vulnerability among women, e.g. [41].

Studies with clinical samples of obese individuals

This section focuses on studies of individuals seeking treatment for obesity, although a parallel literature has investigated weight status in clinically depressed individuals. It appears that different types of depressive symptom are associated with different patterns of weight change. For example, patients with more melancholic features tend to lose weight, while those with atypical features appear to gain weight, although a large-scale study found that increasing BMI was related to a linear decrease in symptoms, 'reduced appetite' and 'pessimistic thoughts' [46]. Understanding this relationship is made problematic by the fact that the majority of currently prescribed antidepressants are associated with weight gain over the course of treatment (see Schwartz *et al.* [47] for a review).

Numerous studies have documented elevated rates of depression among obese individuals seeking treatment (typically gastric surgery), although the degree to which findings are genuinely informative depends upon the groups with whom the treatment-seekers have been compared. Studies have variously employed published norms [48–51], normal-weight controls [52–54], non-treatment-seeking obese controls [53–57] and even seekers of different types of obesity treatment [57,58] as comparison groups.

More recent studies of obese patients have generally confirmed the older literature in finding large excesses of lifetime prevalence of depression [49] and current depression as measured by the Beck Depression Inventory (BDI) [48,51] or the Brief Symptom Inventory (BSI) [50] (see Table 11.3 for details of cross-sectional studies in clinical populations). Friedman and Brownell's [16] meta-analysis of three studies [52,59,60] found a moderate effect size (mean $d = 0.52$) that was consistent across studies. A more recent study [53] compared obese adolescent and young adult in-patients with both normal-weight controls and obese controls. A far greater percentage of in-patients met *Diagnostic and Statistical Manual of Mental Disorders*, 4th edn (DSM-IV) criteria for a mood disorder compared with either obese or normal-weight controls, who did not differ from each other. However, the BMI of in-patients was significantly higher than that of obese controls, making it impossible to ascertain whether their elevated rates of mood disorder related to their treatment-seeking status or the severity of their obesity.

Table 11.3 Cross-sectional studies of clinical samples, 1995–2004

Ref.	Sample details	Measure of obesity	Measure of depression	Main findings	Other results	Obese treatment seekers more depressed than non-obese controls or population norms	Obese treatment seekers more depressed than obese controls
Britz et al. [53]	n = 47 obese in-patients n = 47 obese controls n = 1608 controls Aged 15–21 years (German)	BMI	M-CIDI (interview)	Clinical group had significantly higher rates of all disorders; no differences between obese controls and population controls	In most, psychiatric disorders emerged after onset of obesity; population-based obese had significantly lower BMI than clinical group	Yes	Yes
Elfhag et al. [48]	n = 120 obese patients (Swedish)	BMI	BDI (questionnaire)	Depression not related to degree of obesity, but high rates overall		Yes	Not tested
Fontaine et al. [55]	n = 312 seeking out-patient weight-loss treatment Mean age 39 years n = 89 obese not seeking treatment Mean age 36.4 years (North American)	BMI	SF-36 (questionnaire)	Treatment seekers no more depressed than non-treatment seekers, although treatment seekers were heavier and experienced more physical problems		N/A	No

Glinski et al. [49]	n = 115 GBP surgery patients (North American)	MMPI-2 (interview)	High prevalence of depression (56% lifetime, 19% current) Significantly higher than prevalence in the general population		Yes	Not tested
Higgs et al. [58]	n = 20 obese surgery candidates Mean age 39.95 years n = 18 seeking dietary intervention Mean age 46.8 years (Australian)	BMI Obese = BMI ≥ 30	Surgery candidates significantly more distressed than those seeking support for dietary restriction	Surgery candidates had higher BMI, but this was controlled in all analyses	Not tested	Not tested
Kolotkin et al. [57]	n = 3353 varying in treatment-seeking status and intensity of treatment sought Aged 18–90 years (North American)	BMI	Obesity-specific QOL most impaired in those with highest BMI, white people and women	Treatment seekers more impaired than non-treatment seekers QOL varied with intensity of treatment sought Most intense = most impairment	Not tested	Yes
Kolotkin et al. [56]	n = 339 surgical cases n = 87 obese controls (North American)	BMI Diagnosis of depression by primary care provider	QOL significantly lower and depression rates higher in surgery candidates	BMI, gender, treatment-seeking status and depression accounted for most variance in QOL	Not tested	Yes

(cont.)

Table 11.3 (cont.)

Ref.	Sample details	Measure of obesity	Measure of depression	Main findings	Other results	Obese treatment seekers more depressed than non-obese controls or population norms	Obese treatment seekers more depressed than obese controls
Laferrere et al. [50]	n = 145 obese women Mean age 46.3 years (African American and white American)	BMI	BSI, LDI (questionnaire)	BSI depression slightly above non-obese control population	No racial differences	Yes	Not tested
Marchesini et al. [51]	n = 207 obese treatment seekers (Italian)	BMI	BDI (questionnaire)	43% had BDI scores indicative of depression	Significantly related to poor QOL	Yes	Not tested
Musante et al. [61]	n = 1184 patients of residential weight-loss programme Mean age 47 years (North American)	BMI Obese = BMI ≥ 30	BDI (questionnaire)	BDI scores above general population norms; those with moderate to severe depression had significantly higher BMI than those with none, mild or moderate depression	Gender differences in predictors of comorbid depression	Yes	Not tested
Ryden et al. [62]	n = 2510 Aged 37–57 years (Swedish)	BMI	Measure of distress devised for the SOS study (questionnaire)	Surgical candidates reported significantly higher levels of distress than conventional treatment seekers		Not tested	Not tested

BDI, Beck Depression Inventory; BMI, body mass index; BSI, Brief Symptom Inventory; GBP, gastric bypass; IWQOL, Impact of Weight on Quality of Life; LDI, Life Distress Inventory; M-CIDI, Munich Composite International Diagnostic Interview; MMPI-2, Minnesota Multiphasic Personality Interview 2; N/A, not applicable; QOL, quality of life; SCL-90-R, Symptom Checklist 90, revised; SF-36, Medical Outcomes Study Short Form Health Survey; SOS, Symptom Onset in Schizophrenia.

There is evidence to show that individuals who seek treatment for their obesity may differ in important ways from those who do not [54–57]. Because of potential problems of interpretation, Fitzgibbon *et al.* [54] matched their three groups demographically. Treatment seekers had higher levels of psychopathology and more binge eating than the obese or normal-weight controls, but both obese groups reported more symptoms of distress than the normal-weight group. Similarly, Kolotkin *et al.* [56] reported higher rates of diagnosed depression in surgery cases than in matched non-treatment-seeking controls. However, Fontaine *et al.* [55] found that although obese individuals who had sought treatment were heavier and had a higher prevalence of chronic disease and pain than those who were not trying to lose weight, they were not more depressed.

Even within groups of treatment seekers there is variation. For example, Musante *et al.* [61] documented increased severity of depression with increasing BMI in 1184 self-admitted patients, although no such effect was observed by Elfhag and colleagues [48], albeit in a much smaller sample ($n = 120$). Most of the research in this area has looked at candidates for gastric surgery, but one study attempted to compare the health-related quality of life of overweight/obese individuals between groups differing in treatment-seeking status and treatment intensity [57]. The study found that the greater the intensity of treatment sought, the greater the impairment in quality of life experienced, although depression itself was not assessed. Two other studies also suggest that those seeking more intensive forms of treatment are significantly more distressed than those enrolled in more conventional weight-management programmes [58,62].

Intervention and treatment studies provide more powerful methods with which to examine causal pathways between obesity and depression, although, with some exceptions, most studies in this area concern outcomes after gastric surgery, which limits the possibility of assessing the impact of more typical (10%) weight losses. In addition, control groups are rarely included, and cases are simply compared with population norms, reducing the usefulness of the findings. Overall there is little doubt that, at least in the immediate post-surgery period, significant improvements in mood accompany substantial weight loss [63–66]. In a two-year follow-up of the Swedish Obese Subjects study, Ryden *et al.* [67] found that the pattern and magnitude of change in distress for individuals who had undergone surgery was the same as for those who had undergone more conventional weight-loss treatment; those who lost weight by whatever means experienced a reduction in distress, whereas weight gainers' distress levels remained the same. Positive long-term effects were documented by Dixon and colleagues [68], whose participants completed the BDI before surgery and annually thereafter. After one year, weight loss was associated with significant reductions in BDI score that were sustained up to four years post-surgery. The greatest reductions were seen in those who lost most weight, were female and were younger.

Longer-term effects may depend upon maintenance of weight loss. Wadden *et al.* [69] observed a reduction in depression following non-surgical weight-loss treatment and that was still seen at one-year follow-up. After three years, however, those who had regained their weight reverted to baseline levels of depression. On the other hand, Waters and colleagues [66] found that patients' initial postoperative improvements in psychosocial functioning had dissipated three years later, even in those who had good weight outcomes. The picture is complicated further by studies that show that a few individuals experience an onset of depression post-surgery despite substantial weight loss, e.g. [70]. This finding is consistent with the view that obesity might be psychologically beneficial to the individual, as a symbol of strength or a barrier to unwanted physical contact with others, but empirical evidence to support this assumption is lacking.

A number of other studies have investigated depression as a predictor of treatment outcomes, with mixed results. Tsushima and colleagues [71] reported no association between pre-surgery depression and post-surgery weight loss in a retrospective analysis of the Minnesota Multiphasic Personality Inventory 2 (MMPI-2) scores of 52 patients undergoing gastric bypass. Curiously, a number of studies report better outcomes in terms of weight loss and lower risk of drop-out for patients with higher levels of depression pre-treatment [72,73]. It may be, as Clark *et al.* [72] conclude, that having previously participated in treatment for psychological disorders has resulted in greater skills for lifestyle change, although no details of previous treatment were given for Inelmen *et al.*'s participants [73]. Whatever the explanation for such findings, it is clear that mental health problems should not necessarily be a barrier to obesity treatment, whether behavioural or surgical.

Moderating variables

The most common research strategy in the literature has been to examine simple associations between obesity and depression. However, both Friedman and Brownell [16] and Faith *et al.* [17] recommended further investigation of moderator/mediator models in which causal pathways within subgroups of individuals can be tested. The search for moderating variables addresses the possibility that some population subgroups might experience greater psychological consequences of obesity than others; for example, obesity might pose more of a psychological hazard for women than for men. Unfortunately, even in the more recent literature, few studies have been designed to test for moderation, and where they do power for these subgroup analyses is often limited. Nevertheless, a number of putative moderators are emerging.

Gender is one such moderator, with some studies reporting stronger associations between obesity and depression in women than in men, e.g. [26,30], although others have found no gender differences [45]. Some studies have found similar effect sizes in both sexes, but with wider confidence intervals (CI) for the male sample, reflecting the lower risk in men of both obesity and depression, e.g. [28]. Overall, the pattern of results is not sufficiently clear to conclude that gender is an important moderating variable.

Age has been examined as a moderator in some studies, with an assumption that obesity in adolescence might be particularly stressful because of the salience of appearance in this age group [74–76]. Surprisingly, there has been little evidence for a moderating effect; neither has there been any sign that the associations tend to be stronger in samples of younger adults. In fact, the effects are probably more consistently negative among adolescents than older adults [77].

Race and socioeconomic status (SES) have often been linked with the social costs of obesity and were identified by Friedman and Brownell [16] as plausible mediators. Obesity appears to carry more adverse social implications in higher-SES and white groups, perhaps because meeting appearance norms is more valued [78] or appearance norms are for smaller body sizes. Ross [79] found that being overweight increased depression among well-educated individuals (those with a college degree) but had an almost non-existent effect among poorly educated individuals; however, others have failed to find an effect of education [20,28]. Carpenter and colleagues [26] are one of the few groups to look at interactions with ethnicity; they found no evidence that obesity had a differential association with depression in African Americans compared with whites. Another study to address demographic moderators directly is an investigation of the psychological correlates of obesity in the Health and Behaviour in Teenagers (HABITS study) [80]. Weights and heights were measured in almost 5000 British adolescents aged 11–12 years and depressed mood was assessed using Goodman's Strengths and Difficulties Scale [81]. In this sample, neither the overall association between obesity and depression, nor any interactions with gender, ethnicity or SES were significant, giving no support for the role of demographic moderating variables in this population.

The severity of obesity has emerged as a moderator in most studies in which it has been addressed [28,29,61]. This could be because recent secular trends in obesity have resulted in greater acceptance of 'normal' obesity, with stigmatisation now limited to the 'super obese' (BMI > 40), although Myers and Rosen [82] found that the experience of stigmatisation increases in proportion to body mass up to a BMI of 40 and levels off thereafter. Possibly more salient is the fact that severe obesity is associated with dramatically higher rates of ill-health, which of itself is known to be linked with higher rates of depression [30,79]. If ill-health is an important mediating mechanism in the obesity-depression association, then there is a need for studies that compare levels of depression in obese patients with other clinical groups suffering comparable functional limitations before concluding that the relationship between obesity and depression has a unique status.

Binge eating

One of the most consistent markers of psychological distress – including depression – in obese patients is binge eating. According to a thorough review of the literature, there is considerable evidence that obese individuals with binge-eating disorder (BED) have higher rates of general psychiatric symptomatology (especially depression) than obese non-binge eaters [83]. More recent research tends to support this conclusion in younger adults [84], patients undergoing gastric bypass surgery [85] and weight-loss treatment seekers [86]. One study has failed to confirm the effect [87], and the authors suggest that this is because they diagnosed BED using strict DSM-IV criteria, unlike most other studies, which have overestimated its prevalence. However, with this one exception, there is general agreement that obese binge eaters are a subgroup who have more psychological difficulties.

Once the association between obesity and depression is established, the search for mediators becomes important. These are variables that lie on the causal pathway from obesity to depression; for example, experiences of social exclusion associated with obesity might be part of the causal process leading to a greater risk of depression.

The pathway through experiences of social rejection or humiliation is one important route, and a significant number of studies have focused on teasing as the marker of adverse social experiences. The literature on teasing is limited by being concerned almost exclusively with children, although some studies have looked at its impact on body dissatisfaction in adulthood [88,89]. Jackson and colleagues [89] found that a history of teasing about physical appearance was associated with both depression and body dissatisfaction. In another study examining the impact of stigmatisation and discrimination on the psychological functioning of obese individuals, more frequent exposure to stigmatisation was associated with greater psychological distress [82]. The problem with reports of teasing as the marker of social adversity is the possibility of reporting bias arising from a general negative affectivity.

Body image and dieting

Body image and dieting are related putative mechanisms. Obese people who are concerned about their weight are likely to feel more dissatisfied with their appearance (poor body image) and to take more steps to control their weight (dieting). Body dissatisfaction itself might lead to depression, or the dieting that it motivates might lead to depression. Several studies confirm that body dissatisfaction is a risk factor for depression in obese individuals. Friedman *et al.* [90] found that body-image satisfaction partially mediated the relationship between degree of overweight and depression for both men and women and was also related directly to negative affect. Likewise, Sarwer *et al.* [91] found an increased risk of depression in treatment-seeking obese individuals with more negative body image. Interestingly, overall their patients did not differ from normal-weight population controls in depression. There is evidence from population samples that body dissatisfaction – at all weight levels – is associated with depression [92], making body dissatisfaction a plausible mechanism for depression in the obese. But again there is difficulty in determining the direction of effect: does body dissatisfaction raise the risk of depression, or does depression promote dissatisfaction, or could the association be another reflection of negative affectivity?

Dieting status has also been implicated in the association between obesity and depression. Ross [79] used data from a telephone interview of a random sample of US adults aged 18–90 years and found that although overweight was related to depression after controlling for sociodemographic variables, dieting was found to increase depression and rendered its relationship with obesity non-significant. A related issue may be that of weight cycling. It is difficult to imagine that repeated failures to maintain weight loss would not have adverse psychological consequences, but the data do not provide strong support. Some cross-sectional studies have reported negative psychological effects of weight fluctuation [69,93] and others no effect [94,95]. A rare prospective study [96] failed to support an association between weight cycling and long-term adverse psychological effects, and a review by the same research group [97] suggests that conclusions that weight cycling is psychologically damaging are premature.

General methodological issues

It is important to acknowledge a number of methodological issues that dog this area of research. Depression may be assessed in many different ways, by clinical interview using DSM criteria or by one of a number of self-report questionnaires. This is not a serious problem as long as all the different measures are well validated, but it could be important if there were some subtypes of depression that were linked more strongly with obesity. There have also been differences in the timescale applied to the experience of depression: in the past month, past year, or any time in the life course. However, within the existing research, it is hard to see any consistent associations between the findings and the particular measures of depression that could make sense of the variation in results.

When defining obesity, some researchers have used BMI percentile cut-offs or BMI points (typically over 30 or greater than the eighty-fifth percentile), while others have used a continuous measure of BMI, percentage overweight or waist/hip ratio. Roberts and colleagues [45] demonstrated that findings are affected by the way in which obesity is defined. Using international BMI cut-offs (overweight > 25, obese > 30) resulted in more individuals being classified obese than age-specific US Public Health Service (USPHS) criteria had allowed and resulted in the prospective association between depression and obesity ceasing to be significant. More importantly, many studies have calculated BMI from self-reported heights and weights. Given the general tendency of individuals to underestimate their weight and overestimate their height, it may be that rates of depression at lower levels of overweight or obesity have been exaggerated.

Conclusions

Large-scale cross-sectional studies of community samples of adults suggest that obesity, and particularly severe obesity, is associated with depressed mood or a diagnosis of depression, with rates of obesity being approximately doubled in obese compared with normal-weight groups. However, the majority of obese individuals are not depressed, and depression in obese individuals should be treated as seriously as in others and not presumed to be a consequence of obesity. Prospective studies are scarce, but support a link between obesity and incident depression. Studies in clinically obese populations generally document higher rates of depression than among either non-treatment-seeking obese or normal-weight control groups. However, those who seek treatment may differ in other important ways from those who do not, and depression itself may be a stimulus for seeking professional help. Moreover, even within clinical groups there is variation, and it cannot be assumed that depression is an inevitable consequence of severe overweight. As two reviews have concluded, the most important area for future research concerns the investigation of the mechanisms underlying depression–obesity covariations [16,17]. Potential mediators are suggested by the literature and, where modifiable, should be targeted for intervention.

REFERENCES

1. World Health Organization, *Obesity and Overweight* (Geneva: World Health Organization, 2003).
2. K. M. Flegal M. D. Carroll, C. L. Ogden, C. L. Johnson, Prevalence and trends in obesity among US adults, 1999–2000. *J. Am. Med. Assoc.* **288** (2002), 1723–7.
3. G. A. Bray, Medical consequences of obesity. *J. Clin. Endocrinol. Metab.* **89** (2004), 2583–9.
4. L. Khaodhiar, K. C. McCowen, G. L. Blackburn, Obesity and its comorbid conditions. *Clin. Cornerstone* **2** (1999), 17–31.
5. F. X. Pi-Sunyer, Medical hazards of obesity. *Ann. Intern. Med.* **119** (1993), 655–60.

6. T. L. Visscher, J. C. Seidell, The public health impact of obesity. *Annu. Rev. Public Health* **22** (2001), 355–75.

7. H. I. Kaplan, H. S. Kaplan, The psychosomatic concept of obesity. *J. Nerv. Ment. Dis.* **125** (1957), 181–201.

8. P. B. Goldblatt, M. E. Moore, A. J. Stunkard, Social factors in obesity. *J. Am. Med. Assoc.* **192** (1965), 1039–44.

9. P. Bjorntorp, Endocrine abnormalities of obesity. *Metabolism* **44** (1995), 21–3.

10. G. Oliver, J. Wardle, E. L. Gibson, Stress and food choice: a laboratory study. *Psychosom. Med.* **62** (2000), 853–65.

11. R. B. Harris, Leptin: much more than a satiety signal. *Annu. Rev. Nutr.* **20** (2000), 45–75.

12. A. Steptoe, S. R. Kunz-Ebrecht, L. Brydon, J. Wardle, Central adiposity and cortisol responses to waking in middle-aged men and women. *Int. J. Obes. Relat. Metab. Disord.* **28** (2004), 1168–73.

13. M. F. Dallman, N. Pecoraro, S. F. Akana, *et al.*, Chronic stress and obesity: a new view of 'comfort food'. *Proc. Natl. Acad. Sci. U. S. A.* **100** (2003), 11 696–701.

14. R. M. Puhl, K. D. Brownell, Psychosocial origins of obesity stigma: toward changing a powerful and pervasive bias. *Obes. Rev.* **4** (2003), 213–27.

15. R. Puhl, K. D. Brownell, Bias, discrimination, and obesity. *Obes. Res.* **9** (2001), 788–805.

16. M. A. Friedman, K. D. Brownell, Psychological correlates of obesity: moving to the next research generation. *Psychol. Bull.* **117** (1995), 3–20.

17. M. S. Faith, P. E. Matz, M. A. Jorge, Obesity-depression associations in the population. *J. Psychosom. Res.* **53** (2002), 935–42.

18. A. J. Stunkard, M. S. Faith, K. C. Allison, Depression and obesity. *Biol. Psychiatry* **54** (2003), 330–37.

19. T. A. Wadden, D. B. Sarwer, L. G. Womble, *et al.*, Psychosocial aspects of obesity and obesity surgery. *Surg. Clin. North Am.* **81** (2001), 1001–24.

20. J. Istvan, K. Zavela, G. Weidner, Body weight and psychological distress in NHANES I. *Int. J. Obes. Relat. Metab. Disord.* **16** (1992), 999–1003.

21. T. A. Wadden, G. D. Foster, A. J. Stunkard, J. R. Linowitz, Dissatisfaction with weight and figure in obese girls: discontent but not depression. *Int. J. Obes.* **13** (1989), 89–97.

22. A. L. Stewart, R. H. Brook, Effects of being overweight. *Am. J. Public Health* **73** (1983), 171–8.

23. M. J. Seegers, C. Mertens, Psychological and bioclinical CHD risk factors: quantitative differences between obese, normal and thin subjects. *J. Psychosom. Res.* **18** (1974), 403–11.

24. M. Sullivan, J. Karlsson J. Sjostrom, *et al.*, Swedish obese subjects (SOS): an intervention study of obesity – baseline evaluation of health and psychosocial functioning in the first 1743 subjects examined. *Int. J. Obes. Relat. Metab. Disord.* **17** (1993), 503–12.

25. R. R. Wing, K. A. Matthews, L. H. Kuller, E. N. Meilahn, P. Plantinga, Waist to hip ratio in middle-aged women: associations with behavioral and psychosocial factors and with changes in cardiovascular risk factors. *Arterioscler. Thromb.* **11** (1991), 1250–57.

26. K. M. Carpenter, D. S. Hasin, D. B. Allison, M. S. Faith, Relationships between obesity and DSM-IV major depressive disorder, suicide ideation, and suicide attempts: results from a general population study. *Am. J. Public Health* **90** (2000), 251–7.

27. E. Johnston, S. Johnson, P. McLeod, M. Johnston, The relation of body mass index to depressive symptoms. *Can. J. Public Health* **95** (2004), 179–83.

28. C. U. Onyike, R. M. Crum, H. B. Lee, C. G. Lyketsos, W. W. Eaton, Is obesity associated with major depression? Results from the Third National Health and Nutrition Examination Survey. *Am. J. Epidemiol.* **158** (2003), 1139–47.

29. C. Dong, L. E. Sanchez, R. A. Price, Relationship of obesity to depression: a family-based study. *Int. J. Obes. Relat. Metab. Disord.* **28** (2004), 790–95.

30. A. F. Jorm, A. E. Korten, H. Christensen, *et al.*, Association of obesity with anxiety, depression and emotional well-being: a community survey. *Aust. N. Z. J. Public Health* **27** (2003), 434–40.

31. A. C. Ahlberg, T. Ljung, R. Rosmond, *et al.*, Depression and anxiety symptoms in relation to anthropometry and metabolism in men. *Psychiatry Res.* **112** (2002), 101–10.

32. R. E. Roberts, S. Deleger, W. J. Strawbridge, G. A. Kaplan, Prospective association between obesity and depression: evidence from the Alameda County Study. *Int. J. Obes. Relat. Metab. Disord.* **27** (2003), 514–21.

33. M. S. Kaplan, N. Huguet, J. T. Newsom, B. H. McFarland, J. Lindsay, Prevalence and correlates of overweight and obesity among older adults: findings from the Canadian National Population Health Survey. *J. Gerontol. A Biol. Sci. Med. Sci.* **58** (2003), 1018–30.

34. L. Z. Bin, H. S. Yin, C. W. Man, *et al.*, Obesity and depressive symptoms in Chinese elderly. *Int. J. Geriatr. Psychiatry* **19** (2004), 68–74.

35. H. Noppa, T. Hallstrom, Weight gain in adulthood in relation to socioeconomic factors, mental illness and personality traits: a prospective study of middle-aged women. *J. Psychosom. Res.* **25** (1981), 83–9.

36. L. DiPietro, R. F. Anda, D. F. Williamson, A. J. Stunkard, Depressive symptoms and weight change in a national cohort of adults. *Int. J. Obes. Relat. Metab. Disord.* **16** (1992), 745–53.

37. G. I. Papakostas, T. Petersen, D. V. Iosifescu, *et al.*, Obesity among outpatients with major depressive disorder. *Int. J. Neuropsychopharmacol.* **8** (2005), 59–63.

38. A. M. Bardone, T. E. Moffitt, A. Caspi, *et al.*, Adult physical health outcomes of adolescent girls with conduct disorder, depression, and anxiety. *J. Am. Acad. Child Adolesc. Psychiatry* **37** (1998), 594–601.

39. D. S. Pine, P. Cohen, J. Brook, J. D. Coplan, Psychiatric symptoms in adolescence as predictors of obesity in early adulthood: a longitudinal study. *Am. J. Public Health* **87** (1997), 1303–10.

40. D. S. Pine, R. B. Goldstein, S. Wolk, M. M. Weissman, The association between childhood depression and adulthood body mass index. *Pediatrics* **107** (2001), 1049–56.

41. L. P. Richardson, R. Davis, R. Poulton, *et al.*, A longitudinal evaluation of adolescent depression and adult obesity. *Arch. Pediatr. Adolesc. Med.* **157** (2003), 739–45.

42. J. C. Barefoot, B. L. Heitmann, M. J. Helms, *et al.*, Symptoms of depression and changes in body weight from adolescence to mid-life. *Int. J. Obes. Relat. Metab. Disord.* **22** (1998), 688–94.

43. G. Hasler, D. S. Pine, A. Gamma, *et al.*, The associations between psychopathology and being overweight: a 20-year prospective study. *Psychol. Med.* **34** (2004), 1047–57.

44. R. E. Roberts, W. J. Strawbridge, S. Deleger, G. A. Kaplan, Are the fat more jolly? *Ann. Behav. Med.* **24** (2002), 169–80.

45. R. E. Roberts, G. A. Kaplan, S. J. Shema, W. J. Strawbridge, Are the obese at greater risk for depression? *Am. J. Epidemiol.* **152** (2000), 163–70.

46. I. Berlin, F. Lavergne, Relationship between body-mass index and depressive symptoms in patients with major depression. *Eur. Psychiatry* **18** (2003), 85–8.

47. T. L. Schwartz, N. Nihalani, S. Jindal, S. Virk, N. Jones, Psychiatric medication-induced obesity: a review. *Obes. Rev.* **5** (2004), 115–21.

48. K. Elfhag, S. Rossner, A. M. Carlsson, Degree of body weight in obesity and Rorschach personality aspects of mental distress. *Eat. Weight Disord.* **9** (2004), 35–43.

49. J. Glinski, S. Wetzler, E. Goodman, The psychology of gastric bypass surgery. *Obes. Surg.* **11** (2001), 581–8.

50. B. Laferrere, S. Zhu, J. R. Clarkson, *et al.*, Race, menopause, health-related quality of life, and psychological well-being in obese women. *Obes. Res.* **10** (2002), 1270–75.

51. G. Marchesini, M. Bellini, S. Natale, *et al.*, Psychiatric distress and health-related quality of life in obesity. *Diabetes Nutr. Metab.* **16** (2003), 145–54.

52. D. W. Black, R. B. Goldstein, E. E. Mason, Prevalence of mental disorder in 88 morbidly obese bariatric clinic patients. *Am. J. Psychiatry* **149** (1992), 227–34.

53. B. Britz, W. Siegfried, A. Ziegler, *et al.*, Rates of psychiatric disorders in a clinical study group of adolescents with extreme obesity and in obese adolescents ascertained via a population based study. *Int. J. Obes. Relat. Metab. Disord.* **24** (2000), 1707–14.

54. M. L. Fitzgibbon, M. R. Stolley, D. S. Kirschenbaum, Obese people who seek treatment have different characteristics than those who do not seek treatment. *Health Psychol.* **12** (1993), 342–5.

55. K. R. Fontaine, S. J. Bartlett, I. Barofsky, Health-related quality of life among obese persons seeking and not currently seeking treatment. *Int. J. Eat. Disord.* **27** (2000), 101–5.

56. R. L. Kolotkin, R. D. Crosby, R. Pendleton, *et al.*, Health-related quality of life in patients seeking gastric bypass surgery vs non-treatment-seeking controls. *Obes. Surg.* **13** (2003), 371–7.

57. R. L. Kolotkin, R. D. Crosby, G. R. Williams, Health-related quality of life varies among obese subgroups. *Obes. Res.* **10** (2002), 748–56.

58. M. L. Higgs, T. Wade, M. Cescato, *et al.*, Differences between treatment seekers in an obese population: medical intervention vs. dietary restriction. *J. Behav. Med.* **20** (1997), 391–405.

59. R. J. Hafner, J. M. Watts, J. Rogers, Psychological status of morbidly obese women before gastric restriction surgery. *J. Psychosom. Res.* **31** (1987), 607–12.

60. E. V. Leckie, R. F. Withers, Obesity and depression. *J. Psychosom. Res.* **11** (1967), 107–15.

61. G. J. Musante, P. R. Costanzo, K. E. Friedman, The comorbidity of depression and eating dysregulation processes in a diet-seeking obese population: a matter of gender specificity. *Int. J. Eat. Disord.* **23** (1998), 65–75.

62. A. Ryden, J. Karlsson, L. O. Persson, *et al.*, Obesity-related coping and distress and relationship to treatment preference. *Br. J. Clin. Psychol.* **40** (2001), 177–88.

63. M. P. Dymek, D. le Grange, K. Neven, J. Alverdy, Quality of life and psychosocial adjustment in patients after Roux-en-Y gastric bypass: a brief report. *Obes. Surg.* **11** (2001), 32–9.

64. J. Karlsson, L. Sjostrom, M. Sullivan, Swedish obese subjects (SOS): an intervention study of obesity – two-year follow-up of health-related quality of life (HRQL) and eating behavior

after gastric surgery for severe obesity. *Int. J. Obes. Relat. Metab. Disord.* **22** (1998), 113–26.

65. S. R. Maddi, S. R. Fox, D. M. Khoshaba, *et al.*, Reduction in psychopathology following bariatric surgery for morbid obesity. *Obes. Surg.* **11** (2001), 680–85.

66. G. S. Waters, W. J. Pories, M. S. Swanson, *et al.*, Long-term studies of mental health after the Greenville gastric bypass operation for morbid obesity. *Am. J. Surg.* **161** (1991), 154–7.

67. A. Ryden, J. Karlsson, M. Sullivan, J. S. Torgerson, C. Taft, Coping and distress: what happens after intervention? A 2-year follow-up from the Swedish Obese Subjects (SOS) study. *Psychosom. Med.* **65** (2003), 435–42.

68. J. B. Dixon, M. E. Dixon, P. E. O'Brien, Depression in association with severe obesity: changes with weight loss. *Arch. Intern. Med.* **163** (2003), 2058–65.

69. T. A. Wadden, A. J. Stunkard, J. Liebschutz, Three-year follow-up of the treatment of obesity by very low calorie diet, behavior therapy, and their combination. *J. Consult. Clin. Psychol.* **56** (1988), 925–8.

70. O. Ryden, S. A. Olsson, A. Danielsson, P. Nilsson-Ehle, Weight loss after gastroplasty: psychological sequelae in relation to clinical and metabolic observations. *J. Am. Coll. Nutr.* **8** (1989), 15–23.

71. W. T. Tsushima, M. P. Bridenstine, J. F. Balfour, MMPI-2 scores in the outcome prediction of gastric bypass surgery. *Obes. Surg.* **14** (2004), 528–32.

72. M. M. Clark, B. M. Balsiger, C. D. Sletten, *et al.*, Psychosocial factors and 2-year outcome following bariatric surgery for weight loss. *Obes. Surg.* **13** (2003), 739–45.

73. E. M. Inelmen, E. D. Toffanello, G. Enzi, *et al.*, Predictors of drop-out in overweight and obese outpatients. *Int. J. Obes. Relat. Metab. Disord.* **29** (2005), 122–8.

74. P. J. Cooper, I. Goodyer, Prevalence and significance of weight and shape concerns in girls aged 11–16 years. *Br. J. Psychiatry* **171** (1997), 542–4.

75. D. Neumark-Sztainer, J. Croll, M. Story, *et al.*, Ethnic/racial differences in weight-related concerns and behaviors among adolescent girls and boys: findings from Project EAT. *J. Psychosom. Res.* **53** (2002), 963–74.

76. P. Packard, K. S. Krogstrand, Half of rural girls aged 8 to 17 years report weight concerns and dietary changes, with both more prevalent with increased age. *J. Am. Diet. Assoc.* **102** (2002), 672–7.

77. J. Wardle, L. Cooke, The impact of obesity on psychological well-being in children. *Best Pract. Res. Clin. Endocrinol. Metab.* **19** (2005), 421–40.

78. J. Wardle, K. A. Robb, F. Johnson, *et al.*, Socioeconomic variation in attitudes to eating and weight in female adolescents. *Health Psychol.* **23** (2004), 275–2.

79. C. E. Ross, Overweight and depression. *J. Health Soc. Behav.* **35** (1994), 63–79.

80. J. Wardle, S. Williamson, F. Johnson, C. Edwards, The psychological consequences of obesity in adolescence: cultural moderators of the obesity-depression association. *Int. J. Obes.* (Lond.) **30** (2006), 634–42.

81. R. Goodman, The Strengths and Difficulties Questionnaire: a research note. *J. Child Psychol. Psychiatry* **38** (1997), 581–6.

82. A. Myers, J. C. Rosen, Obesity stigmatization and coping: relation to mental health symptoms, body image, and self-esteem. *Int. J. Obes. Relat. Metab. Disord.* **23** (1999), 221–30.

83. M. de Zwaan, Binge eating disorder and obesity. *Int. J. Obes. Relat. Metab. Disord.* **25**: Suppl 1 (2001), 51–5.

84. T. Reichborn-Kjennerud, C. M. Bulik, P. F. Sullivan, K. Tambs, J. R. Harris, Psychiatric and medical symptoms in binge eating in the absence of compensatory behaviors. *Obes. Res.* **12** (2004), 1445–54.

85. M. Malone, S. Alger-Mayer, Binge status and quality of life after gastric bypass surgery: a one-year study. *Obes. Res.* **12** (2004), 473–81.

86. J. A. Linde, R. W. Jeffery, R. L. Levy, *et al.*, Binge eating disorder, weight control self-efficacy, and depression in overweight men and women. *Int. J. Obes. Relat. Metab. Disord.* **28** (2004), 418–25.

87. M. de Zwaan, J. E. Mitchell, L. M. Howell, *et al.*, Characteristics of morbidly obese patients before gastric bypass surgery. *Compr. Psychiatry* **44** (2003), 428–34.

88. C. M. Grilo, D. E. Wilfley, K. D. Brownell, J. Rodin, Teasing, body image, and self-esteem in a clinical sample of obese women. *Addict. Behav.* **19** (1994), 443–50.

89. T. D. Jackson, C. M. Grilo, R. M. Masheb, Teasing history, onset of obesity, current eating disorder psychopathology, body dissatisfaction, and psychological functioning in binge eating disorder. *Obes. Res.* **8** (2000), 451–8.

90. K. E. Friedman, S. K. Reichmann, P. R. Costanzo, G. J. Musante, Body image partially mediates the relationship between obesity and psychological distress. *Obes. Res.* **10** (2002), 33–41.

91. D. B. Sarwer, T. A. Wadden, G. D. Foster, Assessment of body image dissatisfaction in obese women: specificity, severity, and clinical significance. *J. Consult. Clin. Psychol.* **66** (1998), 651–4.

92. F. Johnson, J. Wardle, Dietary restraint, body dissatisfaction, and psychological distress: a prospective analysis. *J. Abnorm. Psychol.* **114** (2005), 119–25.

93. J. P. Foreyt, R. L. Brunner, G. K. Goodrick, *et al.*, Psychological correlates of weight fluctuation. *Int. J. Eat. Disord.* **17** (1995), 263–75.

94. S. J. Bartlett, T. A. Wadden, R. A. Vogt, Psychosocial consequences of weight cycling. *J. Consult. Clin. Psychol.* **64** (1996), 587–92.

95. T. A. Wadden, S. Bartlett, K. A. Letizia, *et al.*, Relationship of dieting history to resting metabolic rate, body composition, eating behavior, and subsequent weight loss. *Am. J. Clin. Nutr.* **56** (1992), 203–8S.

96. G. D. Foster, T. A. Wadden, P. C. Kendall, A. J. Stunkard, R. A. Vogt, Psychological effects of weight loss and regain: a prospective evaluation. *J. Consult. Clin. Psychol.* **64** (1996), 752–7.

97. G. D. Foster, D. B. Sarwer, T. A. Wadden, Psychological effects of weight cycling in obese persons: a review and research agenda. *Obes. Res.* **5** (1997), 474–88.

Part 3

Biological and behavioural processes

12

Inflammation, sickness behaviour and depression

Robert Dantzer, Nathalie Castanon, Jacques Lestage, Maite Moreau and Lucile Capuron

Introduction

The prevalence of depression in medically ill patients is high, ranging from 5% to 20% versus 3–5% in the general population. The comorbidity of depressive disorders in general hospital patients or in-patients with chronic pathologies who consult general practitioners (GPs) is about 40% [1,2]. The rates are similar in women with breast cancer [3]. Several studies have shown that patients with chronic diseases, including arthritis and coronary heart disease (CHD), are more at risk than healthy subjects for developing mood disorders [4–7]. In most of these studies, depression was identified as a significant risk factor for mortality and health/treatment complications. Depression was associated with greater physical limitation, more frequent subjective health complaints, lower treatment compliance and satisfaction, and reduced perceived quality of life. In addition, the prevalence of major depression in later life was also found to be more frequent among people with chronic illnesses [8].

Psychological factors are usually put forward to explain the comorbidity of depression with medical illnesses. Medically ill patients often suffer from physical limitations and have difficulties maintaining positive social relationships. They frequently report feelings of hopelessness, since they cannot cope with the problems they are confronted with, especially in situations of poor social support. These factors increase the risk for the occurrence of depressive disorders. Lack of compliance with medical treatments, decreased social support and the consequences of biological changes associated with depression (e.g. impaired cellular immune functions) are believed to account for the association between depression and increased morbidity and mortality.

The objective of this chapter is to provide an alternative perspective on the intricate relationships that exist between depressive disorders and a large number

Depression and Physical Illness, ed. A. Steptoe.
Published by Cambridge University Press. © Cambridge University Press 2006.

of chronic medical pathologies. We propose that alterations in mood occurring in somatic patients reflect the neural consequences of the molecular and cellular events that play a pivotal role in the evolution of the disease. This hypothesis is based on findings generated by two convergent lines of research originating from both bench and bedside. The first line of research indicates that immune mediators participating in the pathophysiology of various chronic somatic disorders have potent influences on brain functions, even when these mediators are produced in peripheral tissues. The second line of research points to an association between depression and activation of the innate immune system.

Inflammation and cytokines

The basic mechanisms that explain why we feel sick and behave in a sick way when we are ill are related closely to the mechanisms of inflammation [9,10]. Acute inflammation is characterised by vasodilation and increased vascular permeability, which leads to leukocytic infiltration into the inflamed tissue. Chronic inflammation can occur as a prolongation of the acute episode of inflammation when the causal agent persists, or without any acute phase. There is a bewildering array of inflammatory mediators, the most prominent of which are known as pro-inflammatory cytokines. These protein mediators are produced by mononuclear phagocytes such as macrophages and monocytes in response either to conserved molecular constituents of microbial pathogens (viruses, bacteria, fungi, protozoa) or to endogenous signals of necrotic cell death. Macrophages act as sentinel cells in the tissues, whereas monocytes patrol in the blood. Macrophages and monocytes are part of the innate immune system and have membrane receptors that recognise pathogen-associated molecular patterns. These receptors belong to the family of Toll-like receptors (TLRs) [11]. Although limited in number (there are different TLRs in humans), they are capable of recognising a large variety of pathogen-associated molecular patterns. They all share the property of having a Toll/interleukin-1 (IL-1) receptor domain that involves adaptor proteins to allow the activation of protein kinases, resulting in the activation of a wide number of genes via a limited set of transcription factors, including the nuclear factor kappa B (NFκB) and mitogen-associated protein (MAP) kinases. Lipopolysaccharide (LPS), the active fragment of endotoxin from Gram-negative bacteria, activates TLR4, resulting in an acute-phase reaction that eventually culminates in sepsis. Viral double-stranded RNA is recognised by TLR3. Activation of TLRs results in the synthesis and release of pro-inflammatory cytokines, including IL-1, interleukin 6 (IL-6) and tumour necrosis factor alpha (TNF-α). Mast cells also release preformed TNF-α in addition to histamine. Pro-inflammatory cytokines are part of a myriad of other cytokines that form what is called the cytokine network.

Within the cytokine network, pro-inflammatory cytokines act to promote inflammation, whereas other cytokines, known as anti-inflammatory cytokines, oppose this response by attenuating the production of pro-inflammatory cytokines or by antagonising their action at the receptor level. Interleukin 10 (IL-10) is an example of the former; the specific antagonist of the IL-1 receptor, IL-1Ra, is an example of the latter. In response to TLR signalling, monocytes and macrophages produce both pro-inflammatory and anti-inflammatory cytokines, although with different time courses, since pro-inflammatory cytokines are produced first. In addition to anti-inflammatory cytokines, the activity of pro-inflammatory cytokines can also be regulated by soluble receptors, i.e. shed extracellular portions of membrane receptors that bind excess cytokines.

Pro-inflammatory cytokines produced by peripheral innate immune cells play a key role in the development of the local and systemic inflammatory responses. They induce the expression of adhesion molecules on both circulating phagocytic cells and endothelial cells, thereby favouring margination and diapedesis, which are necessary for leukocytic infiltration. In addition to this local response, pro-inflammatory cytokines are also responsible for the systemic inflammatory response by their actions on peripheral cellular targets such as hepatocytes for the production of acute-phase proteins, synovial cells in the joints and myoblasts in muscles. Pro-inflammatory cytokines play a pivotal role in the mounting of the adaptive immune response that involves T- and B-lymphocytes.

The systemic inflammatory response involves the brain, which triggers a set of metabolic and behavioural adjustments. These adjustments appear in the form of increased thermogenesis and reduced thermolysis, which are characteristic of fever, activation of the hypothalamic-pituitary-adrenocortical (HPA) axis and alterations in behaviour referred to as 'sickness behaviour'. Sickness behaviour can be characterised in experimental animals by depressed locomotion and exploratory activity, lack of interest in social activities, and reduced food and water intake. Systemic and intracerebral administration of either the cytokine inducer LPS or recombinant pro-inflammatory cytokines to rats and mice induces sickness behaviour [9]. Furthermore, sickness behaviour induced by peripheral administration of IL-1 can be abrogated by intracerebroventricular administration of IL-1Ra, indicating that the peripherally injected IL-1 acts in the brain to induce these behavioural changes [12]. The possibility that IL-1 acts in the brain is confirmed by the observation that IL-1 receptors are expressed in the central nervous system and that brain IL-1 signals via the same mechanisms as those mediating its actions in peripheral immune and non-immune cells [13]. Receptors of other pro-inflammatory cytokines such as IL-6 and TNF-α are also expressed in the brain.

Cytokines are relatively large protein molecules that are hydrophilic and do not readily cross the blood–brain barrier. In addition (with the exception of IL-6, which can act on distant targets), cytokines are usually active in the microenvironment in which they are produced and function as autocrine and paracrine factors rather than as hormones. An important finding is the observation that the production of IL-1 and other pro-inflammatory cytokines by peripheral innate immune cells is associated with the production of the same cytokines in the brain by macrophage-like cells in the meninges and around blood vessels and by microglial cells within the brain parenchyma [14,15]. In the brain, IL-1 acts as a pivotal cytokine, since it regulates not only its own synthesis but also the synthesis of other pro-inflammatory cytokines, including TNF-α and IL-6 [16].

All these findings point to the existence of a brain compartment of cytokines that reflects at the cellular and molecular levels the activation of peripheral innate immune cells, the induction of which is responsible for the central component of the acute-phase reaction. This cannot be possible without communication pathways allowing peripheral immune messages to be transmitted from the periphery to the brain. There are at least three communication pathways that transmit the peripheral immune message to the brain. These pathways include blood transfer of cytokines and pathogen-associated molecular patterns, specific transporters supporting passage of cytokines across the blood–brain barrier, and activation of afferent neural pathways. The exact nature of these communication pathways varies with the physiological endpoint under consideration, probably because of the spatial location of the neuronal circuits that underlie its expression. Afferent neural pathways play a major role in the development of cytokine-induced sickness behaviour [17]. In contrast, the humoral route appears to play a more important role for the fever response than for sickness behaviour [18].

The brain cytokine message originates in the choroid plexus and the circumventricular organs, which are devoid of a functional blood–brain barrier. Subsequently, cytokines propagate into the brain parenchyma by volume diffusion and act on brain structures that, for some of them, certainly need to be sensitised by the afferent neural message [17]. It is not yet known whether cytokines ultimately act on brain functions by targeting neuronal cells or whether they act indirectly by modifying the neural environment that is formed by glial and endothelial cells. The generation of molecular intermediates such as prostaglandins and nitric oxide (NO) may be involved in these actions, but the detailed molecular mechanisms of cytokine actions in the brain still need to be elucidated [19]. These mechanisms involve complex relationships between endothelial cells of blood vessels and glial cells, including macrophages surrounding the blood vessels and macrophages in the meninges. Within the brain parenchyma, microglial cells are also involved. Astrocytes interposed between blood vessels and neurons play an important role in the regulation of glutamate metabolism and ionic equilibrium and function as both targets and sources of cytokines.

In summary, when the innate immune system is activated, the brain forms a molecular and cellular image of the peripheral inflammatory response. It is this neural representation of the peripheral immune events that organises the host's response in its subjective, behavioural and metabolic components.

Cytokine-induced sickness behaviour is an adaptive response to infection

Typical symptoms of sickness include weakness, malaise, listlessness and inability to concentrate. Sick individuals are lethargic, show little interest in their surroundings and stop eating and drinking. This constellation of non-specific symptoms is referred to collectively as 'sickness behaviour' [20]. Since symptoms of sickness behaviour do not help us to recognise which pathological process a patient is suffering from, most clinicians do not pay much attention to such symptoms compared with the disease-specific signs that permit diagnosis. At best, sickness behaviour is considered as an uncomfortable but rather banal component of the pathogen-induced debilitative process. In contrast to this commonly held view, it has been proposed that, together with the fever response, behavioural symptoms of sickness represent a highly organised strategy of the organism to fight infection [20,21]. When it was first put forward, this hypothesis was coherent with the already recognised role of fever in the host response to pathogens [22]. In physiological terms, fever corresponds to a new homeostatic state characterised by a raised set-point of body-temperature regulation. A feverish individual feels cold at usual thermoneutral environments. Therefore, the febrile individual not only seeks warmer temperatures but also actively tries to enhance heat production (increased thermogenesis) and reduce heat loss (decreased thermolysis). The higher body temperature that is achieved during fever stimulates proliferation of immune cells and is unfavourable for the growth of many bacterial and viral pathogens. In addition, the reduction of zinc and iron plasma levels that occurs during fever decreases the availability of these vital elements for proliferation of microorganisms. The adaptive nature of the fever response is apparent from studies showing that organisms infected with a bacterium or virus and unable to mount an appropriate fever response (because they have been treated with an antipyretic drug or their fur has been shaved) have a lower survival rate than organisms that develop a normal fever [23].

The amount of energy that is required to increase body temperature during the febrile process is high: in humans, the metabolic rate needs to be increased by 13% to allow a raise of 1 °C in body temperature. Because of the high metabolic cost of fever, there is little room for activities and attitudes other than those favouring heat production (e.g. shivering) and minimising thermal losses (e.g. rest, curl-up posture, piloerection). Since sickness behaviour is often accompanied by pain, it has been proposed that pain is an integral part of, if not the main determinant of, sickness behaviour [24]. According to Watkins and Maier [24], cytokine-induced hyperalgesia would be advantageous to the survival of the organism by directing recuperative behaviours (e.g. licking and protection of the affected bodily site) to the site of injury or infection. Furthermore, by encouraging the organism to curl up and remain immobile, exaggerated pain would also serve to save energy.

Within this context, sickness behaviour can be seen as the behavioural expression of a highly organised strategy that is critical to the survival of the organism in the face of microbial pathogens, just like fear in the face of a predator. If this hypothesis is correct, then sickness should have motivational properties, i.e. sick individuals should be able to reorganise their behaviour depending on its consequences and the internal and external constraints they are exposed to. This flexibility is characteristic of motivated behaviour. Motivation is defined here as a central state that reorganises perception and action. In order to escape a potential threat, a fearful individual must be attentive to everything that can occur in its environment in order to be able to exhibit at the right time the most appropriate defensive behavioural pattern that is available in the individual's repertoire. In other words, a motivational state does not manifest itself by fixed behavioural patterns; on the contrary, motivation uncouples action from stimulus conditions and enables selection of the appropriate strategy depending on the eliciting situation.

The first evidence that sickness behaviour is the expression of a motivational state rather than a consequence of weakness and physical debilitation was provided by Miller's [25] observation that thirsty rats injected with endotoxin stopped bar-pressing for water but, when given water, drank it, although to a lesser extent than normally. This effect was not specific to the thirst motivation, since the endotoxin treatment also reduced the amount of food eaten and even blocked responding in rats trained to press a bar for the rewarding effects of electrical stimulation in the lateral hypothalamus. Interestingly, when rats were trained to turn off an aversive electrical stimulation in this neural structure, endotoxin also reduced the rate of responding, but to a lesser extent than bar-pressing for a rewarding brain stimulation. To demonstrate that this range of responses to endotoxin was the result of the elicitation of a sickness motivational state, Miller administered endotoxin to rats that were trained to obtain restful periods by pressing a lever when placed in a rotating drum. In this situation, endotoxin-treated rats increased their response rate instead of decreasing it. The fact that endotoxin treatment decreased or increased behavioural output depending on its consequences gives strong support to the motivational interpretation of the behavioural effects of such a treatment. Unfortunately, these findings were reported in a review paper but never published as original results.

The motivational interpretation of sickness behaviour was not submitted to test for 30 years after these insightful observations, before Aubert and colleagues [26–28] initiated an extensive series of experiments to validate the concept. An important characteristic of a motivational state is that it competes with other motivational states for behavioural output. It is normally not possible to search for food and court a potential sexual partner at the same time, since the behavioural patterns of foraging and courtship are not compatible. The normal expression of behaviour therefore requires a hierarchical structure of motivational states, which is updated contingent on urgencies that occur in the environment and internal milieu. When an infection occurs, the sick individual is at a life-or-death juncture, and its physiology and behaviour must be altered in order to overcome the disease. However, this is a relatively long-term process that needs to make room for more urgent needs when necessary. As an analogy, it is clear that if a sick person lying in bed hears a fire alarm ringing in the house and sees flames and smoke coming out of the basement, then he or she will momentarily overcome the sickness behaviour in order to escape danger. In motivational terms, fear competes with sickness and, in behavioural terms, fear-motivated behaviour takes precedence over sickness behaviour. An example of this competition between sickness and other motivational states comes from a series of experiments on the effects of LPS on maternal behaviour [28]. Lactating mice injected with an appropriate dose of LPS display a typical sickness behaviour, i.e. they remain immobile without eating or drinking, and do not respond to their pups' solicitations. However, their behaviour changes dramatically when their maternal motivation is challenged by removing the nest and dispersing the pups in the cage. In this situation, LPS-treated mice become active to retrieve their pups and bring them back one after the other to where the nest was. However, provision of cotton wool does not trigger nest building, another manifestation of maternal behaviour, unless the mice are tested at an ambient temperature of 6 °C, in which case mice engage not only in pup retrieval but also in nest building in order to build a near-perfect nest.

From an adaptive point of view, the anorexic effect of cytokines is difficult to re-concile with their pyrogenic activity. Intuitively, one could propose that the enhanced energy requirement of thermogenesis requires increased rather than decreased food intake. One way of resolving this paradox is to pretend that cytokine-induced anorexia spares the energy required for foraging and prevents a weakened organism running the risk of being exposed to a predator during the search for food. Accordingly, cytokines should be more effective in suppressing the foraging than the consummatory components of food intake. This appears to be the case, since, as mentioned previously, LPS- or IL-1-treated animals stopped pressing a lever for food but still ate the food pellets that were delivered independently of their behaviour [27]. Another possibility is that cytokines modify the utility of food, for example by impairing the metabolic utilisation of some of the nutrients they contain. This is particularly the case for lipids, which can no longer be used by an organism exposed to cytokines, since lipogenesis is disrupted and lipids enter a futile cycle. According to this hypothesis, animals treated with cytokines should reorganise their diet to eat fewer lipids and more carbohydrates. To determine whether this is the case, rats were submitted to a dietary self-selection protocol in which they had free access to separate carbohydrate, protein and fat diets for four hours a day [26]. After a ten-day habituation to this regimen that allowed stabilisation of macronutrient intake, rats were injected with LPS or IL-1β. Under the effect of this treatment, they decreased their total food intake but reorganised their self-selection pattern in order to ingest relatively more carbohydrate and less fat, but protein intake remained unchanged. This change in macronutrient intake contrasted with the increased fat intake that occurs in healthy rats exposed to cold.

From cytokine-induced sickness behaviour to depression

Since cytokine-induced sickness behaviour is the expression of a motivational state that is triggered by activation of the peripheral innate immune system, it is not pathological per se but as normal as the fear response that occurs in individuals exposed to the threat of a predator. Like fear, sickness behaviour can become abnormal or pathological when it occurs out of context, i.e. in the absence of any inflammatory stimulus or when exaggerated in intensity and/or duration. This situation may take place if the opposing processes that normally down-regulate activation of the molecular and cellular components of the sickness response are faulty or if the neuronal circuits that are the targets of inflammatory mediators and organise sickness behaviour become sensitised [29].

Another way in which sickness behaviour can become abnormal is when it occurs in response to secondary reinforcers rather than to the primary inflammatory stimulus. One can imagine, for instance, a situation in which the sickness behaviour that is normally triggered by microbial pathogens or by inflammation is associated with beneficial consequences for the subject (e.g. leave of absence with financial compensation), so that its probability of occurrence independently of the initial triggering conditions will increase by virtue of the law of effect.

Although all of these situations can occur in theory, one case that has received special attention during recent years is chronic activation of the innate immune system. This condition occurs in patients receiving repeated injections of recombinant cytokines, mainly interleukin-2 (IL-2) and/or interferon alfa (IFN-α), for the treatment of viral infections (e.g. hepatitis C) or cancer. During the first stages of cytokine therapy, patients develop a full-blown episode of sickness behaviour, characterised by the symptoms of fever, malaise, anorexia, pain and fatigue. At later stages of treatment, up to a third of patients develop alterations in mood that are characteristic of depression, including sadness, inability to feel, depressed mood and even suicidal ideation [30]. The onset of depressive symptoms depends on the cytokine and treatment modalities (e.g. dosage, administration route). Interestingly, the occurrence of depression can be prevented by pretreatment with paroxetine, a selective serotonin reuptake inhibitor (SSRI) with antidepressant properties. Nevertheless, pretreatment with paroxetine has a minimal or null effect on the development of neurovegetative symptoms of sickness, including fever, fatigue and anorexia, confirming the dissociation between sickness behaviour and depression [31].

These findings are important because they can be interpreted to suggest that depressive disorders develop from cytokine-induced sickness behaviour only in vulnerable patients. Vulnerability, in the present context, refers to an innate or acquired predisposition to develop a given pathology when the causal factors are present. Dysfunction in genes controlling key proteins in serotoninergic neurotransmission, e.g. activity of the serotonin transporter [32], and childhood trauma [33] have been identified as vulnerability factors for depression. Vulnerability to cytokine-induced depression can be revealed by psychological features. Indeed, patients with a relatively high score on depression scales, including the Montgomery Asberg Depression Rating Scale (MADRS) and the Hamilton Depression Rating Scale, at the start of cytokine treatment are more likely to develop depressive syndrome in response to cytokine treatment than patients who have a relatively low score at baseline [34,35]. Vulnerability can also be revealed by physiological features. Patients who respond to the first injection of IFN-α by an exaggerated pituitary-adrenal response are more likely to become depressed in response to repeated administration of IFN-α than patients who display a lower pituitary-adrenal response [36]. These two different characteristics are markers of vulnerability. They help us to identify patients who are at risk, but they do not explain why patients having these characteristics are more vulnerable than those who do not have them. In particular, it remains to be elucidated whether the risk factors for developing depression during cytokine therapy are the same as those accounting for depressive disorders in psychiatric patients, or whether these risk factors are specific to cytokines and involve, for instance, polymorphisms in genes involved in cytokine production.

The model of cytokine-induced depression has the advantage of providing clinicians with the possibility of observing the development of depressive symptoms in a longitudinal manner in a relatively large number of patients who can be monitored closely from the time they start receiving immunotherapy. Furthermore, patients who develop depression can be compared transversally with patients who remain free of any mood disorder. The model of cytokine-induced depression provides valuable insights into the relationship between cytokines and depression. At the clinical level, there is some evidence that symptoms of mood disorder are more polymorphic than simply depression. A study on patients with hepatitis C treated with IFN-α showed that dysphoria and mixed states dominate the clinical presentation of patients, with increases in irritability and anxiety as the main symptoms [37]. The reasons for the differences between patients with hepatitis C and those with cancer, who present mainly with depressed mood, are not known. They could be due to the medical context (cytokine immunotherapy is only palliative in cancer, but it is usually curative in hepatitis C), to the immunological context (immune responses of patients infected by a virus are different from those of patients with cancer) or simply to variations in treatment modalities (high doses of IFN-α administered intravenously and daily to patients with malignant melanoma versus low doses of pegylated IFN-α administered once a week to patients with chronic hepatitis C). These variations may also be due to differences in affective/psychiatric background, since a large number of patients with chronic hepatitis C have a history of substance abuse.

At the pathophysiological level, an important insight into the chain of events linking cytokines to mood alterations has emerged from the observation that cancer patients treated with cytokines develop a drastic decrease in plasma tryptophan levels that correlates with depression scores at four weeks of treatment [38]. This decrease in plasma trytophan levels had already been noted, but in a qualitative rather than a quantitative manner [39]. These findings are important, since bioavailability of tryptophan is the limiting factor for the synthesis of serotonin. The acute depletion of tryptophan produced by feeding excess amounts of large neutral amino acids that compete with tryptophan for entry into the brain results in the development of depressed mood in subjects at risk for depression. A likely candidate for this decrease in plasma tryptophan in patients submitted to cytokine immunotherapy is the enzyme indoleamine-2,3-dioxygenase, which degrades tryptophan into kynurenine and quinolinic acid. This enzyme is present in macrophages, monocytes, endothelial cells and brain glial cells. It is potently activated by pro-inflammatory cytokines such as TNF-α and interferon gamma (IFN-γ), both at the periphery and in the brain [40]. Its activation results in a decrease in tryptophan bioavailability for the synthesis of serotonin and in the formation of neuroactive compounds such as kynurenine and quinolinic acid that act at the level of glutamate receptors. The interference of pro-inflammatory cytokines with serotoninergic neurotransmission can certainly explain some of the clinical signs that develop in vulnerable patients, such as impulsivity and depressed mood. However, it does not account for the anhedonia, fatigue and psychomotor retardation that are also observed in cytokine-treated patients [30]. These symptoms probably reflect a decrease in dopaminergic neurotransmission. This hypothesis is supported by neuroimaging studies showing alterations in the activity of the basal ganglia during cytokine therapy [41,42]. A possible mechanism for this effect is the alteration of tyrosine hydroxylase activity, which is associated with cytokine administration. Tyrosine hydroxylase is the rate-limiting enzyme in the synthesis of dopamine. It makes use of tetrahydrobiopterin as a cofactor [43]. Tetrahydrobiopterin is also needed for the activation of the inducible form of nitric oxide synthase (NOS) that is responsible for the synthesis of NO, an important effector for actions of cytokines on their target cells [44,45]. If the production of NO consumes most of the tetrahydrobiopterin that is available locally, then there will not be enough left for the synthesis of dopamine, which could explain the relative deficit in dopaminergic neurotransmission. Such a possibility still needs to be tested.

Despite its heuristic value, the clinical relevance of the model of cytokine-induced depression could be questioned, since it is a rather extreme situation. However, there is evidence that overproduction of pro-inflammatory cytokines is also associated with mood disorders in chronic inflammatory medical conditions, including CHD. Of course, the relationship between cytokines and depression is much less easy to reveal, since patients with such medical conditions are examined at different stages of their disease process. This may result in much higher interindividual variability. Despite these constraints, it has been possible to observe higher levels of myocardial cytokines and higher antibody titres against microbial pathogens possibly involved in the pathophysiology of CHD in patients suffering from vital exhaustion at the time of coronary bypass [46]. In the same manner, depressive disorders that developed over time in post-ischaemic coronary patients were found to be associated with endothelial cell activation and probably inflammation, although the therapeutic use of statins that have anti-inflammatory actions certainly attenuated differences between cases and controls [47].

Conclusions and perspectives

Pro-inflammatory cytokines that are produced by activated innate immune cells induce sickness behaviour by promoting the synthesis and release of the same inflammatory mediators in the brain. The possibility that brain cytokines mediate the non-specific components of sickness that develop in patients with a medical condition is gaining more and more plausibility. For instance, patients with cancer report fatigue, pain, anorexia, sleep disorders, altered cognition and mood disorders. It has been proposed that the diversity of these symptoms certainly masks a common molecular mechanism represented by the central nervous system actions of pro-inflammatory cytokines produced by the host cells in response to the tumour itself or to radiotherapy and/or chemotherapy [48]. In the same vein, there is evidence that cognitive deterioration (and probably behavioural and mood disorders) occurs in patients with Alzheimer's disease who experience an infectious episode in addition to the already rampant neuro-inflammation that is associated with the disease [49]. This view is in accordance with the postulated role of chronic neuro-inflammation in the non-specific symptoms of sickness that can be observed in individuals with Alzheimer's disease providing one searches for them [50]. What applies to the various medical conditions that are listed here as examples certainly applies to other medical conditions that are associated with chronic inflammation and in which a higher prevalence of mood disorders has already been noted. Based on the data that have been collected in patients treated with cytokine immunotherapy, it is now possible to go beyond an educated guess and submit this hypothesis to test by measuring and relating to each other the inflammatory status, tryptophan metabolism, mood changes and other non-specific symptoms in depressed and non-depressed patients, preferably at the same stage of the disease process. Various methodologies can be used for this purpose. In view of the progress that has been made since the mid 1990s, the time is certainly ripe for developing some form of consensus on the selection of the best techniques available to engage in this type of research. At the same time, it should be possible to look for possible cytokine or neurotransmitter candidate genes to account for the vulnerability that has been alluded to earlier and that represents a key element in the understanding of cytokine-induced depression.

Acknowledgements

Supported by the Institute National de la Recherche Agronomique (INRA), the Centre National de la Recherche Scientifique (CNRS), French Ministry of Research (ACI Neurosciences intégrées et computationnelles to NC) and National Institutes of Health (NIH) 1 R01 MH071349-01 to RD.

REFERENCES

1. S. M. Consoli, Depression and associated organic pathologies, a still under-estimated comorbidity: results of the DIALOGUE study. *Presse Med.* **32** (2003), 10–21.

2. M. A. Abidi, A. A. Gadit, Liaison psychiatry and referral rates among hospitalized patients. *J. Coll. Physicians Surg. Pak.* **13** (2003), 274–6.

3. D. W. Kissane, B. Grabsch, A. Love, *et al.*, Psychiatric disorder in women with early stage and advanced breast cancer: a comparative analysis. *Aust. N. Z. J. Psychiatry* **38** (2004), 320–26.

4. D. D. Dunlop, J. S. Lyons, L. M. Manheim, J. Song, R. W. Chang, Arthritis and heart disease as risk factors for major depression: the role of functional limitation. *Med. Care* **42** (2004), 502–11.

5. P. P. Katz, E. H. Yelin, Prevalence and correlates of depressive symptoms among persons with rheumatoid arthritis. *J. Rheumatol.* **20** (1993), 790–96.

6. T. A. Murberg, E. Bru, T. Aarsland, S. Svebak, Functional status and depression among men and women with congestive heart failure. *Int. J. Psychiatr. Med.* **28** (1998), 273–91.

7. J. A. Spertus, M. McDonell, C. L. Woodman, S. D. Fihn, Association between depression and worse disease-specific functional status in outpatients with coronary artery disease. *Am. Heart J.* **140** (2000), 105–10.

8. A. M. Addington, J. J. Gallo, D. E. Ford, W. W. Eaton, Epidemiology of unexplained fatigue and major depression in the community: the Baltimore ECA follow-up, 1981–1994. *Psychol. Med.* **31** (2001), 1037–44.

9. R. Dantzer, Cytokine-induced sickness behaviour: where do we stand? *Brain Behav. Immun.* **15** (2001), 7–24.

10. R. Dantzer, Innate immunity at the forefront of psychoneuroimmunology. *Brain Behav. Immun.* **18** (2004), 1–6.

11. B. Beutler, Innate immunity: an overview. *Mol. Immunol.* **40** (2004), 845–59.

12. S. Kent, R. M. Bluthe, R. Dantzer, *et al.*, Different receptor mechanisms mediate the pyrogenic and behavioural effects of interleukin 1. *Proc. Natl. Acad. Sci. U. S. A.* **89** (1992), 9117–20.

13. P. Parnet, K. W. Kelley, R. M. Bluthe, R. Dantzer, Expression and regulation of interleukin-1 receptors in the brain: role in cytokines-induced sickness behaviour. *J. Neuroimmunol.* **125** (2002), 5–14.

14. A. M. van Dam, M. Brouns, S. Louisse, F. Berkenbosch, Appearance of interleukin-1 in macrophages and in ramified microglia in the brain of endotoxin-treated rats: a pathway for the induction of non-specific symptoms of sickness? *Brain Res.* **588** (1992), 291–6.

15. S. Laye, P. Parnet, E. Goujon, R. Dantzer, Peripheral administration of lipopolysaccharide induces the expression of cytokine transcripts in the brain and pituitary of mice. *Brain Res. Mol. Brain Res.* **27** (1994), 157–62.

16. S. Laye, G. Gheusi, S. Cremona, *et al.*, Endogenous brain IL-1 mediates LPS-induced anorexia and hypothalamic cytokine expression. *Am. J. Physiol. Regul. Integr. Comp. Physiol.* **279** (2000), R93–8.

17. R. Dantzer, J. P. Konsman, R. M. Bluthe, K. W. Kelley, Neural and humoral pathways of communication from the immune system to the brain: parallel or convergent? *Auton. Neurosci.* **85** (2000), 60–65.

18. G. N. Luheshi, R. M. Bluthe, D. Rushforth, *et al.*, Vagotomy attenuates the behavioural but not the pyrogenic effects of interleukin-1 in rats. *Auton. Neurosci.* **85** (2000), 127–32.

19. J. P. Konsman, P. Parnet, R. Dantzer, Cytokine-induced sickness behaviour: mechanisms and implications. *Trends Neurosci.* **25** (2002), 154–9.

20. B. L. Hart, Biological basis of the behaviour of sick animals. *Neurosci. Biobehav. Rev.* **12** (1988), 123–37.

21. R. Dantzer, K. W. Kelley, Stress and immunity: an integrated view of relationships between the brain and the immune system. *Life Sci.* **44** (1989), 1995–2008.

22. M. J. Kluger, Temperature regulation, fever, and disease. *Int. Rev. Physiol.* **20** (1979), 209–51.

23. M. J. Kluger, Is fever beneficial? *Yale J. Biol. Med.* **59** (1986), 89–95.

24. L. R. Watkins, S. F. Maier, The pain of being sick: implications of immune-to-brain communication for understanding pain. *Annu. Rev. Psychol.* **51** (2000), 29–57.

25. N. E. Miller, Some psychophysiological studies of motivation and of the behavioural effects of illness. *Bull. Br. Psychol. Soc.* **17** (1964), 1–20.

26. A. Aubert, G. Goodall, R. Dantzer, Compared effects of cold ambient temperature and cytokines on macronutrient intake in rats. *Physiol. Behav.* **57** (1995), 869–73.

27. A. Aubert, C. Vega, R. Dantzer, G. Goodall, Pyrogens specifically disrupt the acquisition of a task involving cognitive processing in the rat. *Brain Behav. Immun.* **9** (1995), 129–48.

28. A. Aubert, G. Goodall, R. Dantzer, G. Gheusi, Differential effects of lipopolysaccharide on pup retrieving and nest building in lactating mice. *Brain Behav. Immun.* **11** (1997), 107–18.

29. H. Anisman, Z. Merali, Cytokines, stress and depressive illness: brain–immune interactions. *Ann. Med.* **35** (2003), 2–11.

30. L. Capuron, A. Ravaud, A. H. Miller, R. Dantzer, Baseline mood and psychosocial characteristics of patients developing depressive symptoms during interleukin-2 and/or interferon-alpha cancer therapy. *Brain Behav. Immun.* **18** (2004), 205–13.

31. L. Capuron, J. F. Gumnick, D. L. Musselman, *et al.*, Neurobehavioural effects of interferon-alpha in cancer patients: phenomenology and paroxetine responsiveness of symptom dimensions. *Neuropsychopharmacology* **26** (2002), 643–52.

32. I. Jones, N. Craddock, Candidate gene studies of bipolar disorder. *Ann. Med.* **33** (2001), 248–56.

33. C. Heim, C. B. Nemeroff, The role of childhood trauma in the neurobiology of mood and anxiety disorders: preclinical and clinical studies. *Biol. Psychiatry* **49** (2001), 1023–39.

34. L. Capuron, A. Ravaud, Prediction of the depressive effects of interferon alfa therapy by the patient's initial affective state. *N. Engl. J. Med.* **340** (1999), 1370.

35. H. Miyaoka, T. Otsubo, K. Kamijima, *et al.*, Depression from interferon therapy in patients with hepatitis C. *Am. J. Psychiatry* **156** (1999), 1120.

36. L. Capuron, G. Neurauter, D. L. Musselman, *et al.*, Interferon-alpha-induced changes in tryptophan metabolism: relationship to depression and paroxetine treatment. *Biol. Psychiatry* **54** (2003), 906–14.

37. C. Constant, L. Castera, R. Dantzer, *et al.*, Mood alterations during interferon-alpha therapy in chronic hepatitis C: evidence for an overlap between manic/hypomanic and depressive symptoms. *J. Clin. Psychiatry* **66** (2005), 1050–57.

38. L. Capuron, A. Ravaud, P. J. Neveu, *et al.*, Association between decreased serum tryptophan concentrations and depressive symptoms in cancer patients undergoing cytokine therapy. *Mol. Psychiatry* **7** (2002), 468–73.

39. M. Maes, S. Bonaccorso, V. Marino, *et al.*, Treatment with interferon-alpha (IFN alpha) of hepatitis C patients induces lower serum dipeptidyl peptidase IV activity, which is related to IFN alpha-induced depressive and anxiety symptoms and immune activation. *Mol. Psychiatry* **6** (2001), 475–80.

40. J. Lestage, D. Verrier, K. Palin, R. Dantzer, The enzyme indoleamine 2,3-dioxygenase is induced in the mouse brain in response to peripheral administration of lipopolysaccharide and superantigen. *Brain Behav. Immun.* **16** (2002), 596–601.

41. F. D. Juengling, D. Ebert, O. Gut, *et al.*, Prefrontal cortical hypometabolism during low-dose interferon alpha treatment. *Psychopharmacology (Berl.)* **152** (2000), 383–9.

42. L. Capuron, G. Pagnoni, D. H. Lawson, *et al.*, Altered fronto-pallidal activity during high-dose interferon-alpha treatment as determined by positron emission tomography. *Abstr. Soc. Neurosci.* (2002), 498.5.

43. R. Hashimoto, T. Nagatsu, T. Ohta, M. Mizutani, I. Omura, Changes in the concentrations of tetrahydrobiopterin, the cofactor of tyrosine hydroxylase, in blood under physical stress and in depression. *Ann. N. Y. Acad. Sci.* **1018** (2004), 378–86.

44. M. Gilchrist, C. Hesslinger, A. D. Befus, Tetrahydrobiopterin, a critical factor in the production and role of nitric oxide in mast cells. *J. Biol. Chem.* **278** (2003), 50 607–14.

45. T. Kitagami, K. Yamada, H. Miura, *et al.*, Mechanism of systemically injected interferon-alpha impeding monoamine biosynthesis in rats: role of nitric oxide as a signal crossing the blood–brain barrier. *Brain Res.* **978** (2003), 104–14.

46. A. Appels, F. W. Bar, J. Bar, C. Bruggeman, M. de Baets, Inflammation, depressive symptomtology, and coronary artery disease. *Psychosom. Med.* **62** (2000), 601–605.

47. F. Lesperance, N. Frasure-Smith, P. Theroux, M. Irwin, The association between major depression and levels of soluble intercellular adhesion molecule 1, interleukin-6, and C-reactive protein in patients with recent acute coronary syndromes. *Am. J. Psychiatry* **161** (2004), 271–7.

48. C. S. Cleeland, G. J. Bennett, R. Dantzer, *et al.*, Are the symptoms of cancer and cancer treatment due to a shared biologic mechanism? A cytokine-immunologic model of cancer symptoms. *Cancer* **97** (2003), 2919–25.

49. C. Holmes, M. El-Okl, A. L. Williams, *et al.*, Systemic infection, interleukin 1beta, and cognitive decline in Alzheimer's disease. *J. Neurol. Neurosurg. Psychiatry* **74** (2003), 788–9.

50. P. Eikelenboom, W. J. Hoogendijk, C. Jonker, W. van Tilburg, Immunological mechanisms and the spectrum of psychiatric syndromes in Alzheimer's disease. *J. Psychiatr. Res.* **36** (2002), 269–80.

13

The hypothalamic–pituitary–adrenal axis: cortisol, DHEA and mental and behavioural function

Ian M. Goodyer

Introduction

Steroids are an extensive family of chemical agents distributed widely in the brain. They include the classical stress hormone cortisol, oestradiol, testosterone and progesterone (collectively known as the sex hormones), aldosterone and dehydroepiandrosterone (DHEA). Cortisol and DHEA are the most implicated in the response to demand. Both have a high density in the limbic system but are also found in the cortex. Circulating levels of steroids can be measured relatively easily in the periphery from blood, urine and saliva. These peripheral levels are correlated with levels in the cerebrospinal and ventricular fluid in the brain [1]. There is clear-cut evidence that certain steroids are manufactured in the brain and play a key role in brain development and plasticity [2]. These steroids include DHEA and its sulphate DHEAS. Within the brain, these neurosteroids modulate the effects of other transmitters, including gamma-aminobutyric acid (GABA) and glutamate. Neurosteroids can, therefore, alter neuronal excitability throughout the brain very rapidly by binding to receptors for inhibitory or excitatory neurotransmitters at the cell membrane. Alterations in levels of the adrenal steroids cortisol and DHEA have important implications for general cognitive and emotional function. These effects are brought about through altered sensitivity in receptors in steroid-sensitive areas of the brain, notably the limbic system, and their related frontal regions.

Cortisol, DHEA and the brain

Since the 1980s it has become increasingly apparent that steroids have key functions in the brain. Cortisol is critically involved in homeostasis and allostasis and is essential for survival when the body has to mobilise metabolic resources following an event, such as acute illness, physical trauma or social change. In contrast, the

Depression and Physical Illness, ed. A. Steptoe.
Published by Cambridge University Press. © Cambridge University Press 2006.

functions of DHEA are not fully understood, but it is known to be involved in two key processes: maintaining healthy blood vessels (vascular integrity) [3] and protecting the brain from the deleterious effects of cortisol [4]. The latter appears important when the levels of cortisol in the brain are high for days. In these circumstances, parts of the limbic system (notably the hippocampus) may be damaged, and DHEA may act as a neuroprotective agent [5,6]. In addition to adrenal steroids having direct effects on the brain and mental functions, they have interactions with the monoamines. Cortisol in particular has powerful bidirectional effects on serotonin systems in the brain. During development, the absence of cortisol results in serotonin down-regulation and depletion, indicating a potentially important set of relations between these two systems and perhaps a more complex role in the chemical adaptation to social adversity than considered hitherto [7,8].

A great deal is known about the control of cortisol secretion in relation to stressful environments. The hypothalamic–pituitary–adrenal (HPA) axis is the neurochemical system through which the release of cortisol is regulated. There is a negative feedback between the level of circulating cortisol in the periphery and receptor regulation at the level of the hippocampus in the brain. Cortisol enters the brain via the blood–brain barrier and attaches to glucocorticoid receptors therein. These receptors are located in a number of brain regions but are densely packed in the limbic system, and in the hippocampus and amygdala in particular. The degree of receptor occupancy acts as a control signal on the whole axis. High occupancy levels increase inhibitory signals to the hypothalamus, diminishing the release of the peptide corticotropin-releasing factor (CRF), which is the chemical signal passing to the pituitary and regulating the release of a second peptide, adrenocorticotropin hormone (ACTH). Diminished ACTH in response results in the adrenal gland diminishing the release of cortisol. This negative feedback system operates in a loop. Thus, as lower cortisol levels enter the brain, occupancy diminishes, CRF is up-regulated (due to loss of inhibition from the hippocampus) and the system releases more cortisol. This is a highly dynamic physiological process (Figure 13.1).

The glucocorticoid (GC) receptor shows polymorphic variation, the functional significance of which remains to be determined fully but appears in part to control individual variations in circulating levels [9,10]. Allelic variations also occur in the CRF peptide that controls the release of ACTH and, hence, cortisol. These receptors may be a target for preventing cortisol hypersecretion found in a significant proportion of depressive illnesses [11]. There is some preliminary evidence that if polymorphisms are present in both the GC receptor and the CRF peptide, then cortisol levels will be markedly different, depending on the inherited characteristics of these variants [9,10,12]. Thus, there are individual differences in cortisol levels due not only to reactivity to events but also to genetic differences. Furthermore,

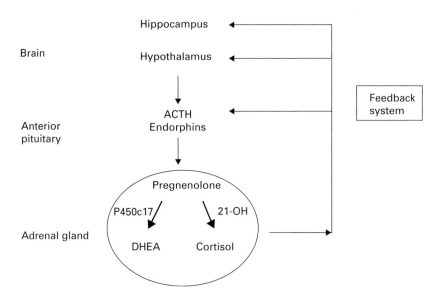

Figure 13.1 The hippocampal-pituitary-adrenal axis ACTH, adrenocorticotropin hormone; DHEA, dehydroepiandrosterone.

it is receptor sensitivity that is most likely to determine the impact of high steroid levels on the tissues in the brain and the subsequent physiological and psychological events. It may be that allelic variation leads to differences in receptor sensitivity and therefore variations in response to corticoids. Thus, the genetic structure of the receptor itself may contribute to modulating the risk for individual differences in behavioural response and psychiatric disorder via its sensitivity to circulating cortisol levels. Finally, allelic variations of CRF may be associated with a wide variety of behavioural characteristics, including the psychological process of behavioural inhibition (a measure of impulse control) [13] and high body mass index (BMI), indicating excess weight gain [14]. This indicates the complex and manifold functions of large peptide molecules in functional activity within an individual.

HPA axis development, dysfunction and psychiatric disorder

In the first nine months of life, the HPA axis is irregular in its function, and cortisol levels fluctuate markedly with no discernible pattern or rhythm. Minor perturbations, such as being picked up, being fed and having clothes changed, result in significant alterations in cortisol levels. By 12 months of age, there is a marked biobehavioural shift in the HPA axis control of cortisol [15]. Social regulation of the axis is now occurring and a rhythm is clearly established, with higher morning levels rising within the first hour after awakening and reaching an apex over the first few hours of the day, followed by a decline over the second half of the day to a low nadir from early evening. This diurnal rhythm remains in this form throughout life.

Investigations of diurnal rhythm of cortisol in twins show that the early-morning levels are significantly more alike in monozygotic twins than in dizygotic twins, whereas evening levels show no such similarity [16]. Other studies have shown that genetic influences on circulating cortisol persist over the 24-hour cycle and may affect the timing of the nadir and the apex [17,18]. This suggests that there is marked genetic control over the switching on of the axis in the morning, but environmental factors exert increasing effects on levels as the day proceeds, although genetic factors remain an influence [16].

As well as diurnal rhythm, levels show reactivity to events. These episodic movements in levels generally show a rapid rise in the presence of a stimulus, regardless of its salience, indicating that this change is related more to surprise or novelty than to personal meaning. Cortisol levels can remain quite high in relation to the behavioural requirements demanded by the stimulus, for example to engage in social conversation with a surprise visitor or to deal with an unpleasant event such as a car crash. Cortisol levels lower gradually as the consequences of the event pass. In general, levels return to baseline about 40 minutes after the cessation of the behavioural response. This rise and fall can occur at any time of the day and appears to be independent of the stage of the diurnal rhythm that the individual is at.

Measurement of circulating adrenal steroids

In contrast to in-dwelling cannulae to obtain blood or 24-hour urine collections, salivary collection allows repeated sampling of large populations. Salivary levels correlate highly with serum levels ($r = 0.6$–0.9), and the latter also correlate highly with levels in the ventricular cerebrospinal fluid (CSF) ($r = 0.8$) [1]. The salivary assays used to measure these steroids are sensitive and specific enough to detect the very low levels present in saliva and alterations in these levels over time. Cortisol levels in saliva (and in CSF) are about 5% of those in serum [19], reflecting the free (unbound to plasma protein) fraction (see below). Cortisol and DHEA in the saliva may reflect levels in the CSF (and, hence, exposure of the brain to these steroids), although there have been no direct studies of the associations between CSF and salivary levels in the same individual. Cortisol is secreted in a pulsatile fashion, and this is reflected in the saliva, with a time lag of about 15 minutes [20].

Cortisol shows marked reactivity to the environment, which is reflected in the amplitude of the diurnal rhythm: in the saliva of 12- to 18-year-olds, this is about ten-fold from 8 a.m. to 8 p.m. In a study of 234 adolescents, the mean ratio of salivary cortisol from 8 a.m. to 8 p.m. was 12.76 (coefficient of variation = 66.8%) [21].

It is important therefore to take sufficient samples, at sufficient time points, in order to define accurately the form of the diurnal pattern of cortisol. Current findings suggest that taking fewer than four samples spread over a 24-hour period is unlikely to provide a reliable index of rhythm, and sampling for less than four days is unlikely to give a valid reflection of mean values. More studies need to be carried out with adequate numbers of normal and mentally ill individuals across the lifespan to define the precise parameters of sampling requirements at different ages. Cortisol reacts to stressful events, e.g. [22], and so precautions should be taken to ensure that subjects are in a basal state, unless the response to stress or demand is an intended feature of the study, e.g. during a behavioural challenge task. Studies have shown that cortisol levels rise markedly following awakening, with the morning apex obtained approximately 45 minutes to an hour later [23,24]. A further consideration is how the data should be treated. A number of derivations can be obtained, which can impact on the sampling procedure. For example, using four samples obtained at the same time of day, it is possible to derive mean group values, compare individual differences in the mean morning awakening apex, or examine the mean maximum secreted level as an index of higher corticoid activity. The precise selection of measurement is related necessarily to the question being investigated. Few studies to date have adequately considered a priori these critical quantitative issues.

There is also a literature using dexamethasone suppression (DST) as an index of cortisol activity across the lifespan [25]. DST is an index of feedback sensitivity, not hypersecretion, and compared with cortisol levels has proved a less consistent index of HPA dysregulation. A more powerful challenge test is the combined dexamethasone/CRF test [26,27]. This has improved sensitivity and specificity and has been shown to identify feedback dysregulation in both patients with acute depression and first-degree relatives at risk for affective disorders. Pharmacological challenge procedures use drugs (e.g. fenfluramine) to probe the HPA axis or neural systems (e.g. serotonin) that impinge upon it [28]. Abnormal responses to such challenge in the form of blunted hormonal responses in the periphery are interpreted as reflecting dysfunctional neurochemical processes in the brain. These techniques provide valuable information about such systems and have been greatly enhanced through the addition of neuroimaging procedures to delineate alterations in blood flow of the brain regions of interest. Such studies have not examined the relations between levels of adrenal steroids, development and the onset of subsequent psychopathology. There is no technical reason why a developmental prospective programme of research monitoring changes in neurosteroid systems, and incorporating neuroimaging and challenge tests, should not be carried out at different points in the lifespan. A key issue for such technology-laden studies is a clear set of a priori hypotheses.

Table 13.1 Proposed protocol for psychoendocrine studies

1. Salivary collections taken at 8 a.m. (or within one hour of awakening), 12 p.m., 4 p.m. and 8 p.m.
2. Samples collected over at least 4 consecutive days
3. Consider negative chemical implications of using salivary aids to salivation
4. Validated assays to a research standard (sensitivity, accuracy, specificity)
5. Sufficient power (sample size) to avoid type 2 errors
6. Control and comparison groups appropriate to the research hypothesis
7. Careful choice of derived measure for analysis (means, peaks, maximum levels, diurnal variation, ratios, interquartile range, etc.)
8. Monitor potential confounds, e.g. steroid therapies including inhalers, prescribed and illicit drugs
9. Record lifestyle factors, including exercise, dieting and smoking
10. Data analytical procedures should take into account sex differences and multiple or repeated comparisons

For DHEA, a second major adrenal steroid, the picture is somewhat different. This steroid is also present in the saliva (and CSF) at about 5% of plasma levels, but there is no known plasma binding protein for DHEA, so the source of this relation remains obscure. The diurnal rhythm in saliva (8 a.m. to 8 p.m.) is also much less (about two-fold) than for cortisol. In adolescents, the mean ratio of salivary DHEA from 8 a.m. to 8 p.m. was 2.07 (coefficient of variation = 33.8%). Interestingly, levels vary with demand, being somewhat higher early in depressive illness but becoming increasingly reduced under conditions of chronicity.

The cortisol/DHEA ratio thus changes during the day from about 5–7 in the morning (8 a.m.) to about 2 at 8 p.m. This ratio is interesting in the light of interactions between the two steroids (see below). From the above, a minimum standard protocol for studies of cortisol and DHEA is proposed (Table 13.1).

Cortisol and unipolar depression

Studies of the HPA axis in psychiatric patients began in the 1970s, with the observation that severely depressed patients showed a sustained elevation of evening cortisol levels, leading to a loss of the expected diurnal rhythm. Such patients showed a sustained high level from around 8 p.m. through to 4 a.m. This observation has been repeated many times, but it is now clear that this dysregulation occurs in no more than about half (and perhaps even fewer) of depressed patients [25]. Until relatively recently, these evening alterations in HPA axis function were considered to be a consequence of being depressed. Thus, the HPA axis dysregulation has been considered an epiphenomenon of acute depressive illness. Two prospective studies have now established that morning cortisol hypersecretion precedes and predicts the onset of major depression in both adult women and adolescents of both sexes [29,30]. These studies measured morning and evening cortisol in adolescents of both sexes and adult women, respectively. Both samples were at high psychosocial risk for unipolar major depression. The participants were prospectively followed and re-evaluated at 12 months. Higher morning cortisol levels were associated with the subsequent onset of major depressive episodes over the follow-up period. In contrast, there was no difference in evening cortisol levels between those who became depressed and those who did not. The association between morning cortisol level and subsequent affective disorder was not a consequence of concurrent recent undesirable events or difficulties, and so it does not appear to be a reactivity effect to immediate or recent negative social experiences. Neither was the hormone–depression relationship a consequence of level of depressive symptoms at the time of cortisol measurement. In the adolescent study there were no sex differences in the liability for subsequent major depression. It appears that higher morning cortisol is a risk factor for both sexes. The findings suggest that this hormonal vulnerability arises from more distal origins rather than recent life events and difficulties. Whether this is a consequence of environmental programming of the HPA axis in early life, genetic factors influencing sensitivity to circulating cortisol, or both, remains unknown.

A further community study failed to establish a direct association between higher cortisol levels and depression in adult women but noted a strong link between cortisol levels and an increase in negative life events [31]. Depressed patients with higher cortisol levels are significantly more likely to experience further negative life events than depressed individuals with normal cortisol levels [32]. These depression-dependent negative life events increase the liability for persistent disorder. Thus, the pathological process that arises from high cortisol levels in currently depressed patients is one that disturbs some aspects of affective-cognitive function that disrupt interpersonal behaviour.

There is increasing evidence that cortisol hypersecretion is also correlated with disturbances in memory [33,34]. A range of factors may influence this cortisol–memory relationship, including social adversity and a previous history of cortisol hypersecretion [35–38]. It seems highly likely that a key cortisol function in the brain of healthy humans is to modulate learning and memory and, perhaps, retrieval of information. This modulation process may have its key focus in the limbic system but is likely to exert an influence on general brain state involving many regions, including the prefrontal and orbitofrontal cortex [39,40].

Overall, the neurochemical coding for responses to social events and the subsequent liability for anxiety and/or depression may be as follows:

1. Occupancy of steroid receptors in the hippocampus and the amygdala triggers a complex cascade of cellular events, leading to subjectively altered mood and organisation of the appraised experiences.
2. Activation and modulation of these affective processes occurs through changes in the level of serotonin (and probably other monoamine systems) in the prefrontal and orbitofrontal cortex.
3. These interrelated physiological changes in the brain, with changes in monoamines as the last chemical step, lead to activation of cognitive controls and behavioural actions.
4. Serotonin-vulnerable individuals will react poorly to the corticoid-driven affective signals arising from deeper in the brain. High cortisol levels will therefore not be responded to adequately and may lead to abnormal psychological processes and psychiatric disorders.

As yet, there are no methodologically sound studies in the community determining how cortisol and serotonin systems interact to cause common anxiety and depressive disorders. Perhaps there will be further advances in understanding the neurochemical basis of response to stress and the onset of psychiatric disorders via modern neuroimaging procedures. Combining this technique with functional activation of brain and chemical systems using chemical and psychological challenge has already shown considerable interplay between the limbic and frontal cortex in volunteers and depressed patients [39,41,42]. These studies are only in their first decade, and much will be learned in the near future.

It remains entirely unclear why only a proportion of depressed individuals or those at risk for depression show higher circulating cortisol levels. It is increasingly apparent that the key process is associated not so much with production but with the tissue sensitivity to circulating cortisol. For example, genotypic variation within the glucocorticoid receptor gene is responsible for variations in response to dexamethasone suppression [43]. There are at least ten polymorphisms in this receptor, which are functionally associated with individual differences in tissue response to circulating cortisol [44]. Further research on the genotype–phenotype relations is likely to cast more light on the associations between HPA axis dysregulation and both physical and mental illnesses [45,46].

DHEA

DHEA shows a very different developmental history to that of cortisol [47]. Unlike cortisol, concentrations of DHEA and its sulphate DHEAS vary with age [48]. DHEA is made by the placenta, and so the fetus is exposed to its action: concentrations decline from the first few months of life until 5 years of age and then rise rapidly from age 7 in girls and around 9 in boys (this is called adrenarche), until levels reach their peak between the ages of 20 and 30 years. Adrenarche is separable from puberty, since gonadotrophins and oestrogen have no effect on DHEA levels and the two events are not linked across time. After age 20–30 years, levels begin to decline in both sexes. By the age of 70–80 years, levels are approximately 10–20% that of a 20-year-old [49]. Unlike cortisol, there is no clear-cut notion of how DHEA is regulated. It is not under the tight control of the HPA axis, and so although levels vary somewhat with the rise and fall of cortisol as the adrenal is stimulated to secrete glucocorticoids, there are clearly other factors involved. DHEA has been shown to act as an antagonist to cortisol at the level of the glucocorticoid receptor [5]. There is also evidence that DHEA promotes neurogenesis [4]. This ability to promote new neuronal growth could, if replicated, be a key neural feature of this hormone. Since high cortisol levels persisting over days are associated with an increase in depression, DHEA may have neuroprotective effects in the brain, diminishing the liability for cortisol to damage neurons and thereby decreasing the risk for psychopathology.

There is also preliminary evidence that increasing DHEA levels lower cortisol in the periphery, providing further support for an antiglucocorticoid effect of DHEA [50]. If this is the action of DHEA, then subjects at risk for psychiatric disorders and showing high cortisol levels would be expected to show high levels of DHEA; this was demonstrated in a prospective study of adolescents. Those who subsequently developed major depression over the next 12 months had significantly higher levels than expected for their age and sex [21,29]. The possibility that this rise is an attempt to offset the increase in cortisol activity is attractive but requires further investigation before firm conclusions can be drawn. For example, there was no clear-cut evidence from the adolescent study that higher DHEA decreased cortisol in some at-risk youths and thereby lowered the liability for subsequent depression. What is clear is that DHEA not only is a passive indicator of a maturational effect of age but also is involved in some active process. The finding requires replication, but DHEA is a promising candidate as a neuroprotective agent at times of acute social adversity.

There is some evidence that although DHEA levels rise during the early phase of a major depression, they may fall if the disorder persists. Two longitudinal studies of depressed patients, one from clinically referred patients and the other from a community-based study, have shown that higher cortisol/DHEA ratios predict persistent disorder and occur due to declining DHEA levels during the illness [32,51]. These findings support the notion that DHEA secretion is vulnerable to chronic illness effects and that its decline is associated with a poor short-term outcome. The reasons for this decline in a potentially helpful neurosteroid are not clear. It may reflect the severity of the metabolic strain that a severe mental illness can produce. Similar findings have been noted in critically medically ill patients, where low DHEA levels predict a poor response to treatment and higher mortality [52,53].

A further difference from cortisol is the absence of any clear-cut associations with psychological processes. DHEA does not appear to be related to memory, learning or self-evaluation measures [54]. By contrast there is quite good evidence that DHEA enhances positive mood and may act as an antidepressant [55–58]. Interestingly, DHEA does not appear to exert effects via testosterone, even though it is in the same metabolic pathway of androgen production. Rather, DHEA appears to have direct effects on the brain, perhaps via its antiglucocorticoid actions in the amygdala and hippocampus, thereby showing a bias for modulating neuroaffective rather than neurocognitive systems. Although definitive studies of sufficient sample size are required to confirm these observations, the evidence that DHEA has mood-enhancing effects is compelling. Following the discovery of an endothelial receptor for DHEA, it may not be too long now before we are able to describe the physiology of this compound. From the psychiatric perspective, DHEA is potentially an important modulator of disordered mood states and deserves to be studied in detail as an adjunct to current treatments, particularly in persistent mood disorders. Much greater precision is required in investigating cognitive–DHEA relations before concluding that there is no association between memory, learning and information retrieval and individual differences in DHEA.

Specific social adversities, steroids and monoamines

Infant stress

Research has implicated a role for infant exposure to adverse early experiences in the formation of HPA axis sensitivity. Animal studies have reported a substantial non-genetic effect of adverse maternal rearing practices on the development of chemical coding systems for behaviour, including HPA axis, hypothalamic and extra-hypothalamic corticotropin-releasing hormone, monoaminergic and GABA/benzodiazepine systems. Loss of maternal care through separation leads to a potential change in the chemical signalling processes between the limbic system and the frontal and prefrontal cortex. Findings in rodents have outlined the neurochemical mechanisms that occur via epigenetic programming as a consequence of variations in maternal care style [59]. The evidence shows that there are major effects on glucocorticoid receptor sensitivity in rodent pups dependent on the degree of positive care obtained. This early environmental effect can be lifelong, with adverse effects on behaviour persisting through to adult rodent life. The pathological mechanisms result in significantly fewer steroid receptors in the limbic system and lower expression of neurotrophic genes involved in brain growth and function. These dysfunctions occur because in pups exposed to adverse rearing, there is methylation of nerve-growth-factor-inducible protein (NGFI) in the presence of high cortisol, effectively silencing this neurotrophic gene, which is a component for activating normal early brain development. Remarkably, the authors of this study showed that in infant rats exposed to poor care, it was possible to alter deleterious effects on brain through demethylation of NGFI via chemical means, thereby switching on the neurotrophic genes that had been switched off by the higher cortisol levels occurring due to the environmental events. This led to a restoration of behaviours no different to those of the normally reared pups. Whether the impact of such experiences varies with genetic variation in glucocorticoid and CRF receptors and shows different effects on levels at different times of the day (or on the 24-hour rhythm as a whole) is not known. Overall, this clear study provides definitive evidence for a key environmental process on the developmental programming of the HPA axis system in a mammalian model. Prospective studies of human infants can now be carried out delineating both the glucocorticoid genetic variation and early rearing environment and examining both the HPA axis stability and behavioural patterns of function.

A partial advance in this direction can be seen in the results of a prospective study of an adolescent cohort followed since birth. Salivary assessment of steroids in adolescents at 13 years of age showed significant increases in morning cortisol levels in those exposed to postnatal depression and difficult early maternal experiences compared with those without such exposure [60]. This long-term association remained even when current adolescent depressive symptoms, puberty and current parental wellbeing were taken into account. This certainly suggests that early adversities may exert long-term effects on HPA axis function and might indicate one familial pathway that results in an increased vulnerability for psychopathology. Whether the liability for higher cortisol levels occurred in those with a particular allelic variation in the glucocorticoid receptor gene is not known.

The extent to which these early effects on brain systems can be moderated via subsequent positive developmental pathways in the environment (such as good peer relations in the preschool and school years) and/or genetic variations in behaviourally sensitive gene pathways is not known. Animal studies on monkeys have shown that offspring that carry the s allele of the serotonin transporter gene and are subject to maternal separation are more likely to show abnormal brain chemistry. These animals have been reported as being more fearful and less prosocial than their mother-reared counterparts with the same genetic makeup [61]. This suggests an important gene–environment interaction in early infancy that leads to a vulnerable animal. These findings are complementary to those reported by Caspi and colleagues showing a significant interaction between the same allelic variation and the increased liability for life events predicting the onset of major depression [62].

Deprivation, maltreatment and traumatic experience

As childhood proceeds, two major negative experiences are, unfortunately, more common than any society would like. First, general deprivation frequently results in low emotional stimulation and a poverty of social experiences required for normal cognitive development, often accompanied by overlooked poor nutrition. Many studies have demonstrated that these privation experiences are associated with an increase in common emotional and behavioural disorders in the school-age years. Severe chronic privations, such as being brought up in an orphanage since birth, are also associated with changes in the sensitivity of the HPA axis, with cortisol hypersecretion frequently (but not inevitably) reported [63]. The multiplicity of factors in chronic deprivation prevents any specific associations being drawn from such studies. Whether social and emotional neglect, poor nutrition, high rates of infection and poor hygiene act separately or in concert to produce HPA axis abnormalities in the early years of life is not clear.

A second major set of events in childhood to influence the HPA axis is that of child maltreatment. Here, the negative experience is focused on physical and/or sexual abuse of children. Invariably in these studies, overt maltreatment is associated with emotionally abusive experiences, such as persistent critical comment, narrow and restricted social opportunities, and a lack of a secure, emotionally consistent confiding relationship. Unfortunately, it has become increasingly apparent that these experiences have significant biological consequences for neural systems and chemical codes for behaviour. Child maltreatment is associated with cortisol hypersecretion in some studies but also with cortisol hyposecretion in others [15]. The latter observation is particularly puzzling but is not confined to maltreatment experiences. Some patients exposed to severe traumas, including war injuries and road-traffic accidents, and diagnosed as suffering from post-traumatic stress disorder (PTSD) also show cortisol hyposecretion [64]. This apparent suppression of HPA axis activity may not arise solely from the recent focal experience but may also be connected either to prior experience or perhaps to genetic vulnerabilities for low cortisol activity. Thus, we do not yet know whether, for some individuals, very severe trauma has a direct and relatively instant suppressive effect on HPA function [64].

Severe conduct disorders

There is a small but increasing literature suggesting that an entirely different group of behaviour disorders also hyposecrete cortisol, even at times of stress. Children, adolescents and young adults with severe conduct disorders have been shown to have remarkably suppressed cortisol levels compared with controls [65,66]. These individuals are known to have high levels of chronic psychosocial adversities, but it is not clear whether low levels of cortisol, suggesting a suppressed HPA axis, are related to a history of adversity, to a particular form of adversity or even to no adversity in this group of behavioural disorders. Indeed, about 10% of the population at large may have flat cortisol levels over the 24-hour period rather than the more common diurnal variation [67]. The implications of a flat cortisol level in the population at large, and the finding that this occurs in some individuals with markedly different disorders, such as PTSD and severe conduct disorder, is a puzzle that requires some considerable sorting out.

The presence of extreme levels (high or low) of cortisol suggests a loss of synchrony or perhaps a blunting between the neurochemical signalling pathways within the brain. For example, experimental studies on conduct-disordered children that induced frustration showed no increase in cortisol levels relative to age-matched controls, who exhibited the predicted rise at the time of stress stimulus [68]. Interestingly, although cortisol levels remained flat during this emotionally charged challenge test, heart rate also remained flat, although the conduct-disordered children reported feeling out of control and angry [69]. These findings showing dissociation between affective-cognitive and physiological responses following induced frustration suggest a potential loss of synchrony at the neurochemical level.

Repeating these studies using neuroimaging techniques may allow us to test whether conduct-disordered individuals do indeed show a different pattern of neural response to that of controls. Lower heart rate in childhood is associated with higher risk for antisocial personality disorder in adult life [70], and behaviourally disordered individuals report fearlessness, even when confronted with fearful stimuli [71,72]. There are also reported reductions in the grey matter of the brain in adults diagnosed with psychopathic disorders [73]. All of these findings support a brain-based aetiology to explain the fact that responses to social adversity are different in behaviourally disordered individuals over the life-span. There are also changes in the serotonin system in severe psychopaths, who show low serotonin function correlated with increased impulsivity compared with controls [74].

What does this impaired serotonin and increased impulsivity response have to do with low or flat cortisol levels at times of stress? Cortisol is part of the chemical coding pathway that accesses personally salient emotional related memories (episodic memories) [35]. Low sensitivity to fearfulness may impair the mobilisation of a fear response through loss of retrieval of fear-related memories. Such memories may not even be kept in memory by behaviour-disordered individuals. This will blunt any signalling processes to cognitive centres in the cortex, and serotonin-vulnerable individuals will be at risk for disinhibited, impulsive non-socially adaptive behavioural responses following adverse experiences. Low or flat cortisol levels during challenge may indicate a defective affectively driven information-processing pathway.

There may also be a developmental connection. The high rate of exposure to chronic adverse life events and difficulties from infancy over the childhood period may suppress or exacerbate the liability for a normal cortisol response to subsequent adversities. Extreme variations in either direction in the cortisol system may induce deleterious changes in monoamine systems in the cortex. The reasons for this may reside in the glucocorticoid rather than the serotonin genes. As described earlier in this chapter, the glucocorticoid receptor gene and the corticotropin-releasing hormone gene possess polymorphisms that influence the regulatory processes controlling the level of circulating cortisol [9,10,75]. These polymorphisms may be functional and may alter the response to circulating levels of cortisol at the level of the receptor. Thus, the glucocorticoid receptor polymorphism may be one of many genes determining the liability for up- or down-regulating the signal from the limbic system to the cortical system following cortisol exposure. It does seem very possible that the level of circulating cortisol varies with experience and that the sensitivity of tissue response is determined by genetic variation and environmental influences in both cortisol and serotonin systems working together to effect the best adaptation possible to environmental demands. The current evidence points to pathophysiology arising from the HPA axis system as due to impairments in the glucocorticoid signalling processes leading to abnormalities of response in the complex cellular cascade following steroid receptor interaction, rather than the over- or under-production of cortisol itself [76]. This process may be, as shown by the work of Weaver and colleagues [59], largely epigenetic in origin, arising from adverse experience but moderated by the nature of genetic variation in key receptor components of this major metabolic system.

Acknowledgements

The author is supported by the Wellcome Trust. He is a member of the Medical Research Council (MRC) Centre for Brain, Behaviour and Neuropsychiatry, Cambridge University.

REFERENCES

1. E. P. Guazzo, P. J. Kirkpatrick, I. M. Goodyer, S. Shiers, J. Herbert, Cortisol, dehydroepiandrosterone (DHEA), and DHEA sulfate in the cerebrospinal fluid of man: relation to blood levels and the effects of age. *J. Clin. Endocrinol. Metab.* **81** (1996), 3951–60.

2. E. E. Baulieu, Neurosteroids: a novel function of the brain. *Psychoneuroendocrinology* **23** (1998), 963–87.

3. D. Liu, J. S. Dillon, Dehydroepiandrosterone activates endothelial cell nitric-oxide synthase by a specific plasma membrane receptor coupled to Galpha(i2,3). *J. Biol. Chem.* **277** (2002), 21 379–88.

4. K. K. Karishma, J. Herbert, Dehydroepiandrosterone (DHEA) stimulates neurogenesis in the hippocampus of the rat, promotes survival of newly formed neurons and prevents corticosterone-induced suppression. *Eur. J. Neurosci.* **16** (2002), 445–53.

5. V. G. Kimonides, M. G. Spillantini, M. V. Sofroniew, J. W. Fawcett, J. Herbert, Dehydroepiandrosterone antagonizes the neurotoxic effects of corticosterone and translocation of stress-activated protein kinase 3 in hippocampal primary cultures. *Neuroscience* **89** (1999), 429–36.

6. V. G. Kimonides, N. H. Khatibi, C. N. Svendsen, M. V. Sofroniew, J. Herbert, Dehydroepiandrosterone (DHEA) and DHEA-sulfate (DHEAS) protect hippocampal neurons against excitatory amino acid-induced neurotoxicity. *Proc. Natl. Acad. Sci. U. S. A.* **95** (1998), 1852–7.

7. D. T. Chalmers, S. P. Kwak, A. Mansour, H. Akil, S. J. Watson, Corticosteroids regulate brain hippocampal 5-HT1A receptor mRNA expression. *J. Neurosci.* **13** (1993), 914–23.

8. S. Wissink, O. Meijers, D. Pearce, B. van der Berg, P. van der Saag, Regulation of the rat serotonin-1A receptor gene by corticosteroids. *J. Biol. Chem.* **275** (2000), 1321–6.

9. R. Rosmond, Y. C. Chagnon, M. Chagnon, *et al.*, A polymorphism of the 5′-flanking region of the glucocorticoid receptor gene locus is associated with basal cortisol secretion in men. *Metabolism* **49** (2000), 1197–9.

10. R. Rosmond, M. Chagnon, C. Bouchard, P. Bjorntorp, A polymorphism in the regulatory region of the corticotropin-releasing hormone gene in relation to cortisol secretion, obesity, and gene–gene interaction. *Metabolism* **50** (2001),1059–62.

11. C. B. Nemeroff, New directions in the development of antidepressants: the interface of neurobiology and psychiatry. *Hum. Psychopharmacol.* **17**: Suppl 1 (2002), 13–16.

12. J. W. Smoller, J. F. Rosenbaum, J. Biederman, *et al.*, Association of a genetic marker at the corticotropin-releasing hormone locus with behavioral inhibition. *Biol. Psychiatry* **54** (2003), 1376–81.

13. J. W. Smoller, J. F. Rosenbaum, J. Biederman, *et al.*, Genetic association analysis of behavioral inhibition using candidate loci from mouse models. *Am. J. Med. Genet.* **105** (2001), 226–35.

14. B. G. Challis, J. Luan, J. Keogh, *et al.*, Genetic variation in the corticotrophin-releasing factor receptors: identification of single-nucleotide polymorphisms and association studies with obesity in UK Caucasians. *Int. J. Obes. Relat. Metab. Disord.* **28** (2004), 442–6.

15. M. R. Gunnar, B. Donzella, Social regulation of the cortisol levels in early human development. *Psychoneuroendocrinology* **27** (2002),199–220.

16. M. Bartels, E. J. de Geus, C. Kirschbaum, F. Sluyter, D. I. Boomsma, Heritability of daytime cortisol levels in children. *Behav. Genet.* **33** (2003), 421–33.

17. P. Linkowski, A. Van Onderbergen, M. Kerkhofs, *et al.*, Twin study of the 24-h cortisol profile: evidence for genetic control of the human circadian clock. *Am. J. Physiol.* **264** (1993), E173–81.

18. A. W. Meikle, J. D. Stringham, M. G. Woodward, D. T. Bishop, Heritability of variation of plasma cortisol levels. *Metabolism* **37** (1988), 514–17.

19. I. M. Goodyer, J. Herbert, P. M. E. Altham, *et al.*, Adrenal secretion during major depression in 8 to 16 year olds: I. Altered diurnal rhythms in salivary cortisol and dehydroepiandrosterone (DHEA) at presentation. *Psychol. Med.* **19** (1996), 245–56.

20. C. Kirschbaum, D. Hellhammer, Salivary cortisol in psychoendocrine research: recent developments and applications. *Psychoneuroendocrinology* **19** (1994), 313–33.

21. I. M. Goodyer, J. Herbert, A. Tamplin, P. M. Altham, First-episode major depression in adolescents: affective, cognitive and endocrine characteristics of risk status and predictors of onset. *Br. J. Psychiatry* **176** (2000), 142–9.

22. M. R. Gunnar, Quality of early care and buffering of neuroendocrine stress reactions: potential effects on the developing human brain. *Prev. Med.* **27** (1998), 208–11.

23. J. C. Pruessner, O. T. Wolf, D. H. Hellhammer, *et al.*, Free cortisol levels after awakening: a reliable biological marker for the assessment of adrenocortical activity. *Life Sci.* **61** (1997), 2539–49.

24. J. C. Pruessner, D. H. Hellhammer, C. Kirschbaum, Burnout, perceived stress, and cortisol responses to awakening. *Psychosom. Med.* **61** (1999), 197–204.

25. P. M. Plotsky, M. J. Owens, C. B. Nemeroff, Psychoneuroendocrinology of depression: hypothalamic-pituitary-adrenal axis. *Psychiatr. Clin. North Am.* **21** (1998), 293–307.

26. M. Deuschle, U. Schweiger, U. Gotthardt, *et al.*, The combined dexamethasone/corticotropin-releasing hormone stimulation test is more closely associated with features of diurnal activity of the hypothalamo-pituitary-adrenocortical system than the dexamethasone suppression test. *Biol. Psychiatry* **43** (1998), 762–6.

27. S. Watson, P. Gallagher, D. Del-Estal, *et al.*, Hypothalamic-pituitary-adrenal axis function in patients with chronic depression. *Psychol. Med.* **32** (2002), 1021–8.

28. S. B. Park, D. J. Williamson, P. J. Cowen, 5-HT neuroendocrine function in major depression: prolactin and cortisol responses to D-fenfluramine. *Psychol. Med.* **26** (1996), 1191–6.

29. I. M. Goodyer, J. Herbert, A. Tamplin, P. M. Altham, Recent life events, cortisol, dehydroepiandrosterone and the onset of major depression in high-risk adolescents. *Br. J. Psychiatry* **177** (2000), 499–504.

30. T. O. Harris, S. Borsanyi, S. Messari, *et al.*, Morning cortisol as a risk factor for subsequent major depressive disorder in adult women. *Br. J. Psychiatry* **177** (2000), 505–10.

31. P. L. Strickland, J. F. Deakin, C. Percival, *et al.*, Bio-social origins of depression in the community: interactions between a. dversity. social, cortisol and serotonin neurotransmission. *Br. J. Psychiatry* **180** (2002), 168–73.

32. I. M. Goodyer, J. Herbert, A. Tamplin, Psychoendocrine antecedents of persistent first-episode major depression in adolescents: a community-based longitudinal enquiry. *Psychol. Med.* **33** (2003), 601–10.

33. J. W. Newcomer, G. Selke, A. K. Melson, *et al.*, Decreased memory performance in healthy humans induced by stress-level cortisol treatment. *Arch. Gen. Psychiatry* **56** (1999), 527–33.

34. S. J. Lupien, C. W. Wilkinson, S. Briere, *et al.*, The modulatory effects of corticosteroids on cognition: studies in young human populations. *Psychoneuroendocrinology* **27** (2002), 401–16.

35. S. J. Lupien, M. Lepage, Stress, memory, and the hippocampus: can't live with it, can't live without it. *Behav. Brain Res.* **127** (2001), 137–58.

36. S. J. Lupien, S. King, M. J. Meaney, B. S. McEwen, Can poverty get under your skin? Basal cortisol levels and cognitive function in children from low and high socioeconomic status. *Devel. Psychopathol.* **13** (2001), 653–76.

37. S. J. Lupien, C. W. Wilkinson, S. Briere, *et al.*, Acute modulation of aged human memory by pharmacological manipulation of glucocorticoids. *J. Clin. Endocrinol. Metab.* **87** (2002), 3798–807.

38. S. J. Lupien, S. King, M. J. Meaney, B. S. McEwen, Child's stress hormone levels correlate with mother's socioeconomic status and depressive state. *Biol. Psychiatry* **48** (2000), 976–80.

39. W. C. Drevets, Neuroimaging abnormalities in the amygdala in mood disorders. *Ann. N. Y. Acad. Sci.* **985** (2003), 420–44.

40. D. A. Seminowicz, H. S. Mayberg, A. R. McIntosh, *et al.*, Limbic-frontal circuitry in major depression: a path modeling metanalysis. *Neuroimage* **22** (2004), 409–18.

41. M. Liotti, H. S. Mayberg, S. K. Brannan, *et al.*, Differential limbic–cortical correlates of sadness and anxiety in healthy subjects: implication for affective disorders. *Biol. Psychiatry* **48** (2000), 30–42.

42. J. H. Meyer, S. Kapur, B. Eisfeld, *et al.*, The effect of paroxetine on 5-HT(2A) receptors in depression: an [(18)F]setoperone PET imaging study. *Am. J. Psychiatry* **158** (2001), 78–85.

43. S. Wust, E. F. Van Rossum, I. S. Federenko, *et al.*, Common polymorphisms in the glucocorticoid receptor gene are associated with adrenocortical responses to psychosocial stress. *J. Clin. Endocrinol. Metab.* **89** (2004), 565–73.

44. A. Stevens, D. W. Ray, E. Zeggini, *et al.*, Glucocorticoid sensitivity is determined by a specific glucocorticoid receptor haplotype. *J. Clin. Endocrinol. Metab.* **89** (2004), 892–7.

45. E. F. Van Rossum, P. G. Voorhoeve, S. J. te Velde, *et al.*, The ER22/23EK polymorphism in the glucocorticoid receptor gene is associated with a beneficial body composition and muscle strength in young adults. *J. Clin. Endocrinol. Metab.* **89** (2004), 4004–4009.

46. E. F. van Rossum, J. W. Koper, A. W. van den Beld, *et al.*, Identification of the BclI polymorphism in the glucocorticoid receptor gene: association with sensitivity to glucocorticoids in vivo and body mass index. *Clin. Endocrinol. (Oxf.)* **59** (2003), 585–92.

47. P. D. Kroboth, F. S. Salek, A. L. Pittenger, T. J. Fabian, R. F. Frye, DHEA and DHEA-S: a review. *J. Clin. Pharmacol.* **39** (1999), 327–48.

48. C. R. Parker, Dehydroepiandrosterone and dehydroepiandrosterone sulfate production in the human adrenal during development and aging. *Steroids* **64** (1999), 640–47.

49. F. Labrie, A. Belanger, L. Cusan, J. L. Gomez, B. Candas, Marked decline in serum concentrations of adrenal C19 sex steroid precursors and conjugated androgen metabolites during aging. *J. Clin. Endocrinol. Metab.* **82** (1997), 2396–402.

50. P. D. Kroboth, J. A. Amico, R. A. Stone, *et al.*, Influence of DHEA administration on 24-hour cortisol concentrations. *J. Clin. Psychopharmacol.* **23** (2003), 96–9.

51. I. M. Goodyer, R. J. Park, J. Herbert, Psychosocial and endocrine features of chronic first-episode major depression in 8–16 year olds. *Biol. Psychiatry* **50** (2001), 351–7.

52. A. Beishuizen, L. G. Thijs, I. Vermes, Decreased levels of dehydroepiandrosterone sulphate in severe critical illness: a sign of exhausted adrenal reserve? *Crit. Care* **6** (2002), 434–8.

53. C. Marx, S. Petros, S. R. Bornstein, *et al.*, Adrenocortical hormones in survivors and nonsurvivors of severe sepsis: diverse time course of dehydroepiandrosterone, dehydroepiandrosterone-sulfate, and cortisol. *Crit. Care Med.* **31** (2003), 1382–8.

54. F. A. Huppert, J. K. Van Niekerk, Dehydroepiandrosterone (DHEA) supplementation for cognitive function. *Cochrane Database Syst. Rev.* **2** (2001), CD000304.

55. P. J. Hunt, E. M. Gurnell, F. A. Huppert, *et al.*, Improvement in mood and fatigue after dehydroepiandrosterone replacement in Addison's disease in a randomized, double blind trial. *J. Clin. Endocrinol. Metab.* **85** (2000), 4650–56.

56. J. K. van Niekerk, F. A. Huppert, J. Herbert, Salivary cortisol and DHEA: association with measures of cognition and well-being in normal older men, and effects of three months of DHEA supplementation. *Psychoneuroendocrinology* **26** (2001), 591–612.

57. O. M. Wolkowitz, V. I. Reus, A. Keebler, *et al.*, Double-blind treatment of major depression with dehydroepiandrosterone. *Am. J. Psychiatry* **156** (1999), 646–9.

58. R. D. Strous, R. Maayan, R. Lapidus, *et al.*, Dehydroepiandrosterone augmentation in the management of negative, depressive, and anxiety symptoms in schizophrenia. *Arch. Gen. Psychiatry* **60** (2003), 133–41.

59. I. C. Weaver, N. Cervoni, F. A. Champagne, *et al.*, Epigenetic programming by maternal behavior. *Nat. Neurosci.* **7** (2004), 847–54.

60. S. L. Halligan, J. Herbert, I. M. Goodyer, L. Murray, Exposure to postnatal depression predicts elevated cortisol in adolescent offspring. *Biol. Psychiatry* **55** (2004), 376–81.

61. M. Champoux, A. Bennett, C. Shannon, *et al.*, Serotonin transporter gene polymorphism, differential early rearing, and behavior in rhesus monkey neonates. *Mol. Psychiatry* **7** (2002), 1058–63.

62. A. Caspi, K. Sugden, T. E. Moffitt, *et al.*, Influence of life stress on depression: moderation by a polymorphism in the 5-HTT gene. *Science* **301** (2003), 386–9.

63. M. R. Gunnar, S. J. Morison, K. Chisholm, M. Schuder, Salivary cortisol levels in children adopted from Romanian orphanages. *Dev. Psychopathol.* **13** (2001), 611–28.

64. R. Yehuda, S. L. Halligan, J. A. Golier, R. Grossman, L. M. Bierer, Effects of trauma exposure on the cortisol response to dexamethasone administration in PTSD and major depressive disorder. *Psychoneuroendocrinology* **29** (2004), 389–404.

65. R. Loeber, S. M. Green, B. B. Lahey, P. J. Frick, K. McBurnett, Findings on disruptive behavior disorders from the first decade of the Developmental Trends Study. *Clin. Child. Fam. Psychol. Rev.* **3** (2000), 37–60.

66. K. Pajer, W. Gardner, R. T. Rubin, J. Perel, S. Neal, Decreased cortisol levels in adolescent girls with conduct disorder. *Arch. Gen. Psychiatry* **58** (2001), 297–302.

67. A. A. Stone, J. E. Schwartz, J. Smyth, *et al.*, Individual differences in the diurnal cycle of salivary free cortisol: a replication of flattened cycles for some individuals. *Psychoneuroendocrinology* **26** (2001), 295–306.

68. S. H. van Goozen, W. Matthys, P. T. Cohen-Kettenis, *et al.*, Salivary cortisol and cardiovascular activity during stress in oppositional-defiant disorder boys and normal controls. *Biol. Psychiatry* **43** (1998), 531–9.

69. S. H. van Goozen, W. Matthys, P. T. Cohen-Kettenis, J. K. Buitelaar, H. van Engeland, Hypothalamic-pituitary-adrenal axis and autonomic nervous system activity in disruptive children and matched controls. *J. Am. Acad. Child. Adolesc. Psychiatry* **39** (2000), 1438–45.

70. A. Raine, P. H. Venables, S. A. Mednick, Low resting heart rate at age 3 years predisposes to aggression at age 11 years: evidence from the Mauritius Child Health Project. *J. Am. Acad. Child. Adolesc. Psychiatry* **36** (1997), 1457–64.

71. A. Raine, C. Reynolds, P. H. Venables, S. A. Mednick, D. P. Farrington, Fearlessness, stimulation-seeking, and large body size at age 3 years as early predispositions to childhood aggression at age 11 years. *Arch. Gen. Psychiatry* **55** (1998), 745–51.

72. R. J. Blair, E. Colledge, L. Murray, D. G. Mitchell, A selective impairment in the processing of sad and fearful expressions in children with psychopathic tendencies. *J. Abnorm. Child Psychol.* **29** (2001), 491–8.

73. A. Raine, T. Lencz, S. Bihrle, L. LaCasse, P. Colletti, Reduced prefrontal gray matter volume and reduced autonomic activity in antisocial personality disorder. *Arch. Gen. Psychiatry* **57** (2000), 119–27.

74. M. Dolan, W. J. Deakin, N. Roberts, I. Anderson, Serotonergic and cognitive impairment in impulsive aggressive personality disordered offenders: are there implications for treatment? *Psychol. Med.* **32** (2002), 105–17.

75. R. DeRijk, M. Schaaf, E. de Kloet, Glucocorticoid receptor variants: clinical implications. *J. Steroid. Biochem. Mol. Biol.* **81** (2002), 103–22.

76. C. L. Raison, A. H. Miller, When not enough is too much: the role of insufficient glucocorticoid signaling in the pathophysiology of stress-related disorders. *Am. J. Psychiatry* **160** (2003), 1554–65.

14

Depression and immunity: biological and behavioural mechanisms

Michael Irwin

Introduction

Depression has a huge impact on individuals and society, with a lifetime prevalence of over 15%. By 2020, depression will be the second leading illness in the world, as projected by the World Health Organization (WHO). In addition to the emotional consequences of depression, the disorder is increasingly implicated in a wide range of medical conditions. Moreover, a growing body of evidence indicates that depression, including even minor depression, has notable immunological consequences. It is important therefore to consider possible immune mechanisms in the detrimental effects of depression on health, particularly in vulnerable individuals such as elderly people and patients with chronic disease.

This chapter provides a review of the research being conducted on the relationship between depression and immunity, beginning with an overview of the clinical importance of depressive disorders for mortality risk. The various immune alterations that occur during depression are examined, with discussion of the role of autonomic, neuroendocrine and behavioural (e.g., sleep) mechanisms. The chapter concludes with consideration of the clinical implications of immune changes in depression for several medical disorders.

Clinical characteristics of depression

Definition of depression

Depression can be defined as a condition that primarily entails a disturbance of mood; this affective disturbance is often characterised by a mood that is sad, hopeless, discouraged or simply depressed [1]. The diagnostic definition of a major depressive disorder states that the depressed mood or loss of pleasure (i.e. anhedonia) must last for at least two weeks, be accompanied by a series of related

Depression and Physical Illness, ed. A. Steptoe.
Published by Cambridge University Press. © Cambridge University Press 2006.

symptoms (e.g. vegetative signs, sleep disturbance) and should not be caused by another psychiatric disorder, general medical condition or substance use/abuse. The symptoms typically experienced during depression include significant weight change ($+/-5\%$), sleep disturbance (insomnia, hypersomnia), psychomotor retardation or agitation, pervasive fatigue, feelings of worthlessness or irrational guilt, mental concentration difficulties and recurrent suicidal ideation.

Although most studies of immune abnormalities have focused on major depression, there appears to be a dose–response relationship between severity of depression and changes of immunity. Thus, several studies have examined the effects of minor depression on immunity, as discussed below. While minor depression is noted as a potential diagnostic category that needs further empirical validation [2], it is essentially characterised by a disturbance in mood or a loss of pleasure, with the presence of two additional symptoms (rather than four for major depressive disorder). Minor depression is also associated with functional impairments and is often viewed as a prodromal state for the occurrence of major depression [2].

Clinical course

The clinical course of major depressive disorder varies markedly with age: its onset is protracted in older adults, with prodromal and progressive elevation of depressive symptoms, in contrast to the relatively short clinical onset in younger patients [3]. Furthermore, in older adults depressive symptoms and stress of physical disability can initiate a continuous decline in physical and psychological health. Even with ongoing clinical management, there are often lingering depressive symptoms and an increased risk of relapse in older adults who are experiencing life stress and chronic disease burden [4]. Together, these data are consistent with the view of depressive disorders as chronic and recurrent with residual disability [5].

Depression, morbidity and mortality

The impact of major depression on disease outcomes and the onset and progression of chronic disease have received increasing attention, due in part to compelling epidemiological data linking depression to mortality [6]. When defined as a taxonomical disorder (e.g. meeting or not meeting diagnostic criteria) or as a continuum (e.g. scores on a depression measure) [7–9], depression is associated with an almost two-fold increased risk of mortality in heterogeneous patient populations typical of a hospitalised setting [8] and in older adults residing in a nursing home [9]. The mortality risk is particularly robust for patients with cardiovascular disease. Patients recovering from myocardial infarction who have a depression show about a two- to three-fold elevated risk of death, even after controlling for the effects of previous cardiovascular severity and extent of cardiac compromise [10,11]. Other data show that behavioural changes that are commonly found in depression, such as disordered sleep, also have independent effects on mortality risk. For example, in older adults, difficulties with sleep initiation and/or maintenance prospectively predicted increased risk of death after controlling for age, gender and medical status [12–15].

Multisystem physiological abnormalities in depression

Central modulation of immunity: effects of corticotropin-releasing hormone

Depressed patients show elevated levels of corticotropin-releasing hormone (CRH) [16]. This key peptide is involved in integrating neural, neuroendocrine and immune responses to stress. Release of CRH in the brain alters a variety of immune processes, including aspects of innate immunity, cellular immunity and in vivo measures of antibody production [17,18]. Peripheral immune measures also change following lesioning of the brain (e.g. hypothalamus) or in response to the stimulation of certain brain regions, which ultimately impact on CRH systems. Autonomic and neuroendocrine pathways are critical links between the brain and the immune system: pharmacological or anatomical (e.g. denervation, adrenalectomy) blockade antagonises the central action of CRH and other peptides (e.g. interleucin1 [IL-1]) on immune function [17–20].

Autonomic nervous system

Consistent with the notion that depression is associated with activation of the peripheral sympathetic nervous system (SNS), depressed patients show elevated levels of circulating catecholamines and neuropeptide Y [21] at rest and in response to acute physical and/or psychological challenge. Such changes in sympathetic activity are thought to regulate aspects of the immune system and to mediate changes of immunity in depression. Sympathetic nerve terminals are juxtaposed with immune cells in organs where the immune system cells develop and respond to pathogens (e.g. bone marrow, thymus, spleen, lymph nodes) [18,22], and receptor binding of noradrenaline and neuropeptide Y serves as 'hard-wire' signal in the connection between the brain and the immune system. Sympathetic nerves also penetrate into the adrenal gland and cause the release of adrenaline into the bloodstream, which circulates to immune cells as another sympathetic regulatory signal.

Under both laboratory and naturalistic conditions including depression, sympathetic activation has been shown to suppress the activity of diverse populations of immune cells including natural killer (NK) cells and T-lymphocytes [18,22]. In contrast, other aspects of the immune response can be enhanced. For example, catecholamines can increase the production of antibodies by B-cells and the ability of macrophages to release cytokines and thereby signal the presence of a pathogen. Additional studies indicate that sympathetic activation can also shunt some immune system cells out of circulating blood and into the lymphoid organs (e.g. spleen, lymph nodes, thymus) while recruiting other types of immune cell into circulation (e.g. NK cells). It is thought that sympathetic activation reduces the immune system's ability to destroy pathogens that live inside cells (e.g. viruses) by decreasing of the cellular immune response, while enhancing the humoral immune response to pathogens that live outside cells (e.g. bacteria) [22].

Neuroendocrine axis

A hallmark of major depression is dysregulation of the hypothalamic-pituitary-adrenal (HPA) axis and the overexpression of cortisol. Cortisol exerts diverse effects on a wide variety of physiological systems and also coordinates the actions of various cells involved in an immune response by altering the production of cytokines or immune messengers [23]. Similar to sympathetic activation, cortisol can suppress the cellular immune response critical to defending the body against viral infections. Cortisol can also prompt some immune cells to move out from circulating blood into lymphoid organs or peripheral tissues such as the skin [24]. The role of HPA dysregulation and abnormal glucocorticoid sensitivity in relation to immune abnormalities in depression is discussed below.

Immunological findings in depression

Converging evidence indicates that depression is associated with alterations of neuroendocrine and autonomic nervous system (ANS) activity, which legitimises the possibility that depression might also alter immune system activity via these pathways. The nature and extent of immune abnormalities found in association with depression are noted for changes in numbers of immune cells, alterations in the function of lymphocytes and dysregulation of the cytokine network.

Enumerative measures

One of the first immunological findings identified in depressed individuals was an increase in the total number of white blood cells and an increase in the numbers and percentages of neutrophils and lymphocytes [25–28]. Inconsistent findings regarding monocyte counts have been garnered, with increases found for depressed individuals in some studies [27] and other depression samples showing decreases or no differences in the absolute or relative numbers of monocytes [25,29]. One population-based cohort study ($n = 11\,367$) revealed an association between recency of depression history and an incremental elevation of white blood cell counts in men but not in women, even with adjustment for age and smoking status [30]. Similar to the findings in adults, depressed adolescents show increased numbers of leukocytes, lymphocytes and monocytes [31].

Cellular enumeration of lymphocyte subsets by the quantification of phenotypic specific cell-surface markers has shown that depression is related negatively to the number and percentages of lymphocytes that are B-cells, T-cells, T-helper cells and T-suppressor/cytotoxic cells [32]. A decrease in circulating number of cells that express the NK cell phenotype has also been reported, which in part is moderated by gender: a decline of NK cell numbers is found in male but not female depressed individuals as compared with gender-matched controls [33]. In depressed adolescents, there is also evidence of a reduced number of NK cells [31]. However, multiple discrepant findings have been reported and, in one of the largest study samples of depressed subjects, no difference in the number of peripheral blood lymphocytes or T-lymphocyte subsets was found between depressed patients and controls [34]. Indeed, with the recent accumulation of studies, it is questionable as to whether there are consistent changes in the number of circulating B-, T- or NK cells in depression [35].

Functional measures

Function of the immune system has typically been evaluated in depressed individuals by assay of non-specific mitogen-induced lymphocyte proliferation, mitogen-stimulated cytokine production and NK cytotoxicity. Some of the first observations evaluating depression and mitogen responses showed reduced proliferation in depressed individuals compared with controls [36,37]. However, subsequent studies failed to replicate these observations, raising questions about the reliability of this immune alteration in depression [34]. Nevertheless, with over a dozen studies that have examined lymphocyte proliferation in depressed adults adolescents [34,38–52), it appears that an impairment in the response of lymphocytes to all three non-specific mitogens predominates in studies of depressed subjects [35].

A reduction of NK activity is now considered to be one of the most reliable and reproducible alterations of ex vivo immune function in depression [35,53]. Irwin and colleagues [29] first reported a decline of NK activity in depressed patients compared with age- and gender-matched comparison controls, and ten subsequent independent samples have replicated this observation [54,55]. Several caveats must be considered when reviewing the associations between NK activity, NK numbers and depression. Compared with controls, decreases in NK counts and NK activity were limited to male but not female depressed individuals [33], and other studies have found no difference of NK activity in depression [34,56]. One study of depressed adolescents found an increase of NK activity [31]. Nevertheless, the meta-analyses of Zorrilla *et al.* [35] and Herbert and Cohen [32] found that depression is associated with a reliable decrease of NK activity. The factors that might moderate or mediate the effects of depression on NK activity are discussed later in this chapter.

Stimulated cytokine production

In contrast with the findings regarding lymphocyte proliferation and NK activity, studies of stimulated cytokine production have not yielded consistent findings. In whole-blood assays, Kronfol and Rennick [57] found increased lipopolysaccharide stimulated production of IL-1β and interleukin 6 (IL-6), but there was no change in the expression of tumour necrosis factor-alpha (TNF-α). Similarly, Bauer *et al.* failed to identify differences in the stimulated production of the T-cell cytokine interleukin 2 (IL-2) [58,59] or in TNF-α in treatment-resistant depressed patients. However, similar to the effects of chronic stress in elderly people, depressed older adults show a dysregulation in the relative balance of Th1 (interferon gamma, IFN-γ) vs. Th2 cytokines (interleukin 10, [IL-10]) as detected by intracellular cytokine assay of CD-8 culture populations incubated with antigens of the anti-influenza vaccine and re-stimulation with a non-specific mitogen [60].

Circulating levels of cytokines: evidence for pro-inflammatory activation

Along with a reduction of non-specific cellular and natural immunity, there is emerging evidence that major depression is associated with immune activation reminiscent of an acute-phase response, including increases in levels of cells bearing activation markers such as HLA-DR+ and CD25+ (interluekin-2 [IL-2] receptor) [61] and increases in humoral factors or plasma proteins (e.g. α1-acid glycoprotein, α1-anti-trypsin, haptoglobin) [62]. There are also reported increases in the circulating concentration of the soluble IL-2 receptor that is released with immune activation [61]. In addition, cytokines such as IL-6, which are typically associated with an inflammatory process, are reportedly elevated in depression, including depressed elderly people [60,63]. Miller *et al.* [64] have suggested that subpopulations of depressed patients, such as individuals with obesity, are likely to show greater elevations of IL-6 than non-obese depressed patients whereas others have suggested that smoking status contributes to increases of IL-6 in depression [65]. However, even after adjustment for socioeconomic status, smoking and body mass index (BMI), elevated levels of IL-6 were more prevalent among people with depressed mood in a community-based sample of older people ($n = 2879$) [66]. Similarly, in a representative sample of the US population ($n = 6149$), a history of major depression was associated with elevated levels of C-reactive protein (CRP), a marker of immune activation, although this relationship was present only in men. In contrast, children with major depression fail to show elevated levels of IL-1β and TNF-α [67]. Together, these data raise the possibility that elderly or older adult populations with depression may be at greater risk for abnormal elevations of pro-inflammatory cytokines. It has been speculated that immune activation is a consequence of depression, although the acute induction of depression by tryptophan depletion of central monoamines failed to alter plasma levels of IL-6 or TNF receptor, and decreases of the Th2 cytokine IL-4 were found [68].

As discussed below, immune activation and the expression of inflammatory cytokines are thought to mediate the link between depression and inflammatory disorders, including cardiovascular disease [69] and rheumatoid arthritis [70]. In addition, pro-inflammatory cytokines are hypothesised to contribute to the occurrence of depressive symptoms in certain medical populations [71], although review of this topic extends beyond the scope of this chapter.

Viral-specific immune measures

Considerable evidence supports the notion that psychological stress and possibly depression are associated with an increased risk of infectious disease [72]. Thus, effort has focused on evaluation of viral-specific immune responses rather than non-specific measures of immunity, with emerging data suggesting that major depression leads to a functional decline of viral-specific memory T-cell responses. Compared with controls, depressed middle-aged adults show a loss in the frequency of peripheral blood immune cells that can respond to challenge with the varicella zoster virus [73]; this loss of memory T-cell function to varicella zoster virus is thought to be a surrogate marker for herpes zoster risk.

Assays of in vivo responses

Another promising strategy to evaluate the effects of depression on immune competence and infectious disease risk focuses on the assessment of in vivo immune responses as measured by delayed-type hypersensitivity (DTH; antigen-specific cell-mediated immune response) or vaccine challenge. In animals, administration of an acute stressor leads to a rapid increase in the DTH response [74], which remains elevated for several days following the challenge. In contrast, chronic stress in animals suppresses the DTH response [74]. In depressed patients, suppression of the DTH response to a panel of antigenic challenges has been found [75]. In contrast, Shinkawa and colleagues [76] found that depressed older people were more likely to show positive tuberculin responses compared with non-depressed people. One small study of ten elderly depressed patients found a modest decline of humoral antibodies to influenza vaccine one month after vaccination compared with controls [60], consistent with observations that psychological stress is associated with declines of hepatitis B antibody responses [77] as well as antibody response to influenza immunisation in elderly [78,79] but not other adult [80] populations.

Clinical moderating factors

Increasing interest has focused on the clinical factors that may identify depressed patients that are vulnerable to the immunological changes found in depression. One such factor is older age, which is associated with marked declines in cellular immunity. Indeed, the presence of comorbid depression, and possibly stress, appears to magnify age-related immune alterations. Gender also exerts differential effects on pituitary, adrenal and immune systems by modulating the sensitivity of target tissues. In response to psychological stress, women show a blunted inhibition of pro-inflammatory cytokine expression [81], which might place them at increased risk for autoimmune disorders compared with men. In contrast, declines of T-cell and NK cell responses appear to be more prominent in depressed men than depressed women [33]. With regard to ethnicity, African American ethnicity interacts with a history of alcohol consumption to exacerbate immune abnormalities [54], although the influence of ethnicity on depression-related changes of immunity is not known. Finally, specific diagnostic comorbidity might moderate immune system functioning in depression. For example, a number of studies have identified sleep in the regulation of some aspects of immune function [82–84], and depressed individuals with somatic symptoms are more likely to show immune changes [85] than those without neurovegetative symptoms.

Treatment of depression

Castanon *et al.* [86] reviewed animal research that focused on the immunological effects of antidepressant medications and concluded that antidepressants decrease pro-inflammatory cytokine expression. Although the specific mechanism(s) involved were not identified, antidepressants modify the expression of glucocorticoids and their receptors [87,88], limit the synthesis of prostaglandin and nitric oxide (NO), which contribute to pro-inflammatory effects [89,90], and act on intracellular messenger pathways, with downstream effects on pro-inflammatory cytokines [91]. However, there are also contradictory findings: in humans, in vitro co-incubation of stimulated immune cells with imipramine, venlafaxine or fluoxetine increased the production of IL-6 but did not affect TNF [92].

Several studies have now investigated the in vivo effects of antidepressant medication on immunity by examining the clinical course of depression along with changes of immunity in relation to antidepressant medication treatment and symptom resolution. In one longitudinal case–control study, Irwin and co-workers [93] found that depressed patients showed a decrease of Hamilton depression scores and an increase in NK activity from the start of treatment to follow-up. Changes of NK activity were related to changes in depressive symptom severity but not treatment status with antidepressant medications. In another longitudinal follow-up study of young adults with unipolar depression involving six weeks of treatment with nortriptyline and alprazolam, clinical improvements in the severity of depressive symptoms was associated with decreased numbers of circulating lymphocytes and decreased responses to phytohaemagglutinin (PHA) and concavalin A (Con A) but not pokeweed mitogen (PWM). In addition, decreases in T-cells, CD4+ and CD29 were found, although there were no changes in B-cell numbers or CD8+ cells. None of these changes was related to nortriptyline blood levels [94]. In addition, Frank *et al.* [95] found that in vivo and in vitro treatment with fluoxetine, a selective serotonin reuptake inhibitor (SSRI), resulted in enhanced NK activity along with changes in depressive symptoms. Finally, one study found that treatment with psychotropic medications reduced pro-inflammatory cytokine interleukin 12 (IL-12) expression in hospitalised psychiatric patients (with schizophrenia, depression or bipolar disorder) compared with controls [96], consistent with the view held by Kenis and Maes [97] that antidepressants decrease pro-inflammatory cytokine expression.

Mechanisms of immune dysfunction in depression

Biological mediators

Depression alters two pathways that have effects on immune system functioning: sympathetic nervous system activity and HPA axis function. Some data are now available to indicate that abnormalities in these efferent mechanisms contribute to immune changes in depression.

Considerable data show that depression is associated with abnormal elevations in sympathetic tone, as measured by increases in resting levels and exaggerated responses to psychological stress. For example, Irwin *et al.* [21] found that plasma concentrations of neuropeptide Y are elevated in depressed patients, aged people and people undergoing severe Alzheimer's disease caregiver stress. In support of the hypothesis that elevated sympathetic activity is associated with immune alterations in depression, further study found that activation of the sympathetic nervous system and release of neuropeptide Y correlated with a reduction of natural cytotoxicity in depression and life stress. Other studies show that excretion of 3-methoxy-4-hydroxy-phenylglycol (MHPG), an index of total body noradrenergic turnover, or sympathetic activity, is related inversely to lymphocyte proliferative responses in depressed patients [48].

An important function of the HPA axis is to shape-immune responses, particularly inflammatory changes such as increases in the production of acute-phase reactants, elevations in circulating levels of pro-inflammatory cytokines (e.g. IL-6 in plasma) and increases in stimulated in vitro peripheral blood monocyte production of proinflammatory cytokines [98]. For example, dexamethsone non-suppression identifies a group of depressed individuals most likely to demonstrate immune activation in which increased concentrations of plasma IL-6 correlate positively with post-DST cortisol levels [99]. Likewise, in a study of 28 in-patients with major depression, Maes and colleagues [100] found a significant positive correlation between mitogen-induced IL-1β production and post-DST cortisol values, which suggested that IL-1β oversecretion may contribute to HPA axis overactivity in depression. Finally, in treatment-resistant depression, cells of non-suppressors produced significantly less TNF compared with suppressors [58].

Unlike the association between markers of immune activation and HPA dysregulation, several studies of patients with major depression have failed to show a relationship between altered T-cell responses or NK cell activity and plasma or urinary concentrations of free cortisol, despite the recognised action of glucocorticoids to suppress multiple aspects of lymphocyte function. For example, in depressed patients, decreased lymphocyte responses to mitogens are not associated with dexamethasone non-suppression [36] or with increased excretion rates of urinary free cortisol [41]. Furthermore, in bereavement complicated by depressive symptoms, changes of NK activity are not associated with plasma cortisol levels [101]. Raison and Miller [102] have suggested that the impairments in T-cell proliferation and NK cell activity frequently reported in major depression might be accounted for by either excessive or insufficient glucocorticoid signalling, which is due in part to the action of pro-inflammatory cytokines to disrupt T-cell signalling pathways and inhibit NK cell activity. One study to our knowledge has shown that low NK cell activity is not associated with increases of circulating levels of IL-6 in the context of major depression [65].

Behavioural mechanisms

In addition to the biological mediators of immune changes in depression, examination of health status and behavioural factors is needed in clinical psychoneuroimmunology. For example, alcohol and tobacco have well-recognised effects on immunity, and yet there is limited empirical information on the processes by which these substances alter immune function in depressed individuals, despite their high rates of use in depressed patients. In the following section, four of the more pertinent behavioural factors linking depression and immune dysfunction are discussed, namely tobacco smoking, alcohol/substance abuse, activity/exercise and sleep disturbance.

Smoking: prevalence and immune effects

Cigarette smoking poses a considerable health risk, with effects on immunity via direct actions or possibly endocrine-mediated mechanisms [103]. Nicotine is reported to affect the HPA axis [104] and humoral and cellular immunity [105]. Additionally, specific immunological alterations occur in adult smokers, affecting a variety of parameters. Adult male smokers have been found to exhibit higher white blood cell (WBC) counts and lower NK activity than non-smoking controls. Jung and Irwin [106] evaluated the interaction between depression status and smoking history, and together these two factors produce greater declines of NK activity than those found in depressed or smoking groups alone. Cigarette use alone, or in combination with depression, might also contribute to the suppression of other non-specific measures of immune function, such as mitogen-induced lymphocyte proliferation. Given the effects of cigarette smoking on markers of immune activation [107], it is also important to address whether smoking status alters the reported relationship between depression and increases in serum levels of IL-6 and acute-phase proteins. Pike and Irwin [65] showed that elevations of IL-6 are found predominantly in depressed smokers, but not in depressed non-smokers, although others have suggested that depression has an independent effect on circulating levels of IL-6 and CRP [64,69]. Importantly, depression appears to interact with cigarette smoking to impact health, rather than there being a unitary link between depression and cancer. In a 12-year follow-up of 2264 adult men and women, depressed mood was found to interact with cigarette smoking, and together depressed mood and cigarette smoking were associated with a marked increase in the relative risk of cancer [108] as compared with the risk associated with smoking or depression status alone.

Alcohol dependence: immune effects in depression

According to Cadoret [109], nearly 30% of individuals with depression also suffer from alcohol dependence and over 30% of depressed individuals escalate their drinking during the depressive episode. Whereas alcohol and substance dependence and depression have a significant negative impact on the immune system, the interaction of alcohol/substance abuse with affective disorders may result in significantly more immune impairment than either condition alone. In a study by Irwin *et al.* [110], individuals with a dual diagnosis of alcoholism and depression have further decreases of NK activity compared with individuals diagnosed with only alcoholism or only depression. Furthermore, these researchers found that depressed individuals with a history of alcoholism had lower NK activity compared with depressed individuals without such a history. Alcoholics with secondary depression showed a further decrease in cytotoxicity compared with alcoholics who were not clinically depressed [111]. Strikingly, this result reflects the effects of a past history of alcohol consumption, rather than the direct pharmacological effect of alcohol, as the alcohol-dependent individuals were free of alcohol for a minimum of two weeks. Consequently, in studies of depressed individuals, the influence of alcohol abuse on immune parameters may not dissipate simply due to a washout period lasting days to weeks.

Activity and exercise: immune consequences in depression

Activity, or a lack thereof, can have negative consequences on the immune system, and some data suggest that older adults with depression may be especially vulnerable to the harmful effects of sedentary lifestyles. Conversely, exercise has been shown to have potent salutary effects on immune measures and has even been found to promote a remission of depressive symptoms in older adults. In the meta-analysis of Herbert and Cohen [32], melancholic depression correlated with greater impairments of cellular immunity, which may be due, at least in part, to an increased predominance of neurovegetative symptoms [54]. Cover and Irwin [85] found that severity of psychomotor retardation uniquely predicted declines of NK activity, similar to the effects of insomnia.

Disordered sleep and immunity: relevance to depression

Disordered sleep and loss of sleep are thought to adversely affect resistance to infectious disease, increase cancer risk and alter inflammatory disease progression. Animal studies show that sleep deprivation impairs influenza viral clearance and increases rates of bacteraemia. In humans, normal sleep is associated with a redistribution of circulating lymphocyte subsets, increases of NK activity, increases of certain cytokines (e.g. IL-2, IL-6) and a relative shift towards Th1 cytokine expression that is independent of circadian processes. Conversely, sleep deprivation suppresses NK activity and IL-2 production, although prolonged sleep loss has been found to enhance measures of innate immunity and pro-inflammatory cytokine expression.

Insomnia is one of the most common complaints of depressed patients, but its role in moderating and/or mediating immune alterations in depression has been relatively unexplored. However, with evidence that subjective insomnia correlates with NK activity in depression, but not with other depressive symptoms, including somatisation, weight loss, cognitive disturbance and diurnal variation [112], the hypothesis has emerged that disordered sleep may be a distinct factor accounting for some of the observed immune alterations found in depression.

In depressed individuals at risk for disordered sleep, alterations of natural and cellular immune function among depressed patients correlate with disturbances of electroencephalography (EEG)-monitored sleep [84,85]. Studies in bereaved subjects have replicated this correlation, and studies have shown by way of causal statistical analyses that disordered sleep also mediates the relationship between severe life stress and a decline of NK responses [113]. Further studies involving subjects with primary insomnia (e.g. no depression, other psychiatric disorder, medical disorder) have found that prolonged sleep latency and fragmentation of sleep are associated with nocturnal elevations of sympathetic catecholamines and declines in daytime levels of NK cell responses [114,115]. A more extensive line of research focused on alcohol-dependent patients with profound disturbances of sleep continuity and sleep architecture [116,117] found that decreases of total sleep time, declines of delta sleep and increases of rapid-eye movement (REM) sleep are associated with increases in the nocturnal and daytime expression of IL-6, possibly with consequences for daytime fatigue [118]. Thus, it appears that disordered sleep may be a critical behavioural factor that mediates the relationship between depression and immune alterations.

Clinical implications of immunity in depression

The factors that account for individual differences in the rate and severity of disease progression are not understood fully. There is, however, increasing evidence to suggest that behaviour and multisystem physiological changes that occur during depression come together to exacerbate the course of many chronic diseases. In the following sections, several pertinent disease examples are presented in relation to relevant psychoneuroimmunology processes in depression.

Cardiovascular disease

Atherosclerosis is now thought to be an inflammatory process that involves a series of steps [119], each of which appears to be impacted by stress and/or depression. Activated macrophages within the vasculature secrete pro-inflammatory cytokines, which in turn leads to expression of adhesion molecules. With recruitment of immune cells to the vascular cell wall or endothelium, and the release of inflammatory cytokines, the vascular endothelium expresses adhesion molecules that facilitate further binding of immune cells. Importantly, psychological and physical stressors increase the release of pro-inflammatory cytokines and expression of adhesion molecules that tether ('slow down') and bind immune cells to the vascular endothelium [120,121]. Moreover, it appears that depression is associated with endothelium activation. Acute coronary patients who are depressed show an increased expression of an adhesion molecule that is released following activation of the vascular endothelium (i.e. soluble intracellular adhesion molecule) [69]. Importantly, this molecular marker of endothelial activation and IL-6 predict risk of future myocardial infarction.

Infectious disease risk

Compelling evidence has shown that inescapable stress, a putative animal model of depression, increases susceptibility to some viral diseases via alterations in immune function [122]. In humans, prospective epidemiological studies and experimental viral challenge studies show that individuals reporting more psychological stress have a higher incidence and a greater severity of certain infectious illness, such as common colds [123]. In most studies, immune correlations were not obtained, although stress-related increases of IL-6 temporally predict greater symptom severity in individuals inoculated with influenza A. Moreover, experimental vaccinations have been used to examine the disease-specific and integrated in vivo action of the immune system in relation to psychological stress.

Human immunodeficiency virus (HIV) infection also shows a highly variable course. Depression, bereavement and maladaptive coping responses to stress (including the stress of HIV infection itself) have all been shown to predict the rate of immune-system decay in patients with HIV. Immune-system decline and HIV replication are particularly rapid in patients living under chronic stress (e.g. gay men who conceal their homosexuality) and in patients with high levels of sympathetic nervous system (SNS) activity (e.g. socially inhibited introverts) [124,125]. Tissue culture studies have shown that SNS neurotransmitters and glucocorticoids can accelerate HIV replication by rendering T-lymphocytes more vulnerable to infection and by suppressing production of the antiviral cytokines that help cells to limit viral replication [126]. Current research is focusing on pharmacological strategies to block the effects of stress neuroendocrine hormones on chronic viral infections such as HIV.

Rheumatoid arthritis: neuroimmune mechanisms

In a negative feedback loop, pro-inflammatory cytokines stimulate the HPA axis, resulting in the secretion of glucocorticoids, which in turn suppresses the immune response. However, in autoimmune disorders such as rheumatoid arthritis (RA), it is thought that the counter-regulatory glucocorticoid response is not achieved fully. In animals that are susceptible to arthritis, there is a central hypothalamic defect in the biosynthesis of CRH, blunted induction of ACTH and adrenal steroids, and decreased adrenal steroid receptor activation in immune target tissues, which together contribute to a weak HPA response (unable to suppress the progression of an autoimmune response) [127]. RA patients also show a relative hypofunctioning of the HPA axis despite the degree of inflammation [128].

In a meta-analysis of RA studies, Dickens *et al.* [129] found that depression was more common in patients with RA than in healthy controls. Stress and depression can lead to HPA axis activation and to increases in pro-inflammatory cytokines, and data suggest that stressful events, particularly interpersonal stressful events, provoke symptoms of disease, such as greater pain and functional limitations in RA patients [130]. For example, negative self-beliefs (e.g. helplessness) predicted greater flare activity in a group of patients undergoing a three-month clinical drug trial. Moreover, the presence of depression in RA patients undergoing stress is associated with exaggerated increases of IL-6, a biomarker predictive of disease progression [70]. Conversely, administration of a psychological intervention that decreases emotional distress produced improvements in clinician-rated disease activity in RA patients, although immunological mediators were not measured [131].

Summary

Substantial evidence generated over two decades of research has found that depression is related to many aspects of immune function, including enumerative changes, functional changes and changes in the expression of cytokines. The relationship between depression and immune changes is complex, and contradictory findings have also been reported, partially due to differences in study populations and methodologies. Nevertheless, meta-analyses confirm that a host of specific immunological changes reliably occur in depressed individuals [35].

Increasing attention is focused on the psychobiological mechanisms that contribute to increased morbidity and mortality in depression. The future of psychoneuroimmunology in the study of depression will likely be led by studies that are sensitive to the nuances of psychological and behavioural symptoms and how these factors alter immunity and ultimately predict individual differences in progression of chronic disease. Understanding the molecular and cellular pathways by which depression and the immune system are interrelated might lead to novel interventions that have the potential to inform management of patients and to promote health in patients recovering from depression.

Acknowledgements

This work was supported in part by grants AA13239, DA16541, MH55253, AG18367, T32-MH19925, AR/AG41867, 1 R01 AR 49840–01 and M01-RR00865 from the General Clinical Research Centers Program and the Cousins Center for Psychoneuroimmunology.

REFERENCES

1. American Psychiatric Association, *Diagnostic and Statistical Manual of Mental Disorders*, 4th edn (Washington, DC: American Psychiatric Association, 2000).

2. M. H. Rapaport, L. L. Judd, P. J. Schettler, *et al.*, A descriptive analysis of minor depression. *Am. J. Psychiatry* **159** (2002), 637–43.

3. A. K. Berger, B. J. Small, Y. Forsell, L. Backman, Preclinical symptoms of major depression in very old age: a prospective longitudinal study. *Am. J. Psychiatry* **155** (1998), 1039–43.

4. J. M. Lyness, E. D. Caine, Y. Conwell, D. King, Depressive symptoms, medical illness, and functional status in depressed psychiatric inpatients. *Am. J. Psychiatry* **150** (1993), 910–15.

5. R. D. Hays, K. B. Wells, C. D. Sherbourne, W. Rogers, K. Spritzer, Functioning and well-being outcomes of patients with depression compared with chronic general medical illnesses. *Arch. Gen. Psychiatry* **52** (1995), 11–19.

6. L. R. Wulsin, G. E. Vailant, V. E. Wells, A systematic review of the mortality of depression. *Psychosom. Med.* **61** (1999), 6–17.

7. M. L. Bruce, P. J. Leaf, G. P. Rozal, L. Florio, R.A. Hoff, Psychiatric status and 9-year mortality data in the New Haven Epidemiologic Catchment Area Study. *Am. J. Psychiatry* **151** (1994), 716–21.

8. C. Herrmann, S. Brand-Driehorst, B. Kaminsky, *et al.*, Diagnostic groups and depressed mood as predictors of 22-month mortality in medical inpatients. *Psychosom. Med.* **60** (1998), 570–77.

9. B. W. Rovner, Depression and increased risk of mortality in the nursing home patient. *Am. J. Med.* **94** (1993), 19–22S.

10. N. Frasure-Smith, F. Lespérance, M. Talajic, Depression following myocardial infarction: impact on 6-month survival. *J. Am. Med. Assoc.* **270** (1993), 1819–25.

11. N. Frasure-Smith, F. Lespérance, M. Talajic, The impact of negative emotions on prognosis following myocardial infarction: is it more than depression? *Health Psychol.* **14** (1995), 388–98.

12. M. A. Dew, C. C. Hoch, D. J. Buysse, *et al.*, Healthy older adults' sleep predicts all-cause mortality at 4 to 19 years of follow-up. *Psychosom. Med.* **65** (2003), 63–73.

13. D. F. Kripke, L. Garfinkel, D. L. Wingard, M. R. Klauber, M.R. Marler, Mortality associated with sleep duration and insomnia. *Arch. Gen. Psychiatry* **59** (2002), 131–6.

14. D. Gottlieb, D. Schulman, B. Nam, R. Agostino, W. Kannel, Sleep duration predicts mortality: the Framingham study. Presented at the 16th Annual Meeting of the Associated Professional Sleep Societies, 8–13 June 2002, Seattle, WA.

15. A. B. Newman, C. F. Spiekerman, P. Enright, *et al.*, Daytime sleepiness predicts mortality and cardiovascular disease in older adults: the Cardiovascular Health Study Research Group. *J. Am. Geriatr. Soc.* **48** (2000), 115–23.

16. M. J. Owens, C. B. Nemeroff, Physiology and pharmacology of corticotropin-releasing factor. *Pharmacol. Rev.* **91** (1991), 425–73.

17. E. M. Friedman, M. A. Irwin, A role for CRH and the sympathetic nervous system in stress-induced immunosuppression. *Ann. N. Y. Acad. Sci.* **771** (1995), 396–418.

18. E. M. Friedman, M. R. Irwin, Modulation of immune cell function by the autonomic nervous system. *Pharmacol. Ther.* **74** (1997), 27–38.

19. M. Irwin, W. Vale, C. Rivier, Central corticotropin-releasing factor mediates the suppressive effect of stress on natural killer cytotoxicity. *Endocrinology* **126** (1990), 2837–44.

20. M. Irwin, Brain corticotropin releasing hormone- and interleukin-1 β-induced suppression of specific antibody production. *Endocrinology* **133** (1993), 1352–60.

21. M. Irwin, M. Brown, T. Patterson, *et al.*, Y. Neuropeptide and natural killer cell activity: findings in depression and Alzheimer caregiver stress. *FASEB J.* **5** (1991), 3100–107.

22. V. M. Sanders, R. H. Straub, Norepinephrine, the beta-adrenergic receptor, and immunity. *Brain Behav. Immun.* **16** (2002), 290–332.

23. J. A. Moynihan, S. Y. Stevens, Mechanisms of stress-induced modulation of immunity in animals. In *Psychoneuroimmunology*, ed. R. Ader, D. L. Felten, N. Cohen (San Diego, CA: Academic Press, 2001), pp. 227–50.

24. F. S. Dhabhar, A. H. Miller, B. S. McEwen, R. L. Spencer, Stress-induced changes in blood leukocyte distribution: role of adrenal steroid hormones. *J. Immunol.* **157** (1996), 1638–44.

25. M. Irwin, T. Patterson, T. L. Smith, *et al.*, Reduction of immune function in life stress and depression. *Biol. Psychiatry* **27** (1990), 22–30.

26. M. Irwin, H. Weiner, Depressive symptoms and immune function during bereavement. In *Biopsychosocial Aspects of Bereavement*, ed. S. Zisook (Washington, DC: APA Press, 1987), pp. 156–74.

27. M. Maes, M. Van der Planken, W. J. Stevens, *et al.*, Leukocytosis, monocytosis, and neutrophilia: hallmarks of severe depression. *J. Psychiatr. Res.* **26** (1992), 125–34.

28. Z. Kronfol, R. Turner, H. Nasrallah, G. Winokur, Leukocyte regulation in depression and schizophrenia. *Psychiatry Res.* **13** (1984), 13–18.

29. M. Irwin, T. L. Smith, J. C. Gillin, Low natural killer cytotoxicity in major depression. *Life Sci.* **41** (1987), 2127–33.

30. P. Surtees, N. Wainwright, N. Day, *et al.*, Association of depression with peripheral leukocyte counts in EPIC-Norfolk-role of sex and cigarette smoking. *J. Psychsom. Res.* **54** (2003), 303–6.

31. S. J. Schleifer, J. A. Bartlett, S. E. Keller, *et al.*, Immunity in adolescents with major depression. *J. Am. Acad. Child Adolesc. Psychiatry* **41** (2002), 1054–60.

32. T. B. Herbert, S. Cohen, Depression and immunity: a meta-analytic review. *Psychol. Bull.* **113** (1993), 472–86.

33. D. L. Evans, J. D. Folds, J. M. Petitto, *et al.*, Circulating natural killer cell phenotypes in men and women with major depression. *Arch. Gen. Psychiatry* **49** (1992), 388–95.

34. S. J. Schleifer, S. E. Keller, R. N. Bond, J. Cohen, M. Stein, Major depressive disorder and immunity: role of age, sex, severity, and hospitalization. *Arch. Gen. Psychiatry* **46** (1989), 81–7.

35. E. P. Zorrilla, L. Luborsky, J. R. McKay, *et al.*, The relationship of depression and stressors to immunological assays: a meta-analytic review. *Brain Behav. Immun.* **15** (2001), 199–226.

36. Z. Kronfol, J. D. House, Depression, hypothalamic-pituitary adrenocortical activity and lymphocyte function. *Psychopharmacol. Bull.* **21** (1985), 476–8.

37. Z. Kronfol, J. Silva, J. Greden, *et al.*, Impaired lymphocyte function in depressive illness. *Life Sci.* **33** (1983), 241–7.

38. J. Albrecht, J. Helderman, M. Schlesser, J. Rush, A controlled study of cellular immune function in affective disorders before and during somatic therapy. *Psychiatry Res.* **15** (1985), 185–93.

39. E. Syvalahti, J. Eskola, O. Ruuskanen, T. Laine, Nonsuppression of cortisol and immune function in depression. *Prog. Neuropsychopharmacol. Biol. Psychiatry* **9** (1985), 413–22.

40. S. J. Schleifer, S. E. Keller, S. G. Siris, K. L. Davis, M. Stein, Depression and immunity: lymphocyte function in ambulatory depressed patients, hospitalized schizophrenic patients, and patients hospitalized for herniorrhaphy. *Arch. Gen. Psychiatry* **42** (1985), 129–33.

41. Z. Kronfol, J. D. House, J. Silva, J. Greden, B. J. Carroll, Depression, urinary free cortisol excretion, and lymphocyte function. *Br. J. Psychiatry* **148** (1986), 70–73.

42. J. R. Calabrese, R. G. Skwerer, B. Barna, *et al.*, Depression, immunocompetence, and prostaglandins of the E-series. *Psychol. Res.* **17** (1986), 41–7.

43. M. T. Lowy, A. T. Reder, G. J. Gormley, H. Y. Meltzer, Comparison of in vivo and in vitro glucocorticoid sensitivity in depression: relationship to the dexamethasone suppression test. *Biol. Psychiatry* **24** (1988), 619–30.

44. M. Maes, E. Bosmans, E. Suy, B. Minner, J. Raus, Impaired lymphocyte stimulation by mitogens in severely depressed patients: a complex interface with HPA axis hyperfunction, noradrenergic activity and the ageing process. *Br. J. Psychiatry* **155** (1989), 793–8.

45. L. L. Altshuler, S. Plaeger-Marshall, S. Richeimer, M. Daniels, L. R. Baxter, Jr, Lymphocyte function in major depression. *Acta Psychiatr. Scand.* **80** (1989), 132–6.

46. D. F. Darko, J. C. Gillin, S. C. Risch, *et al.*, Mitogen-stimulated lymphocyte prolif-eration and pituitary hormones in major depression. *Biol. Psychiatry* **26** (1989), 145–55.

47. Z. Kronfol, M. Nair, J. Goodson, *et al.*, Natural killer cell activity in depressive illness: a preliminary report. *Biol. Psychiatry* **26** (1989), 753–6.

48. P. Cosyns, M. Maes, M. Vandewoude, *et al.*, Impaired mitogen-induced lymphocyte responses and the hypothalamic-pituitary-adrenal axis in depressive disorders. *J. Affect. Disord.* **16** (1989), 41–8.

49. C. Bartoloni, L. Guidi, L. Antico, *et al.*, Psychological status of institutionalized aged: influ-ences on immune parameters and endocrinological correlates. *Int. J. Neurosci.* **51** (1990), 279–81.

50. C. McAdams, B. E. Leonard, Neutrophil and monocyte phagocytosis in depressed patients. *Prog. Neuropsychopharmacol. Biol. Psychiatry* **17** (1993), 971–84.

51. B. Birmaher, B. S. Rabin, M. R. Garcia, *et al.*, Cellular immunity in depressed, conduct disorder, and normal adolescents: role of adverse life events. *J. Am. Acad. Child Adolesc. Psychol.* **33** (1994), 671–8.

52. S. J. Schleifer, S. E. Keller, J. A. Bartlett, Panic disorder and immunity: few effects on circu-lating lymphocytes, mitogen response, and NK cell activity. *Brain Behav. Immun.* **16** (2002), 698–705.

53. M. Stein, A. H. Miller, R. L. Trestman, Depression, the immune system, and health and illness. *Arch. Gen. Psychiatry* **48** (1991), 171–7.

54. M. Irwin, C. Miller, Decreased natural killer cell responses and altered interleukin-6 and interleukin-10 production in alcoholism: an interaction between alcohol dependence and African-American ethnicity. *Alcohol Clin. Exp. Res.* **24** (2000), 560–69.

55. M. Irwin, Effects of sleep and sleep loss on immunity and cytokines. *Brain Behav. Immun.* **16** (2002), 503–12.

56. P. C. Mohl, L. Huang, C. Bowden, *et al.*, Natural killer cell activity in major depression. *Am. J. Psychiatry* **144** (1987), 1619.

57. Z. Kronfol, D. G. Remick, Cytokines and the brain: implications for clinical psychiatry. *Am. J. Psychiatry* **157** (2000), 683–94.

58. M. E. Bauer, A. Papadopoulos, L. Poon, *et al.*, Altered glucocorticoid immunoregulation in treatment resistant depression. *Psychoneuroendocrinology* **28** (2003), 49–65.

59. A. Seidel, V. Arolt, M. Hunstiger, *et al.*, Cytokine production and serum proteins in depres-sion. *Scand. J. Immunol.* **41** (1995), 534–8.

60. P Trzonkowski, J. Mysliwska, B. Godlewska, *et al.*, Immune consequences of the spontaneous pro-inflammatory status in depressed elderly patients. *Brain Behav. Immun.* **18** (2004), 135–48.

61. M. A. Maes, review on the acute phase response in major depression. *Rev. Neurosci.* **4** (1993), 407–16.

62. M. Maes, S. Scharpe, L. Van Grootel, *et al.*, Higher alpha 1-antritrypsin, haptoglobin, ceruloplasmin and lower retinol binding protein plasma levels during depression: further evidence for the existence of an inflammatory respose during that illness. *J. Affect. Disord.* **24** (1992), 183–92.

63. D. L. Musselman, A. H. Miller, M. R. Porter, *et al.*, Higher than normal plasma interleukin-6 concentrations in cancer patients with depression: preliminary findings. *Am. J. Psychiatry* **158** (2001), 1252–7.

64. G. E. Miller, C. A. Stetler, R. M. Carney, K. E. Freedland, W. A. Banks, Clinical depression and inflammatory risk markers for coronary heart disease. *Am. J. Cardiol.* **90** (2002), 1279–83.

65. J. L. Pike, M. R. Irwin, Dissociation of inflammatory markers and natural killer cell activity in major depressive disorder. *Brain Behav. Immun.* **20** (2006), 169–74.

66. B. W. Penninx, S. B. Kritchevsky, K. Yaffe, *et al.*, Inflammatory markers and depressed mood in older persons: results from the health, aging and body composition study. *Biol. Psychiatry* **54** (2003), 566–72.

67. F. Brambilla, P. Monteleone, M. Maj, Interleukin-1beta and tumor necrosis factor-alpha in children with major depressive disorder or dysthymia. *J. Affect. Disord.* **78** (2004), 273–7.

68. J. Stastny, A. Konstantinidis, M. J. Schwarz, *et al.*, Effects of tryptophan depletion and catecholamine depletion on immune parameters in patients with seasonal affective disorder in remission with light therapy. *Biol. Psychiatry* **53** (2003), 332–7.

69. F. Lesperance, N. Frasure-Smith, P. Theroux, M. Irwin, The association between major depression and levels of soluble intercellular adhesion molecule 1, interleukin-6, and C-reactive protein in patients with recent acute coronary syndromes. *Am. J. Psychiatry* **161** (2004), 271–7.

70. A. J. Zautra, D. C. Yocum, I. Villanueva, *et al.*, Immune activation and depression in women with rheumatoid arthritis. *J. Rheumatol.* **31** (2004) 457–63.

71. A. H. Miller, Cytokines and sickness behavior: implications for cancer care and control. *Brain Behav. Immun.* **17**: Suppl 1 (2003), 132–4.

72. G. E. Miller, S. Cohen, S. Pressman, *et al.*, Psychological stress and antibody response to influenza vaccination: when is the critical period for stress, and how does it get inside the body? *Psychosom. Med.* **66** (2004), 215–23.

73. M. Irwin, C. Costlow, H. Williams, *et al.*, Cellular immunity to varicella-zoster virus in patients with major depression. *J. Infect. Dis.* **178** (1998), 104–8.

74. F. S. Dhabhar, Acute stress enhances while chronic stress suppresses skin immunity: the role of stress hormones and leukocyte trafficking. *Ann. N. Y. Acad. Sci.* **917** (2000), 876–93.

75. I. Hickie, C. Hickie, A. Lloyd, D. Silove, D. Wakefield, Impaired in vivo immune responses in patients with melancholia. *Br. J. Psychiatry* **162** (1993), 651–7.

76. M. Shinkawa, K. Nakayama, H. Hirai, M. Monma, H. Sasaki, Depression and immunore-activity in disabled older patients. *J. Am. Geriatr. Soc.* **50** (2002), 198–9.

77. R. Glaser, J. K. Kiecolt-Glaser, R. H. Bonneau, *et al.*, Stress-induced modulation of the immune response to recombinant hepatitis B vaccine. *Psychosom. Med.* **54** (1992), 22–9.

78. J. K. Kiecolt-Glaser, R. Glaser, S. Gravenstein, W. B. Malarkey, Chronic stress alters the immune response to influenza virus vaccine in older adults. *Proc. Natl. Acad. Sci. U. S. A.* **93** (1996), 3043–7.

79. K. Vedhara, N. K. Cox, G. K. Wilcock, *et al.*, Chronic stress in elderly carers of dementia patients and antibody response to influenza vaccination. *Lancet* **353** (1999), 627–31.

80. K. Vedhara, M. P. McDermott, T. G. Evans, *et al.*, Chronic stress in nonelderly caregivers: psychological, endocrine and immune implications. *J. Psychosom. Res.* **53** (2002), 1153–61.

81. N. Rohleder, N. C. Schommer, D. H. Hellhammer, R. Engel, C. Kirschbaum, Sex differences in glucocorticoid sensitivity of proinflammatory cytokine production after psychosocial stress. *Psychosom. Med.* **63** (2001), 966–72.

82. M. Irwin, A. Mascovich, J. C. Gillin, *et al.*, Partial sleep deprivation reduces natural killer cell activity in humans. *Psychosom. Med.* **56** (1994), 493–8.

83. M. Irwin, J. McClintick, C. Costlow, *et al.*, Partial night sleep deprivation reduces natural killer and cellular immune responses in humans. *FASEB J.* **10** (1996), 643–53.

84. M. Irwin, T. L. Smith, J. C. Gillin, Electroencephalographic sleep and natural killer activity in depressed patients and control subjects. *Psychosom. Med.* **54** (1992), 107–26.

85. H. Cover, M. Irwin, Immunity and depression: insomnia, retardation, and reduction of natural killer cell activity. *J. Behav. Med.* **17** (1994), 217–23.

86. N. Castanon, B. E. Leonard, P. J. Neveu, R. Yirmiya, Effects of antidepressants on cytokine production and actions. *Brain Behav. Immun.* **16** (2002), 569–74.

87. E. Goujon, P. Parnet, S. Laye, *et al.*, Stress downregulates lipopolysaccharide-induced expression of proinflammatory cytokines in the spleen, pituitary, and brain of mice. *Brain Behav. Immun.* **9** (1995), 292–303.

88. N. Barden, Regulation of corticosteroid receptor gene expression in depression and antidepressant action. *J. Psychiatry Neurosci.* **24** (1999), 25–39.

89. R. Yirmiya, J. Weidenfeld, Y. Pollak, *et al.*, Cytokines, 'depression due to a general medical condition', and antidepressant drugs. *Adv. Exp. Med. Biol.* **461** (1999), 283–316.

90. I. Yaron, L. Shirazi, R. Judovich, *et al.*, Fluoxetine and amitriptyline inhibit nitric oxide, prostaglandin E2, and hyaluronic acid production in human synovial cells and synovial tissue cultures. *Arthritis Rheum.* **42** (1999), 2561–8.

91. F. Hindmarch, Expanding the horizons of depression: beyond the monoamine hypothesis. *Hum. Psychopharm.* **16** (2001), 203–18.

92. M. Kubera, G. Kenis, E. Bosmans, *et al.*, Stimulatory effect of antidepressants on the production of IL-6. Int. *Immunopharmacol.* **4** (2004), 185–92.

93. M. Irwin, U. Lacher, C. Caldwell, Depression and reduced natural killer cytotoxicity: a longitudinal study of depressed patients and control subjects. *Psychol. Med.* **22** (1992), 1045–50.

94. S. J. Schleifer, S. E. Keller, J. A. Bartlett, Depression and immunity: clinical factors and therapeutic course. *Psychiatry Res.* **85** (1999), 63–9.

95. M. G. Frank, S. E. Hendricks, D. R. Johnson, J. L. Wieseler, W. J. Burke, Antidepressants augment natural killer cell activity: in vivo and in vitro. *Neuropsychobiology* **39** (1999), 18–24.

96. Y. Kim, I. B. Suh, H. Kim, *et al.*, The plasma levels of interleukin-12 in schizophrenia, major depression, and bipolar mania: effects of psychotropic drugs. *Mol. Psychiatry* **7** (2002), 1107–14.

97. G. Kenis, M. Maes, Effects of antidepressants on the production of cytokines. *Int. J. Neuropsychopharmacol.* **5** (2002), 401–12.

98. A. Sluzewska, Indicators of immune activation in depressed patients. *Adv. Exp. Med. Biol.* **461** (1999), 59–73.

99. M. Maes, S. Scharpe, H. Y. Meltzer, *et al.*, Relationships between interleukin-6 activity, acute phase proteins, and function of the hypothalamic-pituitary-adrenal axis in severe depression. *Psychiatry Res.* **49** (1993), 11–27.

100. M. Maes, E. Bosmans, H. Y. Meltze, S. Scharpe, E. Suy, Interleukin-1 beta: a putative mediator of HPA axis hyperactivity in major depression. *Am. J. Psychiatry* **150** (1993), 1189–93.

101. M. Irwin, M. Daniels, S. C. Risch, E. Bloom, H. Weiner, Plasma cortisol and natural killer cell activity during bereavement. *Biol. Psychiatry* **24** (1988), 173–8.

102. C. Raison, A. H. Miller, When not enough is too much: the role of insufficient glucocorticoid signaling in the pathophysiology of stress-related disorders. *Am. J. Psychiatry* **160** (2003), 1554–65.

103. M. L. Sopori, W. Kozak, Immunomodulatory effects of cigarette smoke. *J. Neuroimmunol.* **83** (1998), 148–56.

104. J. A. Rosecrans, L. D. Karin, Effects of nicotine on the hypothalamic-pituitary-axis (HPA) and immune function: introduction to the Sixth Nicotine Round Table Satellite, American Society of Addiction Medicine Nicotine Dependence Meeting. *Psychoneuroendocrinology* **23** (1998), 95–102.

105. C. G. McAllister-Sistilli, A. R. Caggiula, S. Knopf, *et al.*, The effects of nicotine on the immune system. *Psychoneuroendocrinology* **23** (1998), 175–87.

106. W. Jung, M. Irwin, Reduction of natural killer cytotoxic activity in major depression: interaction between depression and cigarette smoking. *Psychosom. Med.* **61** (1999), 263–70.

107. M. A. Mendall, P. Patel, M. Asante, *et al.*, Relation of serum cytokine concentrations to cardiovascular risk factors and coronary heart disease. *Heart* **78** (1997), 273–7.

108. R. W. Linkins, G. W. Comstock, Depressed mood and development of cancer. *Am. J. Epidemiol.* **132** (1990), 962–72.

109. M. A. Schuckit, J. E. Tipp, M. Bergman, *et al.*, Comparison of induced and independent major depressive disorders in 2945 alcoholics. *Am. J. Psychiatry* **54** (1997), 948–57.

110. M. Irwin, C. Caldwell, T. L. Smith, *et al.*, Major depressive disorder, alcoholism, and reduced natural killer cell cytotoxicity: role of severity of depressive symptoms and alcohol consumption. *Arch. Gen. Psychiatry* **47** (1990), 713–19.

111. M. Irwin, M. Schuckit, T. L. Smith, Clinical importance of age at onset in Type 1 and Type 2 primary alcoholics. *Arch. Gen. Psychiatry* **47** (1990), 320–24.

112. M. Irwin, G. Rinetti, L. Redwine, S. Motivala, C. Ehlers, Pro-inflammatory cytokines and disordered sleep in alcohol dependence. *Psychosom. Med.* **65** (2003), A-4.

113. M. Hall, A. Baum, D. J. Buysse, *et al.*, Sleep as a mediator of the stress-immune relationship. *Psychosom. Med.* **60** (1998), 48–51.

114. M. Irwin, C. Clark, B. Kennedy, J. Christian Gillin, M. Ziegler, Nocturnal catecholamines and immune function in insomniacs, depressed patients, and control subjects. *Brain Behav. Immun.* **17** (2003), 365–72.

115. J. Savard, L. Laroche, S. Simard, H. Ivers, C. M. Morin, Chronic insomnia and immune functioning. *Psychosom. Med.* **65** (2003), 211–21.

116. M. Irwin, J. C. Gillin, J. Dang, *et al.*, Sleep deprivation as a probe of homeostatic sleep regulation in primary alcoholics. *Biol. Psychiatry* **51** (2002), 632–41.

117. M. Irwin, C. Miller, J. C. Gillin, A. Demodena, C. L. Ehlers, Polysomnographic and spectral sleep EEG in primary alcoholics: an interaction between alcohol dependence and African-American ethnicity. *Alcohol Clin. Exp. Res.* **24** (2000), 1376–84.

118. L. Redwine, J. Dang, M. Hall, M. Irwin, Disordered sleep, nocturnal cytokines, and immunity in alcoholics. *Psychosom. Med.* **65** (2003), 75–85.

119. P. H. Black, L. D. Garbutt, Stress, inflammation and cardiovascular disease. *J. Psychosom. Res.* **52** (2002), 1–23.

120. L. Redwine, S. Snow, P. Mills, M. Irwin, Acute psychological stress: effects on chemotaxis and cellular adhesion molecule expression. *Psychosom. Med.* **65** (2003), 598–603.

121. M. U. Goebel, P. J. Mills, M. R. Irwin, M. G. Ziegler, Interleukin-6 and tumor necrosis factor-alpha production after acute psychological stress, exercise, and infused isoproterenol: differential effects and pathways. *Psychosom. Med.* **62** (2000), 591–8.

122. J. F. Sheridan, C. Dobbs, D. Brown, B. Zwilling, Psychoneuroimmunology: stress effects on pathogenesis and immunity during infection. *Clin. Microbiol. Rev.* **7** (1994), 200–12.

123. S. Cohen, G. Miller, Stress, immunity and susceptibility to upper respiratory infection. In *Psychoneuroimmunology*, 3rd edn, ed. R. Ader, D. Felten, N. Cohen (San Diego, CA: Academic Press, 2000), pp. 499–509.

124. S. W. Cole, B. D. Naliboff, M. E. Kemeny, *et al.*, Impaired response to HAART in HIV-infected individuals with high autonomic nervous system activity. *Proc. Natl. Acad. Sci. U. S. A.* **98** (2001), 12 695–700.

125. S. W. Cole, M. E. Kemeny, S. E. Taylor, Social identity and physical health: accelerated HIV progression in rejection-sensitive gay men. *J. Pers. Soc. Psychol.* **72** (1997), 320–35.

126. S. W. Cole, Y. D. Korin, J. L. Fahey, J. A. Zack, Norepinephrine accelerates HIV replication via protein kinase A-dependent effects on cytokine production. *J. Immunol.* **161** (1998), 610–16.

127. E. M. Sternberg, G. P. Chrousos, R. L. Wilder, P. W. Gold, The stress response and the regulation of inflammatory disease. *Ann. Intern. Med.* **117** (1992), 854–66.

128. L. J. Crofford, K. T. Kalogeras, G. Mastorakos, *et al.*, Circadian relationships between inter-leukin (IL)-6 and hypothalamic-pituitary-adrenal axis hormones: failure of IL-6 to cause sustained hypercortisolism in patients with early untreated rheumatoid arthritis. *J. Clin. Endocrinol Metab.* **82** (1997), 1279–83.

129. C. Dickens, L. McGowan, D. Clark-Carter, F. Creed, Depression in rheumatoid arthritis: a systematic review of the literature with meta-analysis. *Psychosom. Med.* **64** (2002), 52–60.

130. A. J. Zautra, B. W. Smith, Depression and reactivity to stress in older women with rheumatoid arthritis and osteoarthritis. *Psychosom. Med.* **63** (2001), 687–96.

131. J. M. Smyth, A. A. Stone, A. Hurewitz, A. Kaell, Effects of writing about stressful experiences on symptom reduction in patients with asthma or rheumatoid arthritis: a randomized trial. *J. Am. Med. Assoc.* **281** (1999), 1304–9.

15

Smoking and depression

Jon D. Kassel and Benjamin L. Hankin

Introduction

Cigarette smoking remains the most preventable cause of illness and death in society today. Upwards of 440 000 smokers die in the USA each year [1,2], and worldwide over 1 200 000 deaths a year are attributable to smoking-related causes [3]. Despite these staggering statistics, smokers and non-smokers alike often do not appreciate fully the health risks of tobacco use, particularly cigarette smoking. The latest epidemiological studies indicate that death rates for smokers are two to three times higher than for non-smokers at all ages. This means that half of all smokers will eventually die as a result of their smoking. If current smoking trends persist, then about 500 million people currently alive – nearly 9% of the world's population – will die as a result of tobacco use [3].

Moreover, tobacco is arguably the most addictive substance known to humankind. Whereas approximately 32% of people who initiate cigarette smoking become nicotine-dependent, only 23%, 17% and 15% of individuals who experiment with heroin, cocaine and alcohol, respectively, become dependent on these drugs [4]. Interestingly, unlike with harder drugs, the subjective effects of smoking are subtle. Rarely does a smoker describe that smoking provides them with anything approaching the euphoria or high often attributed to other drugs. And yet, as Shiffman [5] observes, 'the addictive potential of nicotine is all the more impressive for its ability to engender such compulsive use without impressive subjective effects' (p. 15).

The pathways to becoming a smoker are no doubt complex [6,7]. However, of the numerous factors believed to heighten vulnerability to both smoking initiation and subsequent development of nicotine dependence, the role played by various forms of psychopathology and emotional distress appears particularly critical: numerous studies have reliably found high smoking rates among selected populations

Depression and Physical Illness, ed. A. Steptoe.
Published by Cambridge University Press. © Cambridge University Press 2006.

of individuals with mental illness. For example, drawing upon a large, nationally representative sample in the USA, Lasser *et al.* [8] found that individuals with a lifetime history of any psychiatric disorder had higher rates of lifetime and current smoking compared with those individuals who had never suffered from mental illness. Other investigations have reported similar findings, demonstrating strong and reliable associations between psychiatric disorders and cigarette smoking among adults [9–11] and, to a lesser extent, among adolescents [12,13], but see [14].

Whereas the largest associations between smoking initiation have typically been found with substance abuse disorders [9,12,15] and various manifestations of externalising disorders [12,16–20], the link between smoking status and depressive symptomatology has also proven to be robust. Put simply, relative to non-smokers, smokers are more likely to experience depression, and those individuals who experience depressive symptoms are more likely to smoke cigarettes relative to those who are depression-free. Questions invariably arise from such associations, the answers to which would likely have a bearing on smoking prevention and treatment. Thus, a thorough understanding of the processes linking smoking and depression is clearly needed.

The focus of this chapter is on exploring the links between smoking behaviour and depressive symptoms. Rather than providing an exhaustive review, we highlight some of the major findings from the literature and address several conceptual and methodological issues that we believe are critical to gaining a better understanding of smoking–depression associations. As such, we begin by providing brief overviews of the constructs of depression and smoking, noting that neither may be as straightforward as many believe. Next, we present the case that delineating the nature of smoking–depression relationships calls for research that goes beyond simple description of cross-sectional correlational data. Indeed, as we have argued previously [21], explorations of the links between smoking and any given affective condition (including depression) call for both between- and within-subject levels of analyses. Next, we review several conceptual models that may lend themselves to further elucidation of the processes underlying associations between smoking and depression. We then highlight several potentially important moderators of the smoking-depression link. Finally, we offer thoughts on future research directions for this important area of inquiry.

Some conceptual and methodological considerations of 'depression'

An important issue is whether the latent structure of depression is best considered as a category or a dimension. When viewed dimensionally, depression differs quantitatively by degree, i.e. individuals are more or less depressed. Hence, there is no clear boundary between individuals viewed as 'normal' or abnormally 'depressed'.

When conceptualised categorically, depression differs in kind in a qualitatively distinct way, such that individuals are viewed as either depressed or not depressed. One of the most influential nosological classification systems, the *Diagnostic and Statistical Manual of Mental Disorders* [22], clearly espouses a categorical perspective and asserts that there exist depressive 'episodes', as opposed to degrees, of depression. Indeed, there has been considerable debate and discussion of this important issue, e.g., see Coyne [23] for the categorical viewpoint and Flett *et al.* [24] for the continuity/dimensional perspective. Fortunately, a few methodologically sophisticated studies have begun to address this question empirically both with adults [25,26] and with youths [27].

For the most part, these investigations have shown that the latent structure of depression is in fact dimensional in children, adolescents and adults, although there is some question as to whether the more extreme forms of the disorder (e.g. melancholic depression) may be qualitatively different from normal mood [28,29]; but see also Ruscio and colleagues [30] for a more methodologically exacting study showing that even extreme forms of depression are dimensional. Thus, the preponderance of extant evidence suggests that depression varies along a continuum of affective severity. Given that the best available evidence supports the dimensional perspective, we consider and review studies on depressed mood, symptoms and disorder among adolescents and adults to further our understanding of the association between smoking and depression and to consider potential aetiological models that ultimately can advance our knowledge of the causal mechanisms underlying any observed association.

Some conceptual and methodological considerations of 'smoking'

It should be acknowledged up front that certain pharmacodynamic aspects of cigarette smoking make the study of its effects on depressive symptoms difficult to assess and interpret. It has been fairly well established that (i) physical dependence often plays a significant role in smoking [31]; (ii) negative affective states, including anxiety, dysphoria and irritability, are among the hallmark symptoms of nicotine withdrawal [32]; (iii) nicotine often appears to relieve these withdrawal symptoms [33]; and (iv) many studies assessing the subjective effects of smoking and/or nicotine have simply compared groups of nicotine-deprived and non-deprived smokers [34,35]. Hence, it is difficult to ascertain whether any observed differences in depressive symptoms between nicotine-deprived and non-deprived smokers are due to withdrawal adversely affecting deprived smokers, or to smoking genuinely improving mood over normal levels [36–38].

It is also important to note that not all smoking is the same. Put another way, there exists tremendous heterogeneity in smoking behaviour between individuals.

Some smokers are clearly nicotine-dependent, such that they experience nicotine withdrawal when they go without nicotine for even short periods of time. But not all smokers meet criteria for nicotine dependence [39]. Thinking about variability in smoking behaviour from a developmental perspective, several investigators have posited that all smokers proceed through a series of stages and transitions on the path towards nicotine dependence. For example, Flay [40] suggests that smokers progress through the following five discrete stages: (i) the *preparatory stage*, in which attitudes towards nicotine and its perceived functions are formed; (ii) the *initial trying stage*, which includes smoking the first two to three cigarettes, usually in a social context, and the resulting physiological and psychosocial reinforcements obtained; (iii) the *experimentation stage*, which includes situational-specific irregular use over an extended period of time; (iv) *regular use*, during which the individual (typically an adolescent) smokes on a regular basis, e.g. at weekends or daily; and (v) *nicotine dependence or addiction*, in which smoking is governed predominantly by an internally regulated need for nicotine. Hence, one important implication of a stage-modelling perspective is that the relationship between smoking and depression may differ as a function of where a smoker falls on this stage continuum. Put another way, whereas smoking at all certainly heightens the risk of eventually becoming nicotine dependent, such an outcome must not be viewed as destiny. Some smokers, for example, remain at an experimentation or intermittent smoking stage for prolonged periods of time.

It is also important to note that some of the processes governing smoking–depression associations are inherently between-person, whereas others are within-person (see Kassel *et al.* [21] for an in-depth discussion of these issues). For example, the question of whether smokers experience heightened depressive symptoms relative to non-smokers necessarily calls for a between-person level of analysis, as groups of people are being compared. On the other hand, ascertaining whether depressive episodes or states actually cue smoking requires a within-person level of analysis, as it must be demonstrated that a given smoker smokes on occasions defined by depressive symptoms. Finally, some questions combine both levels of analysis. For example, the popular notion that some smokers smoke in order to alleviate unpleasant affect – such as depression or dysphoria – suggests that certain between-person variables are involved in within-person attempts to regulate depressive negative affect when it occurs. We believe that these distinctions have been largely overlooked in previous analyses of smoking–depression relationships.

Thus, in order to understand thoroughly the relationship between cigarette smoking and depression, several distinct but frequently blurred questions must be asked: First, does depression promote smoking? Specifically, are there valid and reliable associations between depression and (i) smoking status (smoker vs. non-smoker) and (ii) actual cueing (prompting) of smoking? Second, even if it was

Table 15.1 Does depression (symptoms and/or episodes) promote smoking?

Smoking stage	Do smokers and non-smokers differ on levels of depression?	Do depressive states cue smoking?	Does smoking reduce symptoms of depression?
Initiation	Cross-sectional studies suggest a tentative yes, although depressive symptoms may not discriminate well between smoking experimentation and non-smoking among adolescents	Unknown, other than self-report data	Unknown, other than retrospective self-report data, suggesting that smoking can alleviate the more generalised state of negative affect
Maintenance	Yes: high levels of comorbidity (although the casual mechanisms underlying these observed associations are not yet clear)	Unclear; laboratory studies and self-report data offer a tentative yes	Rarely, if ever, investigated empirically
Relapse	Not applicable	A tentative yes: both self-report and real-time data show that whereas stress and negative affect often precipitate lapses, few data have implicated depressive symptoms per se	Few data; trend towards smoking worsening or having no effect on depressive symptoms

established that depression is linked to smoking (at either or both of these levels of analysis), this does not mean that smoking necessarily relieves depressive symptoms. This often ignored point leads to another, very different, question: Does smoking genuinely reduce depressive symptoms? Moving beyond the self-report of smokers, what do experimental studies reveal regarding the influence of smoking on depressive symptomatology? In sum, then, the following three questions are addressed regarding smoking–depression relationships: (i) Do smokers and non-smokers differ on levels of depression? (ii) Do depressive symptoms genuinely cue smoking? (iii) Does smoking alleviate symptoms of depression? Moreover, and as noted earlier, these questions ideally should be asked across different stages of smoking experience, as the answers may vary across smoking stages. Here, we address these questions across the smoking initiation (irregular, experimental smoking) maintenance (regular, daily smoking) and relapse (resumption of smoking after a period of abstinence) stages (see Table 15.1 for a summary of our review).

Are smokers more depressed than non-smokers?

Initiation stage

A bevy of cross-sectional and longitudinal studies have demonstrated beyond a doubt that there is a significant association between smoking and depression. We pay particular attention to studies investigating smoking and depression among youths because adolescence is the age when most individuals exhibit increases in depressive symptoms or become clinically depressed for the first time [41–44]. Moreover, adolescence is also the time of life when most individuals initiate smoking and risk becoming nicotine dependent [6,45].

A number of large-scale longitudinal studies have yielded data showing that depressive symptoms are linked to, and precede the onset of, smoking initiation and experimentation [12,46–49]. At the same time, several investigations have (i) been unable to demonstrate a prospective link between depression and smoking uptake [50–53], or (ii) found differential effects for boys and girls (depression predicts smoking uptake for girls but not for boys [54] or depression predicts initiation for boys but not girls [55]), or (iii) reported that ethnicity moderates the association between depression and smoking initiation (depression predicts smoking uptake among white people and Hispanic people but not among African American people [56]).

While it is difficult to reconcile such differential findings, some of the variance is likely attributable to utilisation of different timeframes, dissimilar cultural contexts, different depression measures, univariate versus multivariate analytic procedures, and varying definitions of smoking behaviour (e.g. any smoking vs. daily smoking). Indeed, a close perusal of the data suggests that whereas depression may be a potent predictor of heavy smoking and nicotine dependence among adolescents and young adults [50,57–59]), it is less consistently successful at differentiating non-smokers from smoking initiators and experimenters [50,52,60]. Results from Patton *et al.* [61] also suggest a mediational mechanism, whereby depressive and anxiety symptoms appear to be associated with higher risk for smoking initiation through an increased susceptibility to peer smoking influences. Killen *et al.* [55] similarly found that, for boys only, those who had both more friends who smoked and higher depressive scores were more likely to have initiated smoking over a three-year follow-up period. Thus, moderator and mediator approaches hold potential in delineating smoking–depression relations among adolescents and are clearly in need of further study.

Finally, several longitudinal reports suggest that the relationship between smoking and depression is reciprocal, such that smoking also predicts the subsequent development of depressive symptoms [12,51,62,63]. Thus, some of the co-variance in smoking status and depressive symptomatology may be attributable to the fact that smoking predisposes to the development of depression (see the discussion of the consequence model below).

In sum, most studies report a positive association between smoking onset and depression. At the same time, links between depression and smoking may be bidirectional, such that smoking also increases the risk for subsequent development of depression. Moreover, evidence suggests that cigarette smoking may also increase the risk of agoraphobia, generalised anxiety disorder and panic disorder during late adolescence and early adulthood [64]. Whereas the most popular interpretation of the smoking–depression link is that it reflects self-medication processes, it is important to note that such comorbidity ultimately says nothing about within-person processes inherent to the self-medication model. This is especially true given findings suggestive of reverse causality, i.e. over time, smoking may lead to increases in depression.

Maintenance stage

As noted with regard to smoking initiation, depressive symptomatology in particular emerges as a strong correlate of smoking status among those in the maintenance stage [65]. In 1978, Waal-Manning and de Hamel [66] reported that smokers had elevated depressive symptoms relative to non-smokers. Similar relationships have been found in studies using large nationally representative samples [11,67]. In a study of 3000 young adults, Breslau and colleagues [9] found that those who met criteria for nicotine dependence were also more likely to meet criteria for major depression. Breslau and colleagues [68] also reported that a history of major depressive disorder produced a two-fold increased risk for progression to nicotine dependence. Importantly, findings from Breslau *et al.* [69] indicated that the association between major depression and smoking was specific to nicotine dependence; non-dependent smokers did not differ from non-smokers in this respect. As observed in the initiation stage, the presence of nicotine dependence also appears to heighten the risk for subsequent development of major depression [68]. In our view, the best studies suggest that the frequently observed link between nicotine dependence and depression may reflect (i) bidirectional causal processes (e.g. smoking to alleviate depressed mood and neuropharmacological effects of nicotine on neural substrates linked to depression), (ii) common factors (e.g. neuroticism) that predispose to both disorders [59,68,70] or (iii) the influence of non-shared (individual) environmental factors [71].

Finally, with respect to whether depressive affect actually cues or prompts smoking, the literature has little to say. Again, there is reason to believe that both smoking status (smokers vs. non-smokers) and the amount smoked co-vary with various indices of depression [71]. In an effort to establish the direction of causality, several laboratory studies have demonstrated that during stressful situations, smoking intensity increases [72–74], smokers tend to smoke more [75–77] and self-reported desire to smoke is heightened [78]. Taken together, these within-person studies make a compelling case that stress – but not necessarily depression – increases (cues) smoking among regular smokers.

Relapse stage

Relapse is the modal outcome among those attempting to quit smoking [79,80]. Whereas the best available treatments yield one-year abstinence rates of about 30%, even among smokers who successfully quit for a full year as many as 40% eventually return to regular smoking [81]. Smokers who attempt to quit on their own fare even less well than those who seek formal treatment, with relapse rates ranging from 90% to 97% [82,83].

With respect to the question of whether depression predisposes to or even prompts smoking relapse, a number of studies point to a strong relationship. Here, we find that the presence of clinically significant levels of negative affect (often depressive symptoms) is frequently predictive of relapse [84,85]. For instance, one study reported that the likelihood of quitting smoking was 40% lower among depressed smokers compared with non-depressed smokers [67]. Glassman *et al.* [84] reported a quitting rate of 14% for smokers meeting criteria for major depression, while 31% of participants with no psychiatric diagnosis successfully quit. In the absence of current symptomatology, history of depression appears to heighten risk for both relapse [86] and recurrence of depressive symptomatology subsequent to cessation [87]. These effects may be more pronounced among women [88]. Importantly, Niaura *et al.* [89] demonstrated that even low levels of depressive symptoms assessed at baseline for smokers enrolled in a cessation programme were predictive of time to first cigarette smoked after attempted quitting.

Despite all of the studies demonstrating a link between depression and propensity to relapse, a meta-analysis revealed that lifetime history of major depression does not appear to be an independent risk factor for cessation failure in smoking cessation treatment [90]. Given the corpus of data previously suggesting otherwise, this study suggests that more work must be done in order to better understand the role of depression in promoting relapse.

Does smoking reduce depressive symptoms?

Initiation stage

Sadly, there has been very little empirical investigation with respect to the effect of smoking on depressive affect or any other affective states among smoking initiates. A small body of self-report data, however, does bear on this issue. McNeill and colleagues [91] found that the most frequently cited motive for smoking among a sample of female adolescent smokers was that smoking is calming. Dozois and colleagues [92] and Nichter and colleagues [93] similarly found that 'smoking to relax' and 'stress reduction' were commonly reported motives among adolescent smoking initiates. Whereas adolescents often attribute their smoking to motives associated with stress reduction, it is not clear that such motives necessarily generalise to states of depressive affect.

One can also turn to the animal literature in order to gain some insight into this question. For example, it has been reported that nicotine had greater activity-stimulating (perhaps antidepressant) effects in adolescent male rats than adult male rats [94]. A study further reported that although nicotine exerted anxiety-reducing effects in adolescent male rats, it increased anxiety among adolescent female rats and adult males and females [95]. Finally, Cheeta and colleagues [96] found that female rats were more sensitive to the anxiety-reducing effects of nicotine than were male rats. Taken together, these and other studies suggest that smoking (nicotine) may yield differential effects on adolescents relative to adults, and that these effects may be moderated by sex. Still unclear, however, is the extent to which smoking offers genuine antidepressant effects among smoking initiates.

Maintenance stage

Once again, the literature reveals a dearth of information regarding the effects of smoking on depressive affect among regular smokers. Given the reliable association between depression and smoking discussed earlier, it is surprising that relatively few studies have directly assessed the effects of smoking or nicotine on depression. Smokers reliably report that they smoke more when they are stressed, angry, anxious or sad [97–100] (but see also [101]) and hold the expectation that smoking will alleviate these negative moods [102,103]. Moreover, a study found that, relative to non-depressed smokers, depressed smokers perceive more benefits from smoking and find cigarettes more appealing than alternative rewards [104]. At the same time, the fact that smokers believe that smoking helps to reduce these manifestations of negative affect does not, in and of itself, render this a valid conceptualisation. Additionally, most of the experimental work to date examining nicotine effects on emotion has assessed anxiety; other emotional states, including depression, have been relatively ignored. As we have argued elsewhere [21], this represents a notable gap in the literature that sorely needs to be addressed.

As observed with the smoking initiation stage, however, the animal literature offers some clues regarding nicotine effects on depressive symptomatology. Several studies have suggested that nicotine may exhibit antidepressant effects in rats [105–107]. For example, Tizabi and colleagues [108] reported that acute and chronic administration of nicotine significantly improved the performance of Flinders Sensitive Line rats (bred for their hyperresponsiveness to cholinergic stimulation and, thus, representing an animal model of depression) on a forced swim test. Djuric *et al.* [109] found that, regardless of whether the rat was 'depressed', those rats that ingested nicotine for 14 days exhibited far fewer depression-like behaviours (less immobility on a forced swim test) relative to rats who were not exposed to nicotine or were exposed to nicotine for shorter periods of time. These findings are consistent with the argument put forth by some authors that nicotine may be a more effective antidepressant than an anxiolytic [110,111].

Relapse stage

The question of whether smoking a cigarette relieves symptoms of depression among those in the throes of relapse has garnered little empirical attention. Brandon *et al.* [112] asked smokers who smoked subsequent to participating in a cessation programme to describe their affective reactions to their initial lapse. Whereas almost 50% described feeling depressed or hopeless, 16% anxious or tense, and 10% angry or irritated, only 8% reported feeling relaxed and 6% happy, celebratory or confident. Using palmtop computers to assess real-time affective antecedents and consequences of smoking lapses, Shiffman *et al.* [113] reported that whereas lapses resulted in increases in negative affect, temptation episodes did not. Correspondingly, relative to temptations, lapses almost inevitably resulted in significant drops in self-efficacy and increases in feelings of guilt and discouragement.

Thus, it appears that smoking a cigarette after having tried to quit smoking results in an exacerbation of depressed mood. However, the finding that smoking lapses appear to increase depressive symptoms likely reflect, at least in part, an abstinence violation effect (AVE). The AVE refers to a frequently observed constellation of negative emotions and disparaging self-evaluation that follows a transgression of one's commitment to abstinence [114].

Another interesting perspective on whether smoking reduces depressive symptoms comes from studies examining the time course of depressive symptomatology among those who successfully quit smoking. Almost all of these studies report that although there is usually an initial increase in dysphoria subsequent to cessation, these symptoms diminish over time to levels lower than observed before quitting [115–118]; but see [119]. Moreover, smokers who were unable to maintain abstinence generally continued to manifest high levels of stress and negative affect over time [115,116]. By implication, it has been suggested that whereas smoking engenders depressive symptomatology [120], quitting results in lower depressive levels over time.

Summary

Based upon a review of the empirical literature, we observed consistent between-person associations between smoking status and various indices of depression across the initiation and maintenance stages of smoking. Thus, based on a population-level of analysis, smokers generally experience more depressive symptoms than do non-smokers. To a lesser extent, smoking rate appears to co-vary with depressive symptoms among those in the initiation and maintenance stages (e.g. the more reported depressive symptoms, the more cigarettes are smoked). The nature of the smoking–depression relationship is such that it is clearly stronger when 'smoking' is operationalised as nicotine dependence rather than experimentation or intermittent smoking. An important implication of this is that the field must continue to explore smoking–depression associations from a developmental perspective, realising that the relationship between smoking and depression may change over the course of the lifetime.

The extent to which smoking genuinely reduces depressive affect remains unclear and relatively unstudied. Thus, although many individuals, including tobacco researchers, infer causal processes from the observed differences in depression levels between smokers and non-smokers, i.e. depressed smokers must smoke as a way of coping with (reducing) their depressive affect, such inferences are clearly premature. Although between-person correlational data justifiably invite interpretation, only through careful laboratory and field investigation can we begin to understand the causal processes underlying smoking–depression associations.

Potential conceptual frameworks of smoking–depression relationships

Perhaps the longest and most methodologically rigorous study to date illustrating the smoking-depression association is a 21-year longitudinal study of a large birth cohort sample from childhood through young adulthood using clinical diagnoses of depression and daily smoking and nicotine-dependence measures [121]. These investigators found that clinically depressed individuals had higher rates of smoking and nicotine dependence, even after controlling for numerous potential child and adolescent confounds. Consistent with this finding, Breslau and colleagues have shown that there is a bidirectional association between smoking and depression, such that a baseline history of major depression increased progression to daily smoking, while, importantly, a history of daily smoking enhanced risk for the subsequent development of major depression. They found this pattern in a large five-year prospective study [59] and in data from the National Comorbidity Study [122]. In sum, these rigorous population-based studies with diagnoses of depression and nicotine dependence, as ascertained by clinical interviews, as well as measures of depressive symptoms and daily smoking levels, illustrate well the current state of knowledge on the lifetime and current association between clinical depression and smoking among youths and adults.

Despite the corpus of cross-sectional and prospective studies that have established an association between smoking and depression, such associations may represent a multitude of different relations, including the presence of other factors influencing both smoking and depression. Highlighting this point, Dierker and colleagues [123] asserted: 'Although the association between depression and smoking has been consistently established, little evidence regarding the mechanisms that influence this association is currently available' (p. 947). Because the theories and claims about causal processes have bearing on smoking prevention, intervention and even policy, determination of the underlying causal mechanisms represents a critically important next step for the tobacco-control research agenda. Hence, the primary focus of this section is to consider a variety of conceptual models that may help to explain the smoking–depression association more formally.

These models, although proposed and examined principally within the personality and psychopathology literature [124], hold promise for advancing a deeper understanding of the causal processes involved in the link between smoking and depression. In general, we focus our empirical review of these models around rigorous prospective longitudinal studies as opposed to cross-sectional research, because the former approach affords the best available evidence with which to evaluate these different models and because prospective studies clearly hold the potential to disentangle some of the methodological problems inherent in purely cross-sectional research, e.g. confusing cause, correlates and consequences [21].

Predisposition model

The predisposition model states explicitly that depression (symptoms or clinical episode) precedes and is causally implicated in smoking initiation, maintenance and relapse. As noted earlier, a wealth of prospective longitudinal studies provides evidence for the predisposition model [12,13,50,55,59,63,122,125–128]. Many of these investigations examined experimental or initial non-smokers who were then followed prospectively to show that they progressed to become regular smokers, and several of the studies prospectively examined elevations in future smoking levels after controlling for initial levels of smoking and other confounds.

Consequence model

The consequence model posits the opposite causal direction: long-term smoking (or even, as some argue, short-term smoking) leaves a direct, aetiological 'scar' that contributes to the risk for developing depression. Longitudinal studies, many of which also examined the predisposition model, provide burgeoning evidence for the consequence model as well [12,50,51,59,63,121,122,125,127,129]. Overall, these studies show that smoking predicts onset of depressive disorder or prospective increases in depressive symptoms over time in both adolescents and adults. Several of these studies tested both the predisposition model and the consequence model with the same data and found evidence for bidirectional associations [12,13,50,59,63,125,127], although other studies exploring the use-to-distress and distress-to-use hypotheses found support for only one direction [51,129,130].

Spectrum model

The spectrum, or common-cause, model states that smoking and depression arise from shared aetiological factors. In essence, the spectrum model posits that the significant co-variation found between smoking and depression, even when examined in prospective longitudinal studies with multiple waves of data, may be explained by a single factor or set of variables that give rise to risk for both smoking and depression. Evidence for this model comes from multiple sources and theoretically proposed vulnerability factors. We consider a few specific examples here; see [121] for a sophisticated longitudinal examination of the common-cause hypothesis. For example, psychosocial influences, such as a child's attachment to his or her parents, have been shown to predict smoking initiation in a four-year prospective study [131]; likewise, parental attachment predicts depression in youth [132]. Behavioural genetic research conducted by Kendler and colleagues [133] found a shared genetic liability to major depression that overlaps with smoking [71,134]. In addition to shared genetic influences, neurotransmitters, including dopamine, serotonin, nonadrenaline, gamma-aminobutyric acid (GABA) and glutamate, appear to be neural substrates that are implicated in the aetiology of both depression and smoking [135]. Personality trait vulnerabilities, such as neuroticism, have also been identified as risks for both depression [136] and smoking [137].

As there are many potential shared aetiological vulnerabilities that could be examined, it should be emphasised that many of the common vulnerabilities giving rise to the co-variation of depression and smoking are likely not completely independent risk factors. For example, a molecular genetic study found that the promotor for the serotonin transporter gene interacted with neuroticism to predict smoking behaviour, such that neuroticism was associated positively with current smoking and associated negatively with smoking cessation among those with poorly transcribed serotonin genotypes [138]. Of interest, results from a prospective birth cohort study showed that this same serotonin transporter gene interacted with stressful life events to predict increases in depression over time [139]. Thus, these two different studies with separate predicted outcomes (smoking [138] and depression [139]) reveal that the same molecular genetic vulnerability (poorly transcribed serotonin transporter genes) interacts with other risk factors, highlighting the importance of considering common-cause models at multiple levels with different outcomes.

Pathoplasticity model

Finally, the pathoplasticity model posits that the influence of smoking and depression on the presentation of each other is bidirectional, such that the presence of depression influences the course and presentation of smoking over time (e.g. initiation, maintenance, relapse) and smoking, or nicotine dependence, affects the course of depression (e.g. severity, recurrence). Consistent with the pathoplasticity perspective, we have already observed that smoking places the individual at risk for subsequent development of depressive symptomatology, and that depression predisposes to smoking behaviour, particularly nicotine dependence. We have also noted that according to a number of studies, a lifetime history of depression puts the individual at heightened risk for smoking relapse, but see [90]. Also of relevance, a study reported that individuals with one of various mental disorders and whose illness had remitted were not at increased risk for daily smoking, in contrast to individuals with active disorders [140]. An important implication of these findings points to the possibility of previously unrecognised public-health benefits of early treatment of mental disorders, i.e. prevention of smoking initiation.

A burgeoning literature on smoking cessation outcome studies of depressed smokers, utilising treatments aimed at reducing depressive symptomatology, also bears on notions derived from the pathoplasticity model. For instance, the antidepressant medication bupropion has received empirical scrutiny within the realm of smoking cessation. Bupropion has demonstrated efficacy for standard smoking treatment [141–143] and in conjunction with nicotine-replacement therapy [144] and for relapse prevention [145]. Importantly, several studies have reported that bupropion was equally efficacious for individuals with a history of major depression [146,147]. Lerman *et al.* [142] found that highly nicotine-dependent smokers who received bupropion were more likely to experience decreases in depressive symptoms during active drug treatment but were also more likely to experience a rebound in depressive symptoms when bupropion was discontinued. Taken together, these findings support the notion that at least one mode of pharmacotherapy specifically designed to treat major depressive disorder also facilitates smoking cessation, regardless of whether the smoker has a history of depression or even current depressive symptoms.

Non-pharmacological approaches to treating depression have also been assessed in the context of smoking cessation. Several studies have incorporated cognitive–behavioural mood-management modules aimed specifically at facilitating cessation among formerly depressed smokers. Brown *et al.* [148] found that although inclusion of a mood-management component did not reduce depressive symptoms in formerly depressed smokers trying to quit smoking, it was more effective than standardised treatment (without mood management) for heavy smokers and for those with a history of recurrent major depressive disorder. Interestingly, about 40% of participants showed a pattern of increasing depressive symptoms during the two weeks subsequent to quitting smoking, a pattern that was associated with poor smoking outcome [149]. Several studies by Hall and colleagues have utilised similar designs and yielded mixed findings regarding the efficacy of cessation programmes incorporating mood-management techniques [150,151].

Summary

Several conceptual models were described that offer potential explanation for the observed associations between smoking and depressive symptomatology. These explanations include (i) smoking predisposes to depression, (ii) depression predisposes to smoking, (iii) shared aetiological factors account for both smoking and depression and (iv) the relationship between smoking and depression is reciprocal, such that each influences the course and development of the other. Indeed, as we have seen, there exists evidence in support of all four perspectives. Nonetheless, much more work needs to be done to understand fully the complex nature of the smoking–depression link.

Potential moderators of smoking–depression associations

We highlight several factors that arose in our review of studies examining the link between smoking and depression because there is reason to believe that they may have important implications for elucidating the relation between smoking and depression. As such, we touch upon the roles that (i) context and social climate, (ii) gender differences and (iii) onset vs. persistence play with respect to seeking an understanding of the aetiological associations between smoking and depression.

First, regarding context and social climate, an historical trends study [152] analysed the association between smoking and depression with multiple age groups between in 1952 and 1992. The study found that the association between smoking and depression was non-significant between 1952 and 1970, whereas a strong and significant effect emerged in the 1992 sample (i.e. odds ratio [OR] of 3 that smoking individuals would experience subsequent depression relative to non-smokers). Murphy and colleagues [152] argue that the link between smoking and depression has increased as the social context has changed over time, during which tobacco use decreased while awareness of smoking risks increased. Certainly, these time trends suggest that social context and climate may be important moderators. Moreover, these findings highlight that the aetiological vulnerability models posited to explain the association between smoking and depression are better viewed as dynamic rather than static conceptualisations. Hence, this observation suggests caution in not over-interpreting evidence for or against one or another conceptual model because any association between smoking and depression is likely to be modified, at least in part, by social context, climate and time.

Second, we reviewed several studies highlighting the influence that sex may play in the association between smoking and depression. In a two-cohort study of 14- to 18-year olds [55], boys at baseline who did not have a smoking history but had higher depression symptom scores were more likely to initiate smoking over the three- to four-year prospective follow-up, whereas depression scores were not found to predict smoking initiation among non-smoking girls. In another longitudinal study with three prospective waves following youth from high school to age 24 years [13], smoking initiation preceded onset of depression and, likewise, lifetime depression was associated with smoking initiation for both sexes, although early-onset smokers had a family history of depression among women but not men. An in-depth prospective electronic diary study with adolescents [128] showed that both boys and girls with depressive symptoms exhibited elevated rates of actual smoking and urges to smoke, but depression increased the risk of smoking among girls with behavioural problems, whereas depression decreased the likelihood of smoking among boys with externalising symptoms. Finally, in a four-year longitudinal study of youths aged 12–19 years [153], smoking predicted greater depressive symptoms over time; this effect was stronger among girls than boys. In sum, these studies show that it is important to consider sex when evaluating both the predisposition and consequence models.

Third, and as we have alluded to throughout this chapter, it is important to consider differences between initiation/onset and persistence/recurrence in understanding the unfolding of both smoking and depression over time. As highlighted in the depression literature, there may be similar and/or different processes that contribute to first onsets of depression compared with maintenance or recurrence [154]. For example, Lewinsohn and colleagues [155] examined numerous psychosocial risk factors for depression onset versus recurrence. They found that whereas major life events predicted onset of first depression, dysfunctional attitudes (rigid extreme thinking) were associated more with depression recurrence. Likewise, a large behavioural genetic study from multiple countries found that the genetic influences for smoking persistence were not exactly the same as those for smoking initiation; indeed, less than 40% of the genetic variance in persistence was the same as that for initiation [134].

Related to the distinction between initiation and persistence, researchers may also have to consider the effect that severity of depression and/or smoking has on causal processes across different etiological models. Severity may be an important variable to take into account based on inconsistent results from two behavioural genetic twin studies examining the genetic links between smoking and depression. In the first of these studies [133], genetic influences accounted for the association between depression diagnosis and liability to smoking over the lifetime, whereas the second study [71] found that non-shared specific environmental influences accounted for the majority of the association between depressive symptoms and lifetime smoking liability. Although the latent variable underlying depression is dimensional (as reviewed earlier), studies measuring clinical levels of diagnosed depression tend to examine the more severe end of the depression continuum compared with those studies assessing depressive symptom variability.

Conclusions and future directions

We have seen that the link between cigarette smoking and depression is strong and generally persists throughout the smoker's lifetime. Data were reviewed that, in sum, provide support for the four aetiological models we discussed: (i) depression is a vulnerability factor for smoking, (ii) smoking predisposes to subsequent development of depression, (iii) shared common causes may render individuals vulnerable to both smoking and depression and (iv) the relationship between the development of smoking and depression appears reciprocal, such that each exerts influence over the developmental trajectory of the other. We also emphasised the potentially important role played by context and moderator variables in shaping smoking–depression associations.

In sum, we believe that an integration and synthesis of social and biological explanations should be undertaken in order to grasp fully the complexity of smoking–depression associations. Furthermore, such an approach should take into account developmental context. That is, attempts should be made to ascertain whether associations between smoking and depression vary over the developmental continuum of smoking behaviour. Recent epigenetic approaches to understanding substance-abuse aetiology among youths espouse similar sentiments and afford the opportunity to characterise the emergence of transitional phenotypes as a function of numerous reciprocal influences, including social, cultural, behavioural, neural, neuroendocrine and genetic [156,157].

Such a developmental perspective also affords the opportunity to draw upon alternative models of understanding smoking and depression. For example, the notion of equifinality, which refers to the observation that in any open system a diversity of pathways may lead to the same outcome, provides a useful heuristic for capturing as yet unstudied aspects of the smoking–depression relationship.

The concept of multifinality suggests that any one factor may function differently depending on the organisation of the system in which it operates and, hence, may be indicative of interaction effects [158].

The bottom line is that in this field, we must move beyond a simple description of cross-sectional associations between smoking and depression towards more sophisticated and theoretically informed methodologies. The smoking problem is not going away soon, and neither is depression. As each disorder exacts its devastating toll in terms of lives interrupted and lives lost, it becomes incumbent upon both tobacco and depression researchers alike to elucidate the underlying nature of the smoking–depression link more accurately.

Acknowledgements

The writing of this chapter was supported, in part, by grant P01 CA98262–01A2 from the National Cancer Institute.

REFERENCES

1. U. S. Department of Health and Human Services, *The Health Consequences of Smoking: A Report of the Surgeon General* (Atlanta, GA: U. S. Department of Health and Human Services, Centers for Disease Control and Prevention, National Center for Chronic Disease Prevention and Health Promotion, Office on Smoking and Health, 2004).
2. A. H. Mokdad, J. S. Marks, D. F. Stroup, J. L. Gerberding, Actual causes of death in the United States. *J. Am. Med. Assoc.* **291** (2004), 1238–45.
3. World Health Organization, *Partnership to Reduce Tobacco Dependence* (Copenhagen: World Health Organization, 2000).
4. J. Anthony, K. Warner, R. Kessler, Comparative epidemiology of dependence on tobacco, alcohol, controlled substances and inhalants: basic findings from the National Comorbidity Survey. *Exp. Clin. Psychopharmacol.* **2** (1994), 244–68.
5. S. Shiffman, Comments on nicotine addiction. *Psychopharmacology* **117** (1995), 14–15.
6. J. D. Kassel, S. Weinstein, S. A. Skitch, J. Veilleux, R. J. Mermelstein, The development of substance abuse in adolescence: correlates, causes, and consequences. In *Development of Psychopathology: A Vulnerability-Stress Perspective*, ed. B. L. Hankin, J. R. Abela (Thousand Oaks, CA: Sage, 2005), pp. 355–84.
7. E. T. Moolchan, M. Ernst, J. E. Henningfield, A review of tobacco smoking in adolescents: treatment implications. *J. Am. Acad. Child Adolesc. Psychiatry* **39** (2000), 682–93.
8. K. Lasser, J. W. Boyd, S. Woolhandler, *et al.*, Smoking and mental illness: a population-based prevalence study. *J. Am. Med. Assoc.* **284** (2000), 2606–10.
9. N. Breslau, M. M. Kilbey, P. Andreski, Nicotine dependence, major depression, and anxiety in young adults. *Arch. Gen. Psychiatry* **48** (1991), 1069–74.

10. L. S. Covey, A. H. Glassman, F. Stetner, Cigarette smoking and major depression. *J. Addict. Dis.* **17** (1998), 35–46.

11. L. Degenhardt, W. Hall, The relationship between tobacco use, substance-use disorders and mental health: results from the National Survey of Mental Health and Well-being. *Nicotine Tob. Res.* **3** (2001), 225–34.

12. R. A. Brown, P. M. Lewinsohn, J. R. Seeley, E. F. Wagner, Cigarette smoking, major depression, and other psychiatric disorders among adolescents. *J. Am. Acad. Child Adolesc. Psychiatry* **35** (1996), 1602–10.

13. P. Rohde, P. M. Lewinsohn, R. A. Brown, J. M. Gau, C. W. Kahler, Psychiatric disorders, familial factors and cigarette smoking: I. Associations with smoking initiation. *Nicotine Tob. Res.* **5** (2003), 85–98.

14. H. P. Upadhyaya, D. Deas, K. T. Brady, M. Kruesi, Cigarette smoking and psychiatric comorbidity in children and adolescents. *J. Am. Acad. Child Adolesc. Psychiatry* **41** (2002), 1294–305.

15. K. S. Kendler, M. C. Neale, P. Sullivan, *et al.*, A population-based twin study in women of smoking initiation and nicotine dependence. *Psychol. Med.* **29** (1999), 299–308.

16. D. B. Kandel, J. G. Johnson, H. R. Bird, *et al.*, Psychiatric disorders associated with substance use among children and adolescents: findings from the methods for the Epidemiology of Child and Adolescent Mental disorders (MECA) Study. *J. Abnorm. Child. Psychol.* **25** (1997), 121–32.

17. S. G. Kellam, J. C. Anthony, Targeting early antecedents to prevent tobacco smoking: findings from an epidemiologically based randomized field trial. *Am. J. Public Health* **88** (1998), 1490–94.

18. M. T. Lynskey, D. M. Ferguson, Childhood conduct problems, attention deficit behaviors, and adolescent alcohol, tobacco, and illicit drug use. *J. Abnorm. Child. Psychol.* **23** (1995), 281–302.

19. R. J. McMahon, Child and adolescent psychopathology as risk factors for subsequent tobacco use. *Nicotine Tob. Res.* **1** (1999), S45–50.

20. S. Miller-Johnson, J. E. Lochman, J. D. Coie, R. Terry, C. Hyman, Comorbidity of conduct and depressive problems at sixth grade: substance use outcomes across adolescence. *J. Abnorm. Child. Psychol.* **26** (1998), 221–32.

21. J. D. Kassel, L. R. Stroud, C. A. Paronis, Smoking, stress, and negative affect: correlation, causation, and context across stages of smoking. *Psychol. Bull.* **129** (2003), 270–304.

22. American Psychiatric Association. *Diagnostic and Statistical Manual of Mental Disorders*, 4th edn (Washington, DC: American Psychiatric Association, 1994).

23. J. C. Coyne, Self-reported distress: analog or ersatz depression. *Psychol. Bull.* **116** (1994), 29–45.

24. G. L. Flett, K. Vrendenburg, L. Krames, The continuity of depression in clinical and non-clinical samples. *Psychol. Bull.* **121** (1997), 395–416.

25. A. M. Ruscio, J. Ruscio, The latent structure of analogue depression: should the Beck Depression Inventory be used to classify groups? *Psychol. Assess.* **14** (2002), 135–45.

26. J. Ruscio, A. M. Ruscio, Informing the continuity controversy: a taxometric analysis of depression. *J. Abnorm. Psychol.* **109** (2000), 473–87.

27. B. L. Hankin, R. C. Fraley, B. B. Lahey, I. Waldman, Is depression best viewed as a continuum or discrete category? A taxometric analysis of childhood and adolescent depression in a population-based sample. *J. Abnorm. Psychol.* **114** (2005), 96–110.

28. P. Ambrosini, D. Bennett, C. M. Cleland, N. Haslam, Taxonicity of adolescent melancholia: a categorical or dimensional construct? *J. Psychiatr. Res.* **36** (2002), 247–56.

29. S. R. H. Beach, N. Amir, Is depression taxonic, dimensional, or both? *J. Abnorm. Psychol.* **112** (2003), 228–36.

30. J. Ruscio, A. M. Ruscio, T. M. Keane, Using taxometric analysis to distinguish a small latent taxon from a latent dimension with positively skewed indicators: the case of involuntary defeat syndrome. *J. Abnorm. Psychol.* **113** (2004), 145–54.

31. U. S. Department of Health and Human Services. *The Health Consequences of Smoking: Nicotine Addiction – a Report from the U. S. Surgeon General* (Washington, DC: U. S. Government Printing Office, 1988).

32. J. R. Hughes, S. T. Higgins, D. Hatsukami, Effects of abstinence from tobacco: a critical review. In *Research Advances in Alcohol and Drug Problems*, ed. L. T. Kozlowski, H. M. Annis, H. D. Cappell, *et al.* (New York: Plenum Publishing, 1990), pp. 317–98.

33. J. R. Hughes, D. K. Hatsukami, R. W. Pickens, *et al.*, Effect of nicotine on the tobacco withdrawal syndrome. *Psychopharmacology* **83** (1984), 82–7.

34. G. H. Cutler, F. X. Barrios, Effects of deprivation on smokers' mood during the operation of a complex computer simulation. *Addict. Behav.* **13** (1988), 379–82.

35. S. E. Fleming, T. W. Lombardo, Effects of cigarette smoking on phobic anxiety. *Addict. Behav.* **12** (1987), 195–8.

36. J. R. Hughes, Distinguishing withdrawal relief and direct effects of smoking. *Psychopharmacology* **104** (1991), 409–10.

37. D. Kalman, The subjective effects of nicotine: methodological issues, a review of experimental studies, and recommendations for future research. *Nicotine Tob. Res.* **4** (2002), 25–70.

38. R. West, Beneficial effects of nicotine: fact or fiction? *Addiction* **88** (1993), 589–90.

39. S. Shiffman, J. A. Paty, J. D. Kassel, M. Gnys, M. Zettler-Segal, Smoking behavior and smoking history of tobacco chippers. *Exp. Clin. Psychopharmacol.* **2** (1994), 126–42.

40. B. R. Flay, Youth tobacco use: risks, patterns, and control. In *Nicotine Addiction: Principles and Management*, ed. J. Slade, C. T. Orleans (New York: Oxford University Press, 1993) pp. 365–84.

41. D. A. Cole, J. M. Martin, L. G. Peeke, A. D. Seroczynski, K. Hoffman, Are cognitive errors of underestimation predictive or reflective of depressive symptoms in children: a longitudinal study. *J. Abnorm. Psychol.* **107** (1998), 481–96.

42. B. L. Hankin, L. Y. Abramson, T. E. Moffitt *et al.*, Development of depression from preadolescence to young adulthood: emerging gender differences in a 10-year longitudinal study. *J. Abnorm. Psychol.* **107** (1998), 128–40.

43. B. L. Hankin, L. Y. Abramson, Development of gender differences in depression: an elaborated cognitive vulnerability-transactional stress theory. *Psychol. Bull.* **127** (2001), 773–96.

44. T. J. Wade, J. Cairney, D. J. Pevalin, Emergence of gender differences in depression during adolescence: national panel results from three countries. *J. Am. Acad. Child Adolesc. Psychiatry* **41** (2002), 190–98.

45. J. D. Kassel, Are adolescent smokers addicted to nicotine? The suitability of the nicotine dependence construct as applied to adolescents. *J. Child Adolesc. Subst. Abuse.* **9** (2000), 27–49.

46. J. S. Brook, P. Cohen, D. W. Brook, Longitudinal study of co-occurring psychiatric disorders and substance use. *J. Am. Acad. Child Adolesc. Psychiatry* **37** (1998), 322–30.

47. L. G. Escobedo, M. Reddy, G. A. Giovino, The relationship between depressive symptoms and cigarette smoking in US adolescents. *Addiction* **93** (1998), 433–40.

48. R. F. Ferdinand, M. Bluem, F. C. Verhulst, Psychopathology in adolescence predicts substance use in young adulthood. *Addiction* **96** (2001), 861–70.

49. D. B. Kandel, M. Davies, D. Karus, K. Yamaguchi, The consequences in young adulthood of adolescent drug involvement: an overview. *Arch. Gen. Psychiatry* **43** (1986), 746–54.

50. L. C. Dierker, S. Avenevoli, K. R. Merikangas, B. P. Flaherty, M. Stolar, Association between psychiatric disorders and the progression of tobacco use behaviors. *J. Am. Acad. Child Adolesc. Psychiatry* **40** (2001), 1159–67.

51. E. Goodman, J. Capitman, Depressive symptoms and cigarette smoking among teens. *Pediatrics* **106** (2000), 748–55.

52. M. Q. Wang, E. C. Fitzhugh, B. L. Green, *et al.*, Prospective social-psychological factors of adolescent smoking progression. *J. Adolesc. Health* **24** (1998), 2–9.

53. H. R. White, R. J. Pandina, P. H. Chen, Developmental trajectories of cigarette use from early adolescence into young adulthood. *Drug Alcohol Depend.* **65** (2002), 167–78.

54. E. Costello, A. Erkanli, E. Federman, A. Angold, Development of psychiatric comorbidity with substance abuse in adolescents: effects of timing and sex. *J. Clin. Child Psychol.* **28** (1999), 298–311.

55. J. D. Killen, T. H. Robinson, K. F. Haydel, *et al.*, Prospective study of risk factors for the initiation of cigarette smoking. *J. Consult. Clin. Psychol.* **65** (1997), 1011–16.

56. E. R. Gritz, A. V. Prokhorov, K. S. Hudmon, *et al.*, Cigarette smoking in a multiethnic population of youth: methods and baseline findings. *Prev. Med.* **27** (1998), 365–84.

57. D. M. Fergusson, M. T. Lynskey, J. Horwood, Comorbidity between depressive disorders and nicotine dependence in a cohort of 16-year-olds. *Arch. Gen. Psychiatry* (1996), 1043–7.

58. D. B. Kandel, M. Davies, Adult sequelae of adolescent depressive symptoms. *Arch. Gen. Psychiatry* **43** (1986), 255–62.

59. N. Breslau, E. L. Peterson, L. R. Schultz, H. D. Chilcoat, P. Andreski, Major depression and stages of smoking: a longitudinal investigation. *Arch. Gen. Psychiatry* **55** (1998), 161–6.

60. J. A. Stein, M. D. Newcomb, P. M. Bentler, Initiation and maintenance of tobacco smoking: changing personality correlates in adolescence and young adulthood. *J. Appl. Soc. Psychol.* **26** (1996), 160–87.

61. G. C. Patton, J. B. Carlin, C. Coffey, *et al.*, Depression, anxiety, and smoking initiation: a prospective study over 3 years. *Am. J. Public Health* **88** (1998), 1518–22.

62. W. S. Choi, C. A. Patten, J. C. Gillin, R. M. Kaplan, J. P. Pierce, Cigarette smoking predicts development of depressive symptoms among US adolescents. *Ann. Behav. Med.* **19** (1997), 42–50.

63. M. Windle, R. C. Windle, Depressive symptoms and cigarette smoking among middle adolescents: prospective associations and intrapersonal and interpersonal influences. *J. Consult. Clin. Psychol.* **69** (2001), 215–26.

64. J. G. Johnson, P. Cohen, D. S. Pine, *et al.*, Association between cigarette smoking and anxiety disorders during adolescence and early adulthood. *J. Am. Med. Assoc.* **284** (2000), 2348–51.

65. N. Breslau, Psychiatric comorbidity of smoking and nicotine dependence. *Behav. Genet.* **25** (1995), 95–101.

66. H. Waal-Manning, F. de Hamel, Smoking habit and psychometric scores: a community study. *N. Z. Med. J.* **88** (1978), 188–91.

67. R. F. Anda, D. F. Williamson, L. G. Escobedo, *et al.*, Depression and the dynamics of smoking. *J. Am. Med. Assoc.* **264** (1990), 1541–5.

68. N. Breslau, M. M. Kilbey, P. Andreski, Nicotine dependence and major depression: new evidence from a prospective investigation. *Arch. Gen. Psychiatry* **50** (1993), 31–5.

69. N. Breslau, M. M. Kilbey, P. Andreski, DSM-III-R nicotine dependence in young adults: prevalence, correlates and associated psychiatric disorders. *Addiction* **89** (1994), 743–54.

70. K. S. Kendler, M. C. Neale, C. J. MacLean, *et al.*, Smoking and major depression: a causal analysis. *Arch. Gen. Psychiatry* **50** (1993), 36–43.

71. J. M. McCaffery, R. Niaura, G. E. Swan, D. Carmelli, A study of depressive symptoms and smoking behavior in adult male twins from the NHLBI twin study. *Nicotine Tob. Res.* **5** (2003), 77–83.

72. D. R. Cherek, Effects of acute exposure to increased levels of background industrial noise on cigarette smoking behavior. *Int. Arch. Occup. Environ. Health* **56** (1985), 23–30.

73. G. L. Mangan, J. F. Golding, *The Psychopharmacology of Smoking* (New York: Cambridge University Press, 1984).

74. C. S. Pomerleau, O. F. Pomerleau, The effects of a psychological stressor on cigarette smoking and subsequent behavioral and physiological responses. *Psychophysiology* **24** (1987), 278–85.

75. L. H. Epstein, F. L. Collins, The measurement of situational influences of smoking. *Addict. Behav.* **2** (1977), 47–53.

76. J. E. Rose, S. Ananda, M. E. Jarvik, Cigarette smoking during anxiety-provoking and monotonous tasks. *Addict. Behav.* **8** (1983), 353–9.

77. S. Schachter, B. Silverstein, D. Perlick, Psychological and pharmacological explanations of smoking under stress. *J. Exp. Psychol. Gen.* **106** (1977), 31–40.

78. K. A. Perkins, J. E. Grobe, Increased desire to smoke during acute stress. *Br. J. Addiction* **87** (1992), 1037–40.

79. A. J. Garvey, R. E. Bliss, J. L. Hitchcock, J. W. Heinold, B. Rosner, Predictors of smoking relapse among self-quitters: a report from the normative aging study. *Addict. Behav.* **17** (1992), 367–77.

80. S. Shiffman, Relapse following smoking cessation: A situational analysis. *J. Consult. Clin. Psychol.* **50** (1982), 71–86.

81. Department of Health and Human Services, *The Health Benefits of Smoking Cessation: A Report of the Surgeon General*, DHHS publication no. CDC 90–8416. (Atlanta, GA: Public Health Service, Centers for Disease Control, National Center for Chronic Disease Prevention and Health Promotion, Office on Smoking and Health, 1990).

82. S. Cohen, E. Lichtenstein, J. O. Prochaska, *et al.*, Debunking myths about self-quitting: evidence from 10 prospective studies of persons who attempt to quit smoking by themselves. *Am. Psychol.* **44** (1989), 1355–65.

83. J. R. Hughes, S. B. Gulliver, J. W. Fenwick, *et al.*, Smoking cessation among self-quitters. *Health Psychol.* **11** (1992), 331–4.

84. A. H. Glassman, J. E. Helzer, L. S. Covey, *et al.*, Smoking, smoking cessation and major depression. *J. Am. Med. Assoc.* **264** (1990), 1546–9.

85. S. M. Hall, R. F. Munoz, V. I. Reus, K. L. Sees, Nicotine, negative affect, and depression. *J. Consult. Clin. Psychol.* **61** (1993), 761–7.

86. L. S. Covey, Tobacco cessation among patients with depression. *Primary Care* **26** (1999), 691–706.

87. L. S. Covey, A. H. Glassman, F. Stetner, Major depression following smoking cessation. *Am. J. Psychiatry* **154** (1997), 263–5.

88. B. Borrelli, B. Bock, T. King, B. Pinto, B. H. Marcus, The impact of depression on smoking cessation in women. *Am. J. Prev. Med.* **12** (1996), 378–87.

89. R. Niaura, D. M. Britt, W. G. Shadel, *et al.*, Symptoms of depression and survival experience among three samples of smokers trying to quit. *Psychol. Addict. Behav.* **15** (2001), 13–17.

90. B. Hitsman, B. Borrelli, D. E. McChargue, B. Spring, R. Niaura, History of depression and smoking cessation outcome: a meta-analysis. *J. Consult. Clin. Psychol.* **71** (2003), 657–63.

91. A. D. McNeill, M. Jarvis, R. West, Subjective effects of cigarette smoking in adolescents. *Psychopharmacologia* **92** (1987), 115–17.

92. D. N. Dozois, J. A. Farrow, A. Miser, Smoking patterns and cessation motivations during adolescence. *Int. J. Addict.* **30** (1995), 1485–98.

93. M. Nichter, M. Nichter, N. Vuckovic, G. Quintero, C. Ritenbaugh, Smoking experimentation and initiation among adolescent girls: qualitative and quantitative findings. *Tobacco Control* **6** (1997), 285–95.

94. M. M. Faraday, B. M. Elliott, N. E. Grunberg, Adult vs. adolescent rats differ in biobehavioral responses to chronic nicotine administration. *Pharmacol. Biochem. Behav.* **70** (2001), 475–89.

95. B. M. Elliott, M. M. Faraday, J. M. Phillips, N. E. Grunberg, Effects of nicotine on elevated plus maze and locomotor activity in male and female adolescent and adult rats. *Pharmacol. Biochem. Behav.* **77** (2004), 21–8.

96. S. Cheeta, E. E. Irvine, S. Tucci, J. Sandhu, S. E. File, In adolescence, female rats are more sensitive to the anxiolytic effect of nicotine than are male rats. *Neuropsychopharmacology* **25** (2001), 601–7.

97. R. Coan, Personality variables associated with cigarette smoking. *J. Pers. Soc. Psychol.* **26** (1973), 86–104.

98. F. F. Ikard, P. E. Green, D. Horn, A scale to differentiate between types of smoking as related to the management of affect. *Int. J. Addict.* **4** (1969), 649–59.

99. McKennell, Smoking motivation factors. *Br. J. Soc. Clin. Psychol.* **9** (1970), 8–22.

100. M. A. H. Russell, J. Peto, U. A. Patel, The classification of smoking by factorial structure of motives. *J. R. Stat. Soc. Ser. A* **137** (1974), 313–33.

101. S. Shiffman, Assessing smoking patterns and motives. *J. Consult. Clin. Psychol.* **61** (1993), 732–42.

102. T. H. Brandon, T. B. Baker, The smoking consequences questionnaire: the subjective expected utility of smoking in college students. *Psychol. Assess.* **3** (1991), 484–91.

103. A. L. Copeland, T. H. Brandon, E. P. Quinn, The Smoking Consequences Questionnaire – Adult: measurement of smoking outcome expectancies of experienced smokers. *Psychol. Assess.* **7** (1995), 484–94.

104. B. Spring, R. Pingitore, D. E. McChargue, Reward value of cigarette smoking for comparably heavy smoking schizophrenic, depressed, and nonpatient smokers. *Am. J. Psychiatry* **160** (2003), 316–22.

105. T. P. George, M. R. Picciotto, C. D. Verrico, R. H. Roth, Effects of nicotine pretreatment on dopaminergic and behavioral responses to conditioned fear stress in rats: dissociation of biochemical and behavioral effects. *Biol. Psychiatry* **49** (2001), 300–306.

106. T. P. George, C. D. Verrico, R. H. Roth, Effects of repeated nicotine pre-treatment on mesoprefrontal dopaminergic and behavioral responses to acute footshock stress. *Brain Res.* **801** (1998), 36–49.

107. J. Semba, C. Mataki, S. Yamada, M. Nankai, M. Toru, Antidepressantlike effects of chronic nicotine on learned helplessness paradigm in rats. *Biol. Psychiatry* **43** (1998), 389–91.

108. Y. Tizabi, D. H. Overstreet, A. H. Rezvani, *et al.*, Antidepressant effects of nicotine in an animal model of depression. *Psychopharmacology (Berl.)* **142** (1999), 193–9.

109. D. J. Djuric, E. Dunn, D. H. Overstreet, A. Dragomir, M. Steiner, Antidepressant effect of ingested nicotine in female rats of Flinders resistant and sensitive lines. *Physiol. Behav.* **67** (1999), 533–7.

110. D. J. K. Balfour, D. L. Ridley, The effects of nicotine on neural pathways implicated in depression: a factor in nicotine addiction? *Pharmacol. Biochem. Behav.* **66** (2000), 79–85.

111. D. J. K. Balfour, The influence of stress on psychopharmacological responses to nicotine. *Br. J. Addiction* **86** (1991), 489–93.

112. T. H. Brandon, S. T. Tiffany, K. M. Obremski, T. B. Baker, Postcessation cigarette use: the process of relapse. *Addict. Behav.* **15** (1990), 105–14.

113. S. Shiffman, M. Hickcox, J. A. Paty, *et al.*, The abstinence violation effect following smoking lapses and temptations. *Cogn. Ther. Res.* **21** (1997), 497–523.

114. G. A. Marlatt, J. R. Gordon *Relapse Prevention: Maintenance Strategies in the Treatment of Addictive Behaviors* (New York: Guilford Press, 1985).

115. M. P. Carey, D. L. Kalra, K. B. Carey, S. Halperin, C. S. Richards, Stress and unaided smoking cessation: a prospective investigation. *J. Consult. Clin. Psychol.* **61** (1993), 831–8.

116. S. Cohen, E. Lichtenstein, Perceived stress, quitting smoking, and smoking relapse. *Health Psychol.* **9** (1990), 466–78.

117. J. R. Hughes, Tobacco withdrawal in self-quitters. *J. Consult. Clin. Psychol.* **60** (1992), 689–97.

118. R. West, P. Hajek, What happens to anxiety levels on giving up smoking? *Am. J. Psychiatry* **154** (1997), 1589–92.

119. D. G. Gilbert, F. J. McClernon, N. E. Rabinovich, *et al.*, Mood disturbance fails to resolve across 31 days of cigarette abstinence in women. *J. Consult. Clin. Psychol.* **70** (2002), 142–52.

120. A. C. Parrott, Does cigarette smoking cause stress? *Am. Psychol.* **54** (1999), 817–20.

121. D. M. Fergusson, R. D. Goodwin, L. J. Horwood, Major depression and cigarette smoking: results of a 21-year longitudinal study. *Psychol. Med.* **33** (2003), 1357–67.

122. N. Breslau, S. P. Novak, R. C. Kessler, Psychiatric disorders and stages of smoking. *Biol. Psychiatry* **55** (2004), 69–76.

123. L. C. Dierker, S. Avenevoli, M. Stolar, K. R. Merikangas, Smoking and depression: an examination of mechanisms of comorbidity. *Am. J. Psychiatry* **159** (2002), 947–53.

124. T. A. Widiger, R. Verheul, W. van den Brink, Personality and psychopathology. In *Handbook of Personality: Theory and Research*, ed. L. A. Pervin, O. P. John (New York: Guilford Press, 1999), pp. 347–66.

125. M. Orlando, P. L. Ellickson, K. Jinnett, The temporal relationship between emotional distress and cigarette smoking during adolescence and young adulthood. *J. Consult. Clin. Psychol.* **69** (2001), 959–70.

126. G. Patton, J. Carlin, C. Coffey, *et al.*, Depression, anxiety, and smoking initiation: a prospective study over 3 years. *Am. J. Public Health* **88** (1998), 1518–22.

127. I. C. Scarinci, J. Thomas, P. J. Brantley, G. N. Jones, Examination of the temporal relationship between smoking and major depressive disorder among low-income women in public primary care clinics. *Am. J. Health Promotion* **16** (2002), 323–30.

128. C. K. Whalen, L. D. Jamner, B. Henkder, R. J. Delfino, Smoking and moods in adolescents with depressive and aggressive dispositions: evidence from surveys and electronic diaries. *Health Psychol.* **20** (2001), 99–111.

129. L. T. Wu, J. C. Anthony, Tobacco smoking and depressed mood in late childhood and early adolescence. *Am. J. Public Health* **89** (1999), 1837–40.

130. G. C. Patton, J. B. Carlin, C. Coffey, *et al.*, The course of early smoking: a population-based cohort study over three years. *Addiction* **93** (1998), 1251–60.

131. C. B. Fleming, H. Kim, T. W. Harachi, R. F. Catalano, Family processes for children in early elementary school as predictors of smoking initiation. *J. Adolesc. Health* **30** (2002), 184–9.

132. J. R. Z. Abela, B. L. Hankin, E. A. P. Haigh, *et al.*, Interpersonal vulnerability to depressive episodes in high risk children: the role of insecure attachment and reassurance seeking. *J. Clin. Child Adolesc. Psychol.* **34** (2005), 182–92.

133. K. S. Kendler, M. C. Neale, C. J. MacLean, *et al.*, Smoking and major depression: a causal analysis. *Arch. Gen. Psychiatry* **50** (1993), 36–43.

134. P. A. F. Madden, A. C. Heath, N. L. Pedersen, *et al.*, The genetics of smoking persistence in men and women: a multicultural study. *Behav. Genet.* **29** (1999), 423–31.

135. E. Quattrocki, A. Baird, D. Hurgelun-Todd, Biological aspects of the link between smoking and depression. *Harv. Rev. Psychiatry* **8** (2000), 99–110.

136. R. F. Krueger, Personality traits in late adolescence predict mental disorders in early adulthood: a prospective-epidemiological study. *J. Pers.* **67** (1999), 39–65.

137. D. G. Gilbert. *Smoking: Individual Differences, Psychopathology, and Emotion* (Washington, DC: Taylor & Francis, 1995).

138. S. Hu, C. L. Brody, C. Fisher, *et al.*, Interaction between the serotonin transporter gene and neuroticism in cigarette smoking behavior. *Mol. Psychiatry* **5** (2000), 181–8.

139. A. Caspi, K. Sugden, T. E. Moffitt, *et al.*, Influence of life stress on depression: moderation by a polymorphism in the 5-HTT gene. *Science* **301** (2003), 386–9.

140. N. Breslau, S. P. Novak, R. C. Kessler, Daily smoking and the subsequent onset of psychiatric disorders. *Psychol. Med.* **34** (2004), 323–33.

141. J. S. Ahluwalia, K. J. Harris, D. Catley, K. S. Okuyemi, M. S. Mayo, Sustained-release bupropion for smoking cessation in African Americans: a randomized controlled trial. *J. Am. Med. Assoc.* **288** (2002), 468–74.

142. C. Lerman, R. Niaura, B. N. Collins, *et al.*, Effect of bupropion on depression symptoms in a smoking cessation clinical trial. *Psychol. Addict. Behav.* **18** (2004), 362–6.

143. R. D. Hurt, D. P. Sachs, E. D. Glover, *et al.*, A comparison of sustained-release bupropion and placebo for smoking cessation. *N. Engl. J. Med.* **337** (1997), 1195–202.

144. D. E. Jorenby, S. J. Leischow, M. A. Nides, *et al.*, A controlled trial of sustained-release bupropion, a nicotine patch, or both for smoking cessation. *N. Engl. J. Med.* **340** (1999), 685–91.

145. J. T. Hays, R. D. Hurt, N. A. Rigotti, *et al.*, Sustained-release bupropion for pharmacologic relapse prevention after smoking cessation: a randomized, controlled trial. *Ann. Intern. Med.* **135** (2001), 423–33.

146. K. E. Hayford, C. A. Patten, T. A. Rummans, *et al.*, Efficacy of bupropion for smoking cessation in smokers with a former history of major depression or alcoholism. *Br. J. Psychiatry* **174** (1999), 173–8.

147. L. Sanderson, C. A. Patten, R. S. Niaura, *et al.*, Efficacy of bupropion for relapse prevention in smokers with and without a past history of major depression. *J. Gen. Intern. Med.* **19** (2004), 828–34.

148. R. A. Brown, C. W. Kahler, R. Niaura, *et al.*, Cognitive-behavioral treatment for depression in smoking cessation. *J. Consult. Clin. Psychol.* **69** (2001), 471–80.

149. E S. Burgess, R. A. Brown, C. W. Kahler, *et al.*, Patterns of change in depressive symptoms during smoking cessation: who's at risk for relapse? *J. Consult. Clin. Psychol.* **70** (2002), 356–61.

150. S. M. Hall, R. F. Munoz, V. I. Reus, Cognitive-behavioral intervention increases abstinence rates for depressive-history smokers. *J. Consult. Clin. Psychol.* **62** (1994), 141–6.

151. S. M. Hall, R. F. Munoz, V. I. Reus, *et al.*, Mood management and nicotine gum in smoking treatment: a therapeutic contact and placebo-controlled study. *J. Consult. Clin. Psychol.* **64** (1996), 1003–1009.

152. J. M. Murphy, N. J. Horton, R. R. Monson, *et al.*, Cigarette smoking in relation to depression: historical trends from the Stirling County Study. *Am. J. Psychiatry* **160** (2003), 1663–9.

153. N. L. Galambos, B. J. Leadbeater, E. T. Barker, Gender differences in and risk factors for depression in adolescence: a 4-year longitudinal study. *Int. J. Behav. Dev.* **28** (2004), 16–25.

154. B. L. Hankin, J. R. Z. Abela, Depression from childhood through adolescence and adulthood: a developmental vulnerability-stress perspective. In *Development of Psychopathology: A Vulnerability–Stress Perspective*, ed. B. L. Hankin, J. R. Z. Abela (Thousand Oaks, CA, Sage, 2005), pp. 245–88.

155. P. M. Lewinsohn, T. E. Joiner, P. Rohde, Evaluation of cognitive diathesis-stress models in predicting major depressive disorder in adolescents. *J. Abnorm. Psychol.* **110** (2001), 203–15.

156. M. A. Dawes, S. M. Antelman, M. M. Vanyukov, *et al.*, Developmental sources of variation in liability to adolescent substance use disorders. *Drug Alcohol Dep.* **61** (2000), 3–14.

157. T. A. Wills, J. M. Sandy, A. Yaeger, Temperament and adolescent substance use: an epigenetic approach to risk and protection. *J. Pers.* **68** (2000), 1127–51.

158. D. Cicchetti, F. A. Rogosch, Equifinality and multifinality in developmental psychopathology. *Dev. Psychopathol.* **8** (1996), 597–600.

16

Depression and physical activity

Andrew Steptoe

Introduction

There is an extensive scientific literature dating back several decades linking lack of physical exercise with depressed mood, limited coping skills and low levels of psychological well-being [1,2]. Physical inactivity is also associated with increased risk for many of the medical problems discussed in this book. In some illnesses, such as coronary heart disease (CHD), physical inactivity is thought to have a causal role in disease risk, mediated through metabolic and other pathways [3]. In other conditions, such as chronic pain, inactivity does not cause the problem but nevertheless it contributes to disability. Physical exercise is also important in the regulation and management of chronic conditions, such as diabetes. The question therefore arises of whether the associations between depression and medical problems are mediated through low levels of physical activity and increased sedentary behaviour. Such possibilities have important implications for prevention and patient care.

This chapter discusses the evidence linking physical activity, depression and medical problems and addresses two general questions: First, is reduced physical activity responsible in part for associations between depression and the medical conditions and disabilities discussed in this book? Second, can increases in physical exercise improve the mood of patients and, therefore, be used in the management of these medical problems? The chapter begins with a discussion of the associations between physical activity, depression and depressed mood in clinical and population studies. There are many studies documenting more positive moods in active compared with inactive people, but it is important to assess the strength of the evidence and to rule out the contribution of underlying or unmeasured psychosocial or clinical factors. The chapter goes on to evaluate the impact of changes in depression and physical activity. Such changes can be evaluated in two ways: assessing the effects of

Depression and Physical Illness, ed. A. Steptoe.
Published by Cambridge University Press. © Cambridge University Press 2006.

treating depression on physical activity levels, and assessing the influence of physical training interventions on depression. This field has been beset with methodological problems, some of which are outlined here. Evaluations of physical training interventions in physically healthy populations are followed by considering the evidence that increased physical activity might alleviate depression in patients with medical problems. Finally, the chapter outlines some of the psychobiological mechanisms that might link physical activity, depression and pathophysiological processes in human disease.

This chapter is not intended to review the evidence that physical activity and exercise training are beneficial for health. There are many settings in which positive effects have been established rather convincingly, such as in cardiac rehabilitation, pain management and the postponement of disability [4,5]. Such findings are important but may have nothing to do with depression; rather, they have direct effects on musculoskeletal or aerobic function. It is probable that there are reciprocal relationships between physical activity and depression: depressed mood leads to inactivity, while in some circumstances exercise can alleviate depression. It is important to try to establish whether both of these pathways operate, but ultimately it may be very difficult in many clinical settings to establish the primacy of one factor over the other. This chapter suggests that understanding of the potential role of exercise training in the management of depressed mood in medical patients requires an evaluation of converging evidence from different types of study: population and clinical observational studies, randomised trials and experimental studies. The nature of associations varies with different clinical conditions, and so there is no definitive study that can answer all the questions. It must also be borne in mind that vigorous physical activity may have adverse as well as beneficial effects in medical conditions and is not entirely risk-free. There is evidence, for example, of a small but significant risk of acute cardiac events during vigorous exercise, particularly in normally sedentary individuals [6]. Physical exercise can also cause musculoskeletal problems. It is important therefore to establish the precise nature and the limits of evidence for effectiveness.

Research concerning physical activity has been carried out both in relation to depressive symptoms in the general population and with clinically depressed individuals. Studies of depressive symptoms have typically assessed mood disturbances with questionnaires such as the Beck Depression Inventory (BDI) and the Center for Epidemiologic Studies Depression Scale (CES-D), while clinical studies use diagnostic interviews and expert assessments to identify severe depression and major depressive disorder. Both types of study are discussed in this chapter. The term 'positive mood' is used in this chapter to indicate states of subjective wellbeing and vigour, while adverse states such as anxiety and depression are described as 'negative mood'.

Population studies of physical activity and depressive symptoms

The psychological benefits of physical activity have been trumpeted for many years by enthusiasts. For example, the author of one popular book categorically stated that he had 'never met a depressed runner' [7]. Early studies compared the mood profiles of elite college athletes with sedentary groups and showed lower tension-anxiety and depression and greater mental vigour in the sports players [8]. Studies of this type involve major selection biases, since athletes tend to be healthy and typically engage in vigorous activity because they enjoy it. Subsequently, research has been carried out with population samples that are less biased, both because the participants have come from a broad range of backgrounds and because data were collected as part of larger surveys not carried out because of a specific interest in exercise or sports. For example, Stephens [9] summarised results from four population studies in the USA and Canada that found regular physical exercise to be associated with low levels of anxiety and depression independently of socioeconomic status and physical health. Analyses of a national representative sample of more than 8000 men and women aged 50–54 years in the USA showed that regular physical activity was associated with a lower prevalence of clinical depression independently of age, gender, race, marital status, education, income, physical illness and comorbid psychiatric illness [10]. A dose–response relationship between physical activity level and likelihood of poor mental health was demonstrated in analyses of some 175 000 adults in the Behavioral Risk Factor Surveillance System in the USA [11].

These studies are based on self-reported physical activity, which may not accurately reflect objective levels of energy expenditure; but investigations using wrist actigraphy monitors have found lower levels of everyday physical activity in people with more depressive symptoms [12]. Low levels of physical activity and physical retardation are characteristic of clinical depression, and associations between low-level daytime activity and severity of clinical symptoms have been described [13].

Population studies of adolescents have generally assessed psychological wellbeing broadly, rather than focusing on depressive symptoms in particular. Steptoe and Butler [14] analysed data from one of the British birth cohort studies, a longitudinal study of all children born within one week in 1970 in England, Wales and Scotland. We found that participation in sports and vigorous recreational activities at age 16 years was related inversely to ratings of psychological symptoms on the Malaise Inventory (a measure based on the Cornell Medical Index) and scores on the General Health Questionnaire (GHQ), independently of gender, parental social class, health status and use of hospital services. More recently, Brodersen et al. [15] analysed data from over 4000 11- to 12-year-old boys and girls recruited from a broad range of schools in the London area. Emotional symptoms measured with the Strengths and Difficulties Questionnaire [16] were associated inversely with vigorous physical exercise in boys and related positively to sedentary behaviours such as television watching in girls, independently of ethnicity, socioeconomic and family background, self-rated health, body mass index (BMI) and environmental factors such as the availability of local sports facilities. Studies of adolescents are interesting, since at these ages much physical activity is not a matter of personal choice but is determined by school policies and parental encouragement. The selection biases caused by personal enjoyment of sports are thereby reduced still further.

Longitudinal studies

The population studies described above have applied extensive statistical controls to bolster the argument that associations between lower levels of depressive symptoms and greater physical activity are not due to confounding factors and co-variates. However, cross-sectional studies cannot tease out causal relationships, and it is not clear whether greater activity reduces depressive symptoms or greater levels of depression lead to inactivity, or whether the two factors are simply correlated. A number of longitudinal population studies have therefore been conducted, assessing whether physical activity at baseline predicts later depressive symptoms independently of current depression. The results for adults are summarised in Table 16.1. Several studies have documented a positive association between exercise and later depressive symptoms, but results have been quite mixed. Two analyses from the Alameda County Study showed positive associations, although in one of these the impact of physical activity on later depressive symptoms was no longer significant after adjustment for all relevant co-variates [17,18]. An eight-year follow-up of the National Health and Nutrition Examination Survey (NHANES) 1 showed positive findings, but curiously not in men who had low levels of depressive symptoms at baseline or in women with high depressive symptoms at baseline [19]. The studies of cohorts aged 65 years or older have all found that physical activity predicts later depressive symptoms over four to eight years independently of confounding factors, although the magnitude of effects has been small in some cases [20–22]. Some other studies of healthy participants have not found associations between baseline physical exercise and subsequent depression [23,24].

Particularly relevant in the context of this book is the analysis of the Medical Outcomes Study [25]. The adult participants in this study had one or more of the following conditions: diabetes, hypertension, congestive heart failure, recurrent myocardial infarction, severe depressive symptoms or current depressive disorder. Over the two-year observational period, baseline levels of physical activity were associated inversely with later depressive symptoms across all medical conditions, with particularly strong effects among diabetics.

Table 16.1 Longitudinal population studies of physical activity and depressive symptoms

Ref.	Sample	Duration of follow-up (years)	Depression measure	Physical activity measure	Baseline PA predicts later depression?
Camacho et al. [17]	1947 men and women aged over 20 years, USA	9	Specially constructed questionnaire	General physical activity	Yes, but not significant after adjustment for all co-variates
Farmer et al. [19]	1900 men and women aged 25–77 years, USA	8	CES-D	Recreational physical activity	Yes, in women with low depression and men with high depression at baseline
Kritz-Silverstein et al. [23]	944 men and women aged 50–89 years, USA	8	BDI	Regular strenuous exercise	No
Lampinen et al. [20]	663 men and women aged 65–84 years, Finland	8	Short BDI	General physical activity	Yes, for walking but not strenuous exercise
Mobily et al. [21]	2084 men and women aged 65–101 years, USA	3	CES-D	Walking	Yes
Morgan and Bath [22]	1042 men and men aged 65+ years, UK	4 and 8	HAD	Outdoor/leisure activity	Yes
Stewart et al. [25]	1758 men and women mean age 56.1 years, USA	2	MOS measure	General physical activity	Yes
Strawbridge et al. [18]	1947 men and women aged 50–94 years, USA	5	Interview	General physical activity	Yes
Weyerer [24]	1536 men and women aged 15+ years, Germany	5	CIS	Exercise for sport	No

BDI, Beck Depression Inventory; CES-D, Center for Epidemiologic Studies Depression Scale; CIS, Clinical Interview Schedule; HAD, Hospital Anxiety and Depression Scale; MOS, Medical Outcomes Survey; PA, physical activity.

One longitudinal study that has not been included in Table 16.1 was a follow-up of former medical students from Johns Hopkins' University, since the depression outcome was self-reported clinical depression [26]. The Reno Diet-Heart Study has also been excluded, even though it described an association between changes in physical activity and changes in depressive symptoms over five years, because it involved a non-validated measure of activity [27]. Only a single study to date has investigated these associations in adolescents. Motl *et al.* [28] assessed more than 4000 adolescents who provided data three times over an 18-month period. Increases in exercise levels were associated with reductions in depressed mood, which were independent of gender, socioeconomic position, smoking and alcohol consumption.

The longitudinal data from population studies therefore provide moderate support for the notion that regular exercise protects against the development of depressive symptoms. It is unfortunate that none of these investigations has tested the reverse proposition that depressive symptoms reduce subsequent physical activity. As noted in Chapter 6, depressive symptoms predict incident disability and deterioration in activities of daily living in older people, but relationships in younger groups have not been studied extensively. There are also sufficient discrepancies in observational studies to suggest that the effects of physical activity on depressive symptoms are quite modest and may be swamped by other factors.

More precise types of investigation involving randomised control trials are therefore required to clarify the relationship between depressive symptoms and physical activity. Two types of intervention trial are theoretically relevant: studies that examine the effects on physical activity of treating depression, and studies of the effects on depression of modifying exercise levels.

Treatment of depression and subsequent physical activity

One logical approach to understanding the relationship between depressive symptoms and physical activity is to examine the impact on physical activity of treating depression pharmacologically or with cognitive–behavioural therapy (CBT). Since low levels of physical activity are characteristic of many forms of clinical depression [29], it would not be surprising if relief from depression stimulated increases in activity. Unfortunately, very few depression-treatment studies have evaluated such responses directly, and investigations involving objective measures of activity suggest that the various classes of antidepressants may have different effects. For example, treatment with tricyclic antidepressants appears to stimulate increased levels of physical activity, while selective serotonin reuptake inhibitors (SSRIs) do not [30,31]. No studies have focused specifically on the impact of CBT for depression on physical activity. Even if physical activity levels do increase following successful treatment of depression, it is not certain whether this would indicate a specific association, since increased physical activity might be part of general re-engagement with everyday life. Thus, despite the theoretical possibility that studies of antidepressant treatment would throw light on associations with physical activity, in practice the inferences that can be drawn are rather limited.

Effects on depression of increasing exercise levels

By contrast, there is a substantial literature on the impact of physical activity training on depressive symptoms and clinical depression [32,33]. There have been more than 30 published studies involving randomising depressed individuals or people with high levels of depressive symptoms to physical activity and no treatment or alternative treatment procedures. It is fair to say that despite many positive results, there is still no scientific consensus about the antidepressant effect of increasing physical activity. Three sets of methodological concerns have limited the conclusions that can be drawn. The first set relates to the selection of appropriate control or comparison conditions in randomised trials [34]. Most physical activity programmes include several components apart from physical exertion per se. These include extra attention from trainers or research workers, distraction from everyday activities and preoccupations, and increased levels of social contact. Physical exercise training is an activity in which participants acquire extra abilities or capacity as they progress through the training schedule, and this itself may be reinforcing and enhance self-concept and self-efficacy [35]. As Lawlor and Hopker [33] have pointed out, taking up physical activity is seen as virtuous, and so depressed patients who exercise may receive praise that boosts their self-esteem. These elements might all have favourable effects on depressed mood, but they are neither intrinsic to nor exclusive to physical activity. Similar non-specific elements might operate with learning a sedentary skill such as playing the piano. Thus, in order to demonstrate that physical exercise itself has a positive effect on depressed mood, comparisons with treatment conditions that match for these components are needed.

A second set of methodological concerns derive from the literature on clinical trials, embodied in guidelines such as the CONSORT consensus (www.consort-statement.org). These guidelines lay down a set of criteria for the adequacy of studies of clinical interventions, and many investigations of physical activity and depression fall short in this respect. In fairness, it should be recognised that some investigators in this field intended their studies to be not effectiveness trials but studies of efficacy. Nonetheless, if research findings are to inform evidence-based healthcare, then there is a growing acceptance that such criteria must be fulfilled. One of the most important is the use of intention-to-treat analyses, in which all entrants to studies are analysed irrespective of whether they completed the trial or dropped out. Physical activity studies are notorious for high drop-out rates. This introduces a selection bias, since the individuals who complete the protocol may be those who have benefited psychologically, while those who drop out have probably not experienced positive changes. There is good evidence that clinical effectiveness is overestimated if analysis is restricted to people who have completed all aspects of the protocol [36]. Additionally, if drop-outs are excluded from analyses, then the allocation of participants to conditions is no longer random and a false-positive impression will emerge. With few exceptions [5,37–40], most studies of physical activity and depression have limited analysis to people who completed the study.

Another methodological problem from the clinical trials perspective is the use of non-blinded assessment. Ideally, the researchers who measure outcomes should not be aware of which treatment the participant has undergone, otherwise their own biases and expectations might influence results. Studies that rely on self-reporting assessment of depressive symptoms inevitably do not satisfy this criterion, and few trials have involved measurements of depression from clinicians blind to group allocation.

A third set of limitations relates to the representativeness of people who participate in randomised trials. Studies of physical activity involve substantial personal commitment from volunteers, and only a proportion of individuals with appropriate levels of depressive symptoms will agree to participate or be randomised. Even in the best trials, the results may therefore be relevant only to the types of people who agree to take part in studies and not to clinical patients or depressed individuals in the population more generally.

The challenges inherent in conducting methodologically rigorous studies are illustrated by the Depression Outcomes Study of Exercise (DOSE), a trial designed to assess dose–response antidepressant effects of exercise in young adults with mild or moderate major depression [41]. The study involved a comparison of low and high 'doses' of physical exercise three or five times per week for 24 weeks, with an attention-placebo condition of very-low-intensity exercise. A rigorous selection procedure was used in recruitment to ensure that participants were sedentary, in the appropriate range for depression, not taking medication or undergoing psychotherapy and not suffering from substance or alcohol abuse. Statistical power was estimated with analysis on an intention-to-treat basis, and it was decided that each of the four treatment groups required 18 participants completing the programme, with 12 in the control group. In order to achieve this sample size, no fewer than 1664 patients were screened. More than 1500 were excluded because they were taking medication or undergoing psychotherapy (even though still depressed), were too active, did not meet depression criteria, changed their minds about participating or some other reason. This represents an enormous expenditure of effort and professional resources on a comparatively small number of participants. This experience is not unique. A study in Scotland of older adults who had responded poorly to standard antidepressant treatment involved evaluation of 1885 patients in order to recruit 86 study participants [38]. Clearly, a dedicated and well-funded research programme is required in order to undertake such a project. The question also arises as to how generalisable the results will be beyond the 5% of patients who finally entered the study.

Literature on the effects of physical activity interventions on depressive symptoms has been reviewed a number of times, with conclusions ranging from the cautious to the very positive, depending on how many of these methodological factors are emphasised. Lawlor and Hopker [33] carried out a meta-analysis of randomised trials published up to 2000, involving clinically depressed patients or adults in the community with high levels of depressive symptoms. They noted that trials were typically small, with only a single study involving more than 100 patients; most involved no follow-up beyond the active intervention period. The standardised mean difference in effect sizes was −1.1 (95% confidence interval (CI) −1.5 to −0.6), favouring physical activity compared with no treatment. This corresponded to a mean difference of just over seven points on the BDI. The comparisons of physical activity with established treatments such as cognitive or pharmacotherapy showed no differences between conditions. There was no convincing evidence at that time of a dose–response relationship between physical activity and depression [42]. However, newer studies suggest that this summary may be overly pessimistic.

Illustrative studies

This chapter describes in more detail three methodologically sound studies to illustrate the impact of increasing physical activity on depressive symptoms. Singh *et al.* [39,43] randomised 32 community-dwelling adults aged over 60 years who had elevated BDI scores to exercise and control groups. Exercise training involved high-intensity resistance training of upper- and lower-body muscle groups three days per week for ten weeks, followed by a further ten weeks of unsupervised exercise at home or at a health club. The control group attended a series of ten weekly health-education lectures. Both groups received weekly telephone calls from the investigators to provide matched attention levels, and depression was not mentioned to participants in either condition as an endpoint of the study. At the end of the 20-week intervention, there was a significantly greater decrease in BDI scores in the physical exercise group. Some 73% of those randomised to exercise training had BDI scores below the threshold for probable clinical depression, compared with 36% of health-education controls. Participants were reassessed after 26 months, and differences between groups were still present. Interestingly, the reduction in BDI was marginally greater in those individuals who continued to be active during the follow-up period, compared with those who stopped exercising. This study is notable because it involved an elderly population (aged 60–84 years) and tested strength and resistance training rather than the more commonly studied aerobic activity.

A second study with important findings involved 156 men and women with major depressive disorder who were randomised to aerobic training or medication with setraline (an SSRI), or a combination of the two [37]. Exercise training was carried out in three supervised sessions per week for 16 weeks, and was based primarily on walking and jogging. Intention-to-treat analyses were incorporated, and psychological state was measured by assessors blind to treatment allocation. Although pharmacologically treated patients showed more rapid therapeutic responses, there were no differences between the conditions in the reductions in depression achieved at the end of 16 weeks. However, a further evaluation six months after the end of the trial showed different results [44]. Interview-based assessments indicated that clinical depression was present in only 30% of participants in the exercise training group, compared with 52% in the medication and 55% in the combination condition. Controlling for age, gender, baseline depression and the use of antidepressant medication, the odds of major depressive disorder at six months post-treatment were 0.49 (C.I 0.32 to 0.74) among individuals who were exercising for 50 minutes or more per week compared with those exercising below this level.

The results of the DOSE study mentioned earlier were published in 2005 [40]. Data were analysed both on an intention-to-treat basis (including all enrolled participants) and as an efficacy trial, including only those who completed the trial. Major depressive disorder was assessed using the Hamilton Rating Scale for Depression (HRSD), completed by trained observers who were blind to the treatment condition. As noted earlier, the study assessed the impact of lower- and higher-intensity physical activity performed either three or five times per week. All physical activity was carried out under supervision in the laboratory in order to ensure that the correct intensity was applied. The results indicate that reductions in depression were stimulated by exercise, with the intensity rather than frequency being more important. Two of the outcomes are summarised in Figure 16.1. Figure 16.1a shows the HRSD scores at the end of the 12-week programme. The groups did not differ at baseline, and so it is apparent that greater average reductions were observed with higher intensity exercise. Figure 16.1b shows the proportion of participants with a decrease in HRSD score of at least 50%, where again the intensity effect is apparent. Follow-up analyses have not yet been published.

The results of these and other studies suggest that physical activity training does have beneficial effects on clinical depression and depressive symptoms in otherwise healthy adults, although corroboration from additional well-controlled trials is certainly needed. There is evidence in older adults at least that strength and

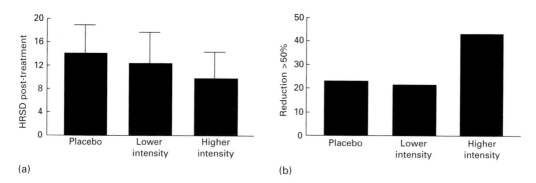

Figure 16.1 (a) Mean scores on the Hamilton Rating Scale for Depression (HRSD) following treatment in the control, lower-intensity and higher-intensity training conditions of the Depression Outcomes Study of Exercise (DOSE) study. Error bars are standard deviations. (b) Proportion of participants in each condition who achieved at least a 50% reduction in HRSD scores from pre- to post-treatment. For details, see Dunn *et al.* [40].

resistance training and aerobic exercise have positive effects, and the impact of all these programmes appears to depend on maintaining regular exercise patterns.

Physical activity interventions in medical conditions

There are fewer studies of the effects of physical exercise interventions on depression and wellbeing in patients with medical conditions than in physically healthy populations. Nevertheless, there are some indications that beneficial effects accrue, although findings are not all positive. One of the earliest studies was a small-scale comparison of 21 patients with advanced renal disease who had been undergoing dialysis for at least six months [45]. Depression is a common problem in patients undergoing haemodialysis and peritoneal dialysis [46,47]. Patients were randomised to an aerobic training programme three times a week for six months, or an attention-control condition involving regular support groups. Over the training period, BDI scores declined to a greater extent with exercise, and these low levels were maintained at 18 months. Similar positive effects have been described in a more recent study of uraemic patients on maintenance haemodialysis [48].

Results for chronic obstructive pulmonary disease have been less clear. Emery and colleagues [49] randomised 79 older patients to 10 weeks of a combination of exercise, education and stress management, or education and stress management only, or a waiting-list control group. The combined condition was intensive, involving five weeks of aerobic exercise for four hours per day, educational lectures on the physiology of the condition, and stress-management groups, followed by a five-week period with less frequent contact. Although some changes in depression were reported over the study, the results were inconclusive. Depressive symptoms were assessed with three measures, but only one showed significant differences between groups. Depressive symptoms on the Derogatis Symptom Checklist (SCL-90) decreased for the combined exercise, education and stress-management condition, and not in the education and stress-management group. However, SCL-90 depressive symptoms also fell in the waiting-list control group. In a subsequent report, patients who continued to exercise one year later were compared with those who did not exercise, and differences on the SCL-90 were again observed [50]. However, the randomised element was no longer present in these analyses.

Another condition in which the effects of exercise interventions have been studied is human immunodeficiency virus (HIV)/acquired immunodeficiency syndrome (AIDS). Aerobic training has been advocated for its effects on immune function, viral load and cardiorespiratory fitness, and a systematic review has been published in the Cochrane Library [51]. Unfortunately, few of these studies have involved systematic assessments of depressive symptoms, but some researchers have shown favourable effects of aerobic exercise training on psychological wellbeing in this group [52].

The largest, and one of the best conducted, studies of exercise training and depression in a medical condition is the trial of patients with osteoarthritis published by Penninx *et al.* [5] (see Chapter 6). More than 400 patients were randomised to a health-education control, or resistance training involving strengthening exercises, or aerobic training with a walking-based programme. Intention-to-treat analysis of depressive symptoms assessed with the CES-D was carried out at 3, 9 and 18 months. Aerobic exercise led to significantly greater reductions in depressive symptoms than did control, after adjustment for age, race, gender, education, baseline disability and baseline depression. Resistance training was no more effective than control. Effects were observed in patients with both high and low depression scores at baseline, although the absolute effects were larger in those who were initially more depressed. Aerobic exercise also produced lower disability ratings and pain at follow-up. Subsequent analyses suggested that the positive effects of aerobic exercise on depression were mediated partly through changes in pain and disability.

Exercise training is an important part of rehabilitation for many painful conditions. However, the fact that aerobic exercise had positive effects on depression in Penninx and colleagues' study does not mean that it is necessarily helpful in other painful conditions. Negative results have been published for problems such as fibromyalgia [53] and chronic neck pain [54]. It is necessary, therefore, to evaluate effects separately in different pain syndromes.

There has been considerable interest in the impact of exercise training on the subjective wellbeing of patients with cancer [55]. Unfortunately, many of the randomised trials in this field appear to have methodological limitations, including high rates of pre-trial exclusion and subsequent drop-out [56]. One well-conducted study involving mixed cancer patients showed that in comparison with group psychotherapy alone, a combination programme of exercise plus group psychotherapy had favourable effects on functional wellbeing and fatigue, but no significant effect on depressed mood [57]. Further studies that are currently in progress may resolve the uncertainty in this area of physical activity research [58].

Chronic heart failure is a condition involving dyspnoea and fatigue and is often associated with an increasingly sedentary lifestyle. The effects of exercise training on functional capacity have been established in controlled trials [59], but less is known about the effects on depression. A report compared a three-month aerobic training programme with standard treatment in patients with stable chronic heart failure [60]. Exercise training improved muscle strength and aerobic capacity and also led to a small but significant reduction in depressive symptoms compared with controls. Interestingly, however, this study also involved objective measurement of everyday physical activity and found no group difference on this measure and no correlation between changes in objective activity and improvement in depression. This suggests that the positive effects on depression were not simply a function of increased activity levels but of some other elements of the training programme.

Understanding the mechanisms

The central question of this chapter is whether variations in physical activity mediate associations between depression and physical illness. It is likely that the answer to this question varies across medical conditions, and that a single conclusion cannot be drawn. It is possible, for instance, that physical activity is more important in mediating depression–illness associations with problems such as chronic heart failure and disability than it is for coronary heart disease or cancer.

Several issues need to be distinguished. First, are depressed individuals in poorer physical health because they are inactive, or because depression leads to inactivity, which in turn has adverse effects on clinical states? Few studies have been analysed in such a way as to address this question directly; nevertheless, the weight of the evidence at present is that lack of physical activity plays only a limited role in the association between depression and poor physical health.

Second, does relief from depression have a positive effect on physical health because it stimulates increased activity levels? As noted earlier, current evidence about the impact of the treatment of depression on physical activity is mixed, and few of these effects have yet been evaluated in patients with diagnosed clinical conditions.

A third issue that has more practical treatment implications is whether increasing physical activity has a positive effect on health because it leads to improvement in depressive symptoms. The evidence summarised in previous sections indicates that physical exercise interventions can impact favourably on psychological wellbeing in patients with chronic health problems. It is less certain, however, whether this antidepressive effect of physical activity is responsible for the more general health benefits of exercise programmes. One study suggests that this mechanism is not very important, at least as far as coronary heart disease and mortality are concerned. Blumenthal *et al.* [61] followed up over 2000 men and women for up to four years after acute myocardial infarction. Self-reports of physical activity were obtained six months after the cardiac admission. It was found that patients who said that they exercised regularly had a reduced risk of dying, with a hazard ratio of 0.69 (95% CI 0.47 to 0.97) in comparison with non-exercisers, after adjusting for co-variates that contribute to mortality. It was also found that people who exercised had lower depression scores on the BDI at the time of infarction and greater reductions in depression between infarction and six months. These results are consistent with physical activity having effects on both cardiac health and depression. However, adding depression to the statistical model did not alter the association between regular exercise and mortality, and so there was no evidence that depression mediated the beneficial effects of exercise.

A further possibility is that shared biological processes underpin some of the associations between physical exercise, depression and physical illness. Increasing physical activity levels might have positive effects on biological responses that are implicated in disease pathology, which are in turn also related to depression. If this were the case, then depression, physical activity and illness might be linked through common biological mechanisms, without depression playing either a causal or a mediating role. Three possible pathways are outlined below.

Inflammation and immunity

The evidence linking depressive symptoms with disturbances of immune function and with activation of inflammatory processes has been detailed in Chapters 12–14. As noted in these chapters and elsewhere in this book, disturbances of inflammation and immune mechanisms may mediate in part the influence of depression on cardiovascular disease, diabetes, arthritic conditions and chronic fatigue. Acute physical activity stimulates many inflammatory and immune responses, with marked increases in circulating interleukin 6 (IL-6) concentration (produced mainly by working muscle), increases in the numbers of circulating leukocytes and increases in the surface expression of adhesion molecules [62,63]. It would appear that if anything, vigorous activity might have deleterious effects on immune- and inflammation-mediated disease. However, by contrast, regular exercise participation has protective effects. Cross-sectional studies indicate that physically more active individuals have lower levels of C-reactive protein (CRP), IL-6 and tumour necrosis factor alpha (TNF-α) [64,65]. One intervention study involving six months of moderate aerobic training in volunteers at high risk of cardiovascular disease showed a decrease of more than 50% in the production from mononuclear cells of atherogenic cytokines such as interleukin 1 beta (IL-1β), TNF-α and interferon gamma (IFN-γ), together with an increase interleukin 4 (IL-4) and interleukin 10 (IL-10) [66]; CRP also decreased by 35%. Several studies have observed favourable effects of training on inflammatory markers in patients with chronic heart failure. For example, LeMaitre *et al.* [67] found that six weeks' training in patients with stable chronic heart failure led to decreases in soluble TNF-α receptor 2 levels and reductions in circulating TNF-α.

A related mechanism that is relevant to depression in coronary heart disease and that also responds to exercise training is vascular endothelial dysfunction. As noted in Chapter 3, endothelial function is associated with the early stages of atherogenesis and is also impaired in depressed patients [68]. In animal studies, physical inactivity has been shown to increase oxidative stress and vascular endothelial dysfunction [69]. Exercise training in patients with coronary artery disease has been found to improve coronary artery endothelial function, as indexed by vasoconstrictive responses to acetylcholine and to improved peripheral arterial function assessed using flow-mediated dilation [70,71].

Neuroendocrine function

The relationship between hormones such as cortisol and dehydroepiandrosterone (DHEA) and depression was reviewed in Chapter 13. Acute exercise increases not only circulating glucocorticoid levels but also tissue sensitivity to glucocorticoids [72]. This is thought to be a protective response designed to limit muscle inflammatory responses and to reduce exercise-induced muscle damage. Exercise training increases circulating levels of DHEA sulphate (DHEAS) at rest, while endurance-trained individuals show a dampened cortisol response to physical activity [73,74].

Cardiovascular stress reactivity

A third mechanism that might be associated with depression, physical illness and exercise levels is cardiovascular stress reactivity. Heightened heart rate and noradrenaline responses to mental stress have been described in healthy women with elevated BDI scores [75]. Cardiovascular stress reactivity or impaired post-stress recovery have in turn been found to predict progression of subclinical atherosclerosis [76] and increased cardiovascular disease risk prospectively [77,78]. By contrast, aerobic exercise training has been shown, at least in some studies, to be associated with reduced levels of cardiovascular activity during stress and post-stress recovery

[79]. Acutely, stress reactivity is reduced in the period following episodes of strenuous exercise [80]. This could be a further mechanism linking regular physical exercise, depression and disease risk.

Conclusions

Discussion of physical exercise, depression and health generates strong feelings on both sides of the argument. Many advocates of regular physical activity regard the issue as settled, while sceptics are much more cautious about the interpretation of observational and intervention studies. There is certainly evidence that increasing physical exercise in people willing to become more active leads to reductions in depression mood and that these effects may be present both in patients with medical disorders and in healthy individuals. There are also plausible biological mechanisms linking physical activity with pathways relevant to both depression and physical illness. The mechanisms reviewed here are those that might specifically relate physical activity with pathophysiology. There is another literature concerned with the psychological processes through which activity influences depressive states, involving factors such as self-efficacy, self-esteem, distraction and coping; this has not been discussed since it does not impinge directly on biological responses [34].

In many circumstances, increasing physical activity is likely to have benefits for health, regardless of whether it influences mood. But there is not yet compelling evidence in most illness groups that relief of depression through promotion of physical activity will have direct effects on disease states. Nevertheless, research in this field is continually developing, so if and when such effects are demonstrated they will undoubtedly have important implications for the management of many physical illnesses.

Acknowledgements

I am grateful to Mark Hamer for his comments on an earlier draft of this chapter. This research was supported by the British Heart Foundation.

REFERENCES

1. V. B. Hammett, Psychological changes with physical fitness training. *Can. Med. Assoc. J.* **96** (1967), 764–9.

2. C. H. Folkins, W. E. Sime, Physical fitness training and mental health. *Am. Psychol.* **36** (1981), 373–89.

3. P. D. Thompson, D. Buchner, I. L. Pina, *et al.*, Exercise and physical activity in the prevention and treatment of atherosclerotic cardiovascular disease a statement from the Council on Clinical Cardiology (Subcommittee on Exercise, Rehabilitation, and Prevention) and the

Council on Nutrition, Physical Activity, and Metabolism (Subcommittee on Physical Activity). *Circulation* **107** (2003), 3109–16.

4. J. A. Jolliffe, K. Rees, R. S. Taylor, *et al.*, Exercise-based rehabilitation for coronary heart disease. *Cochrane Database Syst. Rev.* (1) (2001), CD001800.

5. B. W. Penninx, W. J. Rejeski, J. Pandya, *et al.*, Exercise and depressive symptoms: a comparison of aerobic and resistance exercise effects on emotional and physical function in older persons with high and low depressive symptomatology. *J. Gerontol. B Psychol. Sci. Soc. Sci.* **57** (2002), P124–32.

6. M. A. Mittleman, M. Maclure, G. H. Tofler, *et al.*, Triggering of acute myocardial infarction by heavy physical exertion: protection against triggering by regular exertion – Determinants of Myocardial Infarction Onset Study Investigators. *N. Engl. J. Med.* **329** (1993), 1677–83.

7. K. W. Johnsgard, *The Exercise Prescription for Depression and Anxiety* (New York: Plenum Press, 1989).

8. W. P. Morgan, S. E. Goldston (eds), *Exercise and Mental Health* (Washington, DC: Hemisphere, 1987).

9. T. Stephens, Physical activity and mental health in the United States and Canada evidence from four population surveys. *Prev. Med.* **17** (1988), 35–47.

10. A. D. Goodwin, Association between physical activity and mental disorders among adults in the United States. *Prev. Med.* **36** (2003), 698–703.

11. D. W. Brown, D. R. Brown, G. W. Heath, *et al.*, Associations between physical activity dose and health-related quality of life. *Med. Sci. Sports Exerc.* **36** (2004), 890–96.

12. M. V. Mendlowicz, G. Jean-Louis, H. von Gizycki, F. Zizi, J. Nunes, Actigraphic predictors of depressed mood in a cohort of non-psychiatric adults. *Aust. N. Z. J. Psychiatry* **33** (1999), 553–8.

13. M. H. Teicher, Actigraphy and motion analysis: new tools for psychiatry. *Harv. Rev. Psychiatry* **3** (1995), 18–35.

14. A. Steptoe, N. Butler, Sports participation and emotional wellbeing in adolescents. *Lancet* **347** (1996), 1789–92.

15. N. H. Brodersen, A. Steptoe, S. Williamson, J. Wardle, Sociodemographic, developmental, environmental, and psychological correlates of physical activity and sedentary behavior at age 11 to 12. *Ann. Behav. Med.* **29** (2005), 2–11.

16. R. Goodman, Psychometric properties of the strengths and difficulties questionnaire. *J. Am. Acad. Child Adolesc. Psychiatry* **40** (2001), 1337–45.

17. T. C. Camacho, R. E. Roberts, N. B. Lazarus, G. A. Kaplan, R. D. Cohen, Physical activity and depression evidence from the Alameda County Study. *Am. J. Epidemiol.* **134** (1991), 220–31.

18. W. J. Strawbridge, S. Deleger, R. E. Roberts, G. A. Kaplan, Physical activity reduces the risk of subsequent depression for older adults. *Am. J. Epidemiol.* **156** (2002), 328–34.

19. M. E. Farmer, B. Z. Locke, E. K. Moscicki, *et al.*, Physical activity and depressive symptoms: the NHANES I Epidemiologic Follow-up Study. *Am. J. Epidemiol.* **128** (1988), 1340–51.

20. P. Lampinen, R. L. Heikkinen, I. Ruoppila, Changes in intensity of physical exercise as predictors of depressive symptoms among older adults: an eight-year follow-up. *Prev. Med.* **30** (2000), 371–80.

21. K. E. Mobily, L. M. Rubenstein, J. H. Lemke, M. W. O'Hara, R. B. Wallance, Walking and depression in a cohort of older adults: The Iowa 65+ Rural Health Study. *J. Aging Phys. Act.* **4** (1996), 119–35.

22. K. Morgan, P. A. Bath, Customary physical activity and psychological wellbeing: a longitudinal study. *Age Ageing* **27**: Suppl 3 (1998), 35–40.

23. D. Kritz-Silverstein, E. Barrett-Connor, C. Corbeau, Cross-sectional and prospective study of exercise and depressed mood in the elderly: the Rancho Bernardo study. *Am. J. Epidemiol.* **153** (2001), 596–603.

24. S. Weyerer, Physical inactivity and depression in the community: evidence from the Upper Bavarian Field Study. *Int. J. Sports Med.* **13** (1992), 492–6.

25. A. L. Stewart, R. D. Hays, K. B. Wells, *et al.*, Long-term functioning and well-being outcomes associated with physical activity and exercise in patients with chronic conditions in the Medical Outcomes Study. *J. Clin. Epidemiol.* **47** (1994), 719–30.

26. L. Cooper-Patrick, D. E. Ford, L. A. Mead, P. P. Chang, M. J. Klag, Exercise and depression in midlife: a prospective study. *Am. J. Public Health* **87** (1997), 670–73.

27. J. P. Foreyt, R. L. Brunner, G. K. Goodrick, S. T. St Jeor, G. D. Miller, Psychological correlates of reported physical activity in normal-weight and obese adults: the Reno diet-heart study. *Int. J. Obes. Relat. Metab. Disord.* **19**: Suppl 4 (1995), 69–72.

28. R. W. Motl, A. S. Birnbaum, M. Y. Kubik, R. K. Dishman, Naturally occurring changes in physical activity are inversely related to depressive symptoms during early adolescence. *Psychosom. Med.* **66** (2004), 336–42.

29. C. Sobin, H. A. Sackeim, Psychomotor symptoms of depression. *Am. J. Psychiatry* **154** (1997), 4–17.

30. N. Raoux, O. Benoit, N. Dantchev, *et al.*, Circadian pattern of motor activity in major depressed patients undergoing antidepressant therapy: relationship between actigraphic measures and clinical course. *Psychiatry Res.* **52** (1994), 85–98.

31. A. C. Volkers, J. H. Tulen, W. W. Van Den Broek, *et al.*, 24-hour motor activity after treatment with imipramine or fluvoxamine in major depressive disorder. *Eur. Neuropsychopharmacol.* **12** (2002), 273–8.

32. S. J. H. Biddle, N. Mutrie, *Psychology of Physical Activity* (London: Routledge, 2001).

33. D. A. Lawlor, S. W. Hopker, The effectiveness of exercise as an intervention in the management of depression: systematic review and meta-regression analysis of randomised controlled trials. *Br. Med. J.* **322** (2001), 763–7.

34. A. Steptoe, Physical activity and psychological well-being. In *Physical Activity and Mental Health*, ed. N. G. Norgan (Cambridge: Cambridge University Press, 1992), pp. 207–29.

35. R. J. Sonstroem, W. P. Morgan, Exercise and self-esteem: rationale and model. *Med. Sci. Sports Exerc.* **21** (1989), 329–37.

36. S. Hollis, F. Campbell, What is meant by intention to treat analysis? Survey of published randomised controlled trials. *Br. Med. J.* **319** (1999), 670–74.

37. J. A. Blumenthal, M. A. Babyak, K. A. Moore, *et al.*, Effects of exercise training on older patients with major depression. *Arch. Intern. Med.* **159** (1999), 2349–56.

38. A. S. Mather, C. Rodriguez, M. F. Guthrie, *et al.*, Effects of exercise on depressive symptoms in older adults with poorly responsive depressive disorder: randomised controlled trial. *Br. J. Psychiatry* **180** (2002), 411–15.

39. N. A. Singh, K. M. Clements, M. A. Fiatarone, A randomized controlled trial of progressive resistance training in depressed elders. *J. Gerontol. A Biol. Sci. Med. Sci.* **52** (1997), M27–35.

40. A. L. Dunn, M. H. Trivedi, J. B. Kampert, C. G. Clark, H. O. Chambliss, Exercise treatment for depression: efficacy and dose response. *Am. J. Prev. Med.* **28** (2005), 1–8.

41. A. L. Dunn, M. H. Trivedi, J. B. Kampert, C. G. Clark, H. O. Chambliss, The DOSE study: a clinical trial to examine efficacy and dose response of exercise as treatment for depression. *Control. Clin. Trials* **23** (2002), 584–603.

42. A. L. Dunn, M. H. Trivedi, H. A. O'Neal, Physical activity dose-response effects on outcomes of depression and anxiety. *Med. Sci. Sports Exerc.* **33** (2001), S587–97, 609–10.

43. N. A. Singh, K. M. Clements, M. A. Singh, The efficacy of exercise as a long-term antidepressant in elderly subjects: a randomized, controlled trial. *J. Gerontol. A Biol. Sci. Med. Sci.* **56** (2001), M497–504.

44. M. Babyak, J. A. Blumenthal, S. Herman, *et al.*, Exercise treatment for major depression maintenance of therapeutic benefit at 10 months. *Psychosom. Med.* **62** (2000), 633–8.

45. R. M. Carney, B. Templeton, B. A. Hong, *et al.*, Exercise training reduces depression and increases the performance of pleasant activities in hemodialysis patients. *Nephron* **47** (1987), 194–8.

46. F. O. Finkelstein, S. H. Finkelstein, Depression in chronic dialysis patients assessment and treatment. *Nephrol. Dial. Transplant* **15** (2000), 1911–13.

47. R. Einwohner, J. Bernardini, L. Fried, B. Piraino, The effect of depressive symptoms on survival in peritoneal dialysis patients. *Perit. Dial. Int.* **24** (2004), 256–63.

48. E. Kouidi, A. Iacovides, P. Iordanidis, *et al.*, Exercise renal rehabilitation program: psychosocial effects. *Nephron* **77** (1997), 152–8.

49. C. F. Emery, R. L. Schein, E. R. Hauck, N. R. MacIntyre, Psychological and cognitive outcomes of a randomized trial of exercise among patients with chronic obstructive pulmonary disease. *Health Psychol.* **17** (1998), 232–40.

50. C. F. Emery, R. L. Shermer, E. R. Hauck, E. T. Hsiao, N. R. MacIntyre, Cognitive and psychological outcomes of exercise in a 1-year follow-up study of patients with chronic obstructive pulmonary disease. *Health Psychol.* **22** (2003), 598–604.

51. S. Nixon, K. O'Brien, R. H. Glazier, A. M. Tynan, Aerobic exercise interventions for adults living with HIV/AIDS. *Cochrane Database Syst. Rev.* (2) (2005), CD001796.

52. W. W. Stringer, M. Berezovskaya, W. A. O'Brien, C. K. Beck, R. Casaburi, The effect of exercise training on aerobic fitness, immune indices, and quality of life in HIV+ patients. *Med. Sci. Sports Exerc.* **30** (1998), 11–16.

53. J. R. Redondo, C. M. Justo, F. V. Moraleda, *et al.*, Long-term efficacy of therapy in patients with fibromyalgia a physical exercise-based program and a cognitive-behavioral approach. *Arthritis Rheum.* **51** (2004), 184–92.

54. J. Ylinen, E. P. Takala, M. Nykanen, *et al.*, Active neck muscle training in the treatment of chronic neck pain in women: a randomized controlled trial. *J. Am. Med. Assoc.* **289** (2003), 2509–16.

55. K. S. Courneya, Exercise in cancer survivors: an overview of research. *Med. Sci. Sports Exerc.* **35** (2003), 1846–52.

56. L. M. Oldervoll, S. Kaasa, M. J. Hjermstad, J. A. Lund, J. H. Loge, Physical exercise results in the improved subjective well-being of a few or is effective rehabilitation for all cancer patients? *Eur. J. Cancer* **40** (2004), 951–62.

57. K. S. Courneya, C. M. Friedenreich, R. A. Sela, *et al.*, The group psychotherapy and home-based physical exercise (group-hope) trial in cancer survivors physical fitness and quality of life outcomes. *Psychooncology* **12** (2003), 357–74.

58. A. J. Daley, N. Mutrie, H. Crank, R. Coleman, J. Saxton, Exercise therapy in women who have had breast cancer: design of the Sheffield women's exercise and well-being project. *Health Educ. Res.* **19** (2004), 686–97.

59. R. Belardinelli, D. Georgiou, G. Cianci, A. Purcaro, Randomized, controlled trial of long-term moderate exercise training in chronic heart failure: effects on functional capacity, quality of life, and clinical outcome. *Circulation* **99** (1999), 1173–82.

60. R. van den Berg-Emons, A. Balk, H. Bussmann, H. Stam, Does aerobic training lead to a more active lifestyle and improved quality of life in patients with chronic heart failure? *Eur. J. Heart Fail.* **6** (2004), 95–100.

61. J. A. Blumenthal, M. A. Babyak, R. M. Carney, *et al.*, Exercise, depression, and mortality after myocardial infarction in the ENRICHD trial. *Med. Sci. Sports Exerc.* **36** (2004), 746–55.

62. R. J. Shephard, Cytokine responses to physical activity, with particular reference to IL-6: sources, actions, and clinical implications. *Crit. Rev. Immunol.* **22** (2002), 165–82.

63. R. J. Shephard, Adhesion molecules, catecholamines and leucocyte redistribution during and following exercise. *Sports Med.* **33** (2003), 261–84.

64. E. S. Ford, Does exercise reduce inflammation? Physical activity and C-reactive protein among US adults. *Epidemiology* **13** (2002), 561–8.

65. D. B. Panagiotakos, C. Pitsavos, C. Chrysohoou, S. Kavouras, C. Stefanadis, The associations between leisure-time physical activity and inflammatory and coagulation markers related to cardiovascular disease: the ATTICA Study. *Prev. Med.* **40** (2005), 432–7.

66. J. K. Smith, R. Dykes, J. E. Douglas, G. Krishnaswamy, S. Berk, Long-term exercise and atherogenic activity of blood mononuclear cells in persons at risk of developing ischemic heart disease. *J. Am. Med. Assoc.* **281** (1999), 1722–7.

67. J. P. LeMaitre, S. Harris, K. A. Fox, M. Denvir, Change in circulating cytokines after 2 forms of exercise training in chronic stable heart failure. *Am. Heart J.* **147** (2004), 100–105.

68. A. J. Broadley, A. Korszun, C. J. Jones, M. P. Frenneaux, Arterial endothelial function is impaired in treated depression. *Heart* **88** (2002), 521–3.

69. U. Laufs, S. Wassmann, T. Czech, *et al.*, Physical inactivity increases oxidative stress, endothelial dysfunction, and atherosclerosis. *Arterioscler. Thromb. Vasc. Biol.* **25** (2005), 809–14.

70. R. Hambrecht, A. Wolf, S. Gielen, *et al.*, Effect of exercise on coronary endothelial function in patients with coronary artery disease. *N. Engl. J. Med.* **342** (2000), 454–60.

71. D. G. Edwards, R. S. Schofield, S. L. Lennon, *et al.*, Effect of exercise training on endothelial function in men with coronary artery disease. *Am. J. Cardiol.* **93** (2004), 617–20.

72. M. Duclos, C. Gouarne, D. Bonnemaison, Acute and chronic effects of exercise on tissue sensitivity to glucocorticoids. *J. Appl. Physiol.* **94** (2003), 869–75.

73. K. Aizawa, T. Akimoto, H. Inoue, *et al.*, Resting serum dehydroepiandrosterone sulfate level increases after 8-week resistance training among young females. *Eur. J. Appl. Physiol.* **90** (2003), 575–80.

74. M. S. Tremblay, J. L. Copeland, W. Van Helder, Effect of training status and exercise mode on endogenous steroid hormones in men. *J. Appl. Physiol.* **96** (2004), 531–9.

75. K. C. Light, R. V. Kothandapani, M. T. Allen, Enhanced cardiovascular and catecholamine responses in women with depressive symptoms. *Int. J. Psychophysiol.* **28** (1998), 157–66.

76. J. R. Jennings, T. W. Kamarck, S. A. Everson-Rose, *et al.*, Exaggerated blood pressure responses during mental stress are prospectively related to enhanced carotid atherosclerosis in middle-aged Finnish men. *Circulation* **110** (2004), 2198–203.

77. F. A. Treiber, T. Kamarck, N. Schneiderman, *et al.*, Cardiovascular reactivity and development of preclinical and clinical disease states. *Psychosom. Med.* **65** (2003), 46–62.

78. A. Steptoe, M. Marmot, Impaired cardiovascular recovery following stress predicts 3-year increases in blood pressure. *J. Hypertens.* **23** (2005), 529–36.

79. T. W. Spalding, L. A. Lyon, D. H. Steel, B. D. Hatfield, Aerobic exercise training and cardio-vascular reactivity to psychological stress in sedentary young normotensive men and women. *Psychophysiology* **41** (2004), 552–62.

80. A. Steptoe, N. Kearsley, N. Walters, Cardiovascular activity during mental stress following vigorous exercise in sportsmen and inactive men. *Psychophysiology* **30** (1993), 245–52.

17

Depression and adherence to medical advice

Douglas A. Raynor, Rena R. Wing and Suzanne Phelan

The coexistence of depression and medical illness has been the focus of a great deal of attention in the past several years. Depression appears to occur in at least 25% of medical patients, although estimates vary based on measurement criteria, type and stage of medical disease, and level of depressive severity [1,2]. Depression has also been associated with poorer health outcomes in these diseases. Depression may influence the development and progression of diseases directly via physiological pathways or indirectly via behavioural pathways [3].

Adherence to treatment regimens is one possible behavioural pathway by which depression affects physical health. Adherence is the degree to which a person's behaviour (e.g. taking medications, attending treatment sessions, executing lifestyle changes) coincides with medical or health advice [4]. Adherence is critical for the prevention and treatment of medical diseases. Unfortunately, adherence is less than optimal across a wide range of medical regimens [5]. Individuals who are depressed may be less likely to adhere to various aspects of their treatment regimens, and this lack of adherence may produce poorer health outcomes.

There is a large literature on predictors of adherence. A substantial number of variables have been associated with adherence, but findings across studies have been inconsistent [6]. Depression has emerged as one of the few promising predictors of treatment adherence among medical patients [7]. There are many reasons to hypothesise that depression may negatively influence an individual's willingness and capacity to adhere to a treatment regimen. For instance, depression tends to reduce concentration, energy, motivation, social support and positive expectations, which in turn may lead to poor treatment adherence. The purpose of this chapter is to discuss the research evaluating the relationship between depression and adherence to medical regimens. We consider methodological issues in the assessment of adherence and depression and then review the empirical studies that have examined whether depressed individuals have poorer treatment adherence.

Depression and Physical Illness, ed. A. Steptoe.
Published by Cambridge University Press. © Cambridge University Press 2006.

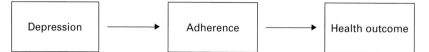

Figure 17.1 Model showing adherence as the mediator of the relationship between depression and health outcome.

Establishing an association between depression and adherence is part of the broader question of whether the relationship between depression and health outcomes is mediated by adherence (Figure 17.1). To establish such mediation, it is necessary to show that (i) depression influences adherence, (ii) adherence influences health outcome, (iii) depression influences health outcome and, most importantly, (iv) the relationship between depression and health outcome is removed by adjusting for adherence. Discussing all of the parts of this model is beyond the scope of this chapter. We focus on the relationship between depression and adherence and identify key studies that address the question of whether adherence mediates the relationship between depression and health outcome.

Adherence to chronic disease regimens

'Adherence' is the term most commonly used to describe a patient's actualisation of health-related behavioural prescriptions. Other terms, primarily 'compliance', have also been used to describe this process. Since the term 'adherence' accentuates the patient's perspective and connotes more voluntary action, this term is used throughout this chapter.

Minimal empirical attention was directed towards understanding adherence to medical regimens before the 1970s. However, this phenomenon has become a central concern in healthcare delivery and research in more recent decades. This increased attention is exemplified by the publication trends over the later half of the twentieth century. From 1943 to 1999, 16 658 English-language research and review articles on the topic of medical adherence (i.e. compliance) were included in the Index Medicus and other bibliographical collections [8]. Interestingly, 534 articles, or 3%, were published between 1943 and 1975, and 16 124 articles, or 97%, were published after 1976.

There are many reasons for the increased attention over time, but the foremost explanation is the often replicated documentation of high levels of poor adherence to medical regimens and its associated costs [9]. Satisfactory adherence across a range of chronic disease regimens is as low as 15–20% [9]. In certain circumstances, failure to adhere to medical regimens may result in serious consequences. For instance, low adherence rates among individuals with chronic medical illnesses have been associated with increased hospital admissions and longer hospital stays

[10]. Non-adherence may play an important role in the re-emergence of drug-resistant organisms, including tuberculosis [11] and human immunodeficiency virus (HIV) [12]. Non-adherence to treatment requirements for chronic diseases, such as end-stage renal disease, is associated with serious medical complications and earlier mortality [13]. The annual cost of non-adherence to medical treatment in the USA has been estimated to be $300 billion [14].

In light of the potentially severe consequences of non-adherence to health regimens, the identification of factors that predict adherence has received considerable attention. When concomitants of non-adherence are identified, appropriate interventions may be developed in order to enhance patient adherence and, ultimately, health outcomes [3].

Defining and assessing adherence

There are several forms of non-adherent behaviour that are usually reported in the chronic disease literature, including missed appointments, premature termination of treatment, errors in medication usage, and irregular implementation of other behaviour changes, such as following a diet and exercise regimen [15]. Most chronic diseases require multicomponent regimens; for instance, the prescribed regimen for diabetes often entails medication use, regular exercise, special diet, and blood or urine glucose self-monitoring [16]. In some studies, these different aspects of self-care behaviours have been associated with each other [17], whereas in other situations adherence to one of these behaviours is unrelated to adherence to other aspects [18]. Given the latter, it is important to assess adherence to different aspects of the treatment regimen.

A major problem in this area is the measurement of adherence. There are a variety of different ways to assess adherence, and the accuracy of these measures varies considerably. For example, in order to assess adherence to medication, techniques range from less reliable approaches such as self-reporting and pill counting to more reliable biological assays and electronic event monitoring. Dunbar-Jacob and colleagues [7] compared various approaches to assessing medication adherence and concluded that electronic event monitoring measures are the most accurate and other measures may overestimate adherence. Self-reporting is the most commonly used approach to assessing adherence to lifestyle aspects of the regimen, such as adherence to diet and physical activity. However, the accuracy of self-reporting measures is problematic. Individuals underreport approximately 20% of actual food intake across different methods of dietary assessment and energy expenditure [19]. Specific populations appear to underreport food intake more than others. In particular, individuals with weight concerns, including overweight and obese individuals, dieters and females, appear to underreport more than others. Moreover, specific foods considered unhealthy in Western culture (e.g. high-fat and high-sugar foods and snacks) appear to be underreported to a greater degree than other foods [19].

Although more advanced methods of measuring food intake are currently limited, several improved measures of exercise and smoking have been developed. For instance, doubly labelled water, pedometers and accelerometers are available to measure physical activity [20]. Expired carbon monoxide and salivary cotinine are two relatively accurate measures of smoking cessation [21]. Each of these measures has advantages and disadvantages in terms of accuracy and validity. However, due to the high costs of these more advanced measures, self-reporting continues to be the most commonly used measure in the adherence literature.

This state of affairs has important implications for evaluating the literature on the effects of depression on adherence. Dunbar-Jacob and colleagues [7] compared a set of predictors across three measurement methods: electronic event monitoring, 24-hour recall and an interview reviewing the previous month. When using 24-hour recall and the interview, psychosocial characteristics did not predict adherence; when using electronic event monitoring, social support and pain significantly predicted adherence. Dunbar-Jacob *et al.* [7] suggested that 'the electronic event monitors cause us to reexamine what we know about predictors of adherence. Our data suggest that many of the findings on adherence predictors may be related to the measurement method rather than the actual behaviour' (p. 110). Given that any single adherence measure is limited in some way, the use of multiple measures within studies (e.g. electronic monitoring, biological assay) would provide the most accuracy and facilitate greater understanding of predictors of adherence. Confidence in the observed association between depression and treatment adherence may thus depend on the type and number of adherence measures.

Another problem in this field has been the tendency to dichotomise adherence. Patients who are taking 80% or more of their prescribed medication are often considered 'adherent' whereas those taking below 80% are deemed 'non-adherent'. The decision of which criterion to select for the cut-off point is typically subjective. Moreover, such a criterion does not allow investigators to examine temporal distributions of adherence. An alternative is to define adherence to chronic disease regimens along a continuum, which avoids the use of arbitrary cut-off scores, maximises statistical power and facilitates the comparison of adherence rates across a range of behaviours, diseases and studies. Still, since relatively complex non-parametric strategies may be necessary in order to take advantage of the entire range of non-normal adherence data [7], the use of dichotomisation is omnipresent in the adherence literature.

Defining and assessing depression

'Depression' is a broad construct with many overlapping meanings in the general population and the mental health field. The construct 'depression' is often used as a synonym for negative mood states, particularly sadness; it also refers to several clinical disorders and their symptoms [22]. Different definitions of depression have been used throughout the literature on the relationship between depression and adherence.

Mental health professionals have developed a taxonomic classification system that is codified in the *Diagnostic and Statistical Manual of Mental Disorders* (DSM). In the current version (DSM-IV) [23], major depressive disorder (MDD) is the most severe unipolar affective disorder. Episodes of major depression are characterised by the presence of depressed mood or anhedonia 'most of the day, nearly every day', persisting for at least two weeks and accompanied by at least four additional symptoms. Although the DSM-IV stipulates a minimum duration of two weeks, patients often experience a depressive episode lasting for at least four to six months [24]. Additionally, recurrence of episodes is common among individuals with MDD.

Dimensional approaches to defining depression primarily rely on rating scales of depressive symptoms, such as the Beck Depression Inventory (BDI) [25] and the Center for Epidemiological Studies–Depression Scale (CES-D) [26]. In general, these instruments are composed of a standardised series of statements or questions based upon typical symptoms of depression. These instruments are dimensional, given that their scoring system consists of summing items into a total score that reflects the overall severity of depressive symptoms along a continuum [27]. Advocates of the dimensional perspective argue that there is a linear relationship between mild, moderate and severe forms of depression [28]. Although individuals with MDD usually have high scores along the dimension of depressive symptomatology, individuals with milder forms of depression may also have relatively high scores due to a period of distress or negative mood. In contrast to major depressive episodes, episodes of depression in non-clinical populations are thought to be more short-lived, with periods lasting hours or days instead of months [22]. The differing lengths of depression that are derived from the taxonomic and dimensional approaches may be an important factor in the interpretation of the depression-treatment adherence literature.

There are two predominant approaches to measuring depression: interview and self-report. Structured and semi-structured interviews have been developed for diagnosing depressive disorders and other psychopathological conditions. Examples of structured diagnostic interviews include the Schedule for Affective Disorders and Schizophrenia (SADS) [29], the Diagnostic Interview Schedule (DIS) [30] and the Structured Clinical Interview for DSM-IV [31]. These interviews are composed of standardised criteria that increase the reliability and generalisability of research findings [32]. Another important attribute of the interview approach is that examiners can differentially diagnose seemingly overlapping disorders. Furthermore, reporting biases by patients are minimised with this approach. A drawback of the interviews is their extended duration and expense of administration. In fact, despite the relative advantages of the interviews, the high costs result in their relatively infrequent use, particularly in cases where psychopathology is not the primary focus of research.

Patient rating scales are the most common approach for measuring depression in the medically ill, largely due to their inexpensiveness and the ease of administration and scoring. Their low cost permits administration to a wide range of patients. This method is also useful for tracking changes of depressive symptoms over time. One of the problems with these instruments is that for the most part they were originally developed for use in specific non-medical populations. For instance, the CES-D was developed for use in non-psychiatric populations in the community, and the BDI was developed to measure depression severity in populations previously diagnosed with major depression [33]. As a result, the instruments often possess adequate sensitivity but relatively poor specificity. Additionally, given that all but a select few of the patient rating scales are collected via patient self-reporting, these measures are subject to accuracy problems. For instance, depressed patients often experience cognitive dysfunction, which may interfere with the patient's ability to understand and respond accurately to scale items [34].

An inherent challenge in the measurement of depression among medical patients is the confounding of somatic and neurovegetative symptoms across the psychological and medical conditions. It is difficult to determine reliably whether depressive symptoms in a medically ill patient are a function of the psychopathological condition or the disease itself, or both. Specific neurovegetative and somatic symptoms that may overlap include fatigue, sleep disturbance, appetite/weight change, loss of libido, and psychomotor retardation.

An additional complication in measuring depression is the problem of psychiatric comorbidity. Depression often coexists with other psychiatric conditions. Among individuals experiencing MDD in the community, 56% were diagnosed with one or more other psychiatric disorders [35]. Anxiety symptoms and disorders are the most commonly reported comorbidity. The fact that depression and anxiety share many symptoms, such as sleep disturbance, worry, guilt and poor concentration, makes differential diagnosis quite difficult. Without controlling for anxiety, an observed association between depression and treatment adherence may actually be due to the effects of anxiety on adherence.

Thus, in evaluating the literature on depression and adherence, it is important to consider the approaches that have been used to measure each of these constructs.

Research on depression and adherence to medical regimens

Methods for identifying, including and evaluating studies

We have conducted a thorough search for articles that examine the relationship between depression and adherence to medical regimens in adult populations.

Articles were identified through electronic database searches and the ancestry approach. First, the PsychLit and MedLine electronic databases were searched from 1968 through 2004. Keywords included 'patient adherence' or 'patient compliance' and 'medical' or 'disease'. Second, references from review or empirical articles were reviewed for applicability. Studies were included in this review if the following criteria were met: (i) adults diagnosed with a chronic medical disease; (ii) patients prescribed medical or health treatment involving some type of behaviour, such as pharmacotherapy, diet, exercise, smoking cessation, behavioural self-monitoring (e.g. checking blood glucose levels) or attending a medical intervention (e.g. chemotherapy); and (iii) measures of depression and treatment adherence were included. Forty-one studies met these criteria and are described in Table 17.1 [36–76].

There were substantial differences across the 41 studies in terms of research location, research design, medical diseases and measures of depression and treatment adherence. As a result, there was no common denominator for computing effect sizes that would facilitate quantitative comparison of results across studies. Thus, Table 17.1 simply indicates whether there was a significant association between depression and adherence. A negative correlation would support the hypothesis that higher levels of depression are associated with poorer levels of adherence. 'Mixed' correlations occur when depression is associated negatively with some but not all adherence measures.

Overview of existing research

Examination of the relationship between depression and adherence has occurred in a variety of medical conditions. The breakdown of medical diseases in Table 17.1 is as follows: four cancer, seven cardiovascular disease (CAD), four diabetes, nine HIV, nine renal disease, one multiple sclerosis, three pulmonary disease, one rheumatoid arthritis, one hypertension and two unspecified chronic diseases. Of particular note is the recent increase of studies of depression and adherence to HIV regimen, with most of these studies being conducted after 2000.

Reviewing the studies in Table 17.1, it is clear that they differ in methodological rigour. For example, sample size in these studies ranges from 20 to over 5000. Some of the studies are prospective, but many assess depression and adherence concurrently. Assessment of adherence varies from simple self-reporting to the use of very objective measures, including electronic blister medication packets and glucometers with memory chips. Some studies focus on depressive symptomatology, whereas others involve diagnostic categories; associated with this difference is the fact that some studies assess depression with self-report questions or with validated questionnaires, whereas others use diagnostic interviews.

Keeping these methodological differences in mind, and the other methodological issues raised in the previous sections of this chapter, we present a brief review of

Table 17.1 Correlational studies on depression and adherence to medical regimens

Study	Sample/design information	Measure of adherence	Measure of depression	Results
Ades et al. [36]	226 patients with recent MI or coronary bypass surgery; 57% male; mean age 70 years, cross-sectional design	Participation in a cardiac rehabilitation programme	Unspecified self-report questions	Participation in cardiac rehabilitation associated with less depression before hospitalisation, but not with depression while hospitalised
Avants et al. [37]	43 patients with HIV, opioid dependence and cocaine abuse; 69% male; mean age 41 years; 48% African American, 38% white, 14% Hispanic; prospective design (4 weeks)	Weekly structured interview of medication adherence	BDI	Depression associated negatively with medication adherence; a composite score of 'emotional functioning,' including depression, negatively associated with medication adherence in multiple regression analysis
Ayres et al. [38]	74 women with breast cancer, 77% African American; prospective design (4–6 months)	Attendance at chemotherapy appointments	Affect Balance Scale	Depression associated positively with chemotherapy adherence
Blumenthal et al. [39]	35 patients with MI; mean age 54 years; 91% male; prospective design (1 year)	Attendance at exercise sessions	MMPI Depression Scale	Depression associated negatively with exercise adherence
Bosley et al. [40]	102 patients with asthma; age 18–70 years; prospective design (12 weeks)	Turbohaler inhalation computers	HADS	Depression but not anxiety associated negatively with medication adherence
Bosley et al. [41]	93 patients with COPD; age 45–77 years; prospective design (4 weeks)	Dataloggers	HADS	Depression and anxiety not associated with medication adherence
Botelho and Dudrak [42]	59 elderly patients with ≥2 chronic diseases; age 65+ years; prospective design (8 weeks)	Home-based pill counts by staff	BDI	Depression not associated with medication adherence
Carney et al. [43]	55 patients with CAD; mean age 69 years; 75% male; prospective design (3 weeks)	Electronic blister medication packets	Diagnostic Interview Schedule with DSM-III-R	Depression associated negatively with medication adherence

Study	Sample	Adherence measurement	Depression measurement	Findings
Carney et al. [44]	92 patients with CAD and MI; mean age 59 years; 82% male; prospective design (8 weeks)	Electronic blister medication packets	BDI	Depression not associated with medication adherence
Carrieri et al. [45]	96 patients with HIV; 69% male; age 18+ years; prospective design (18 months)	Self-reporting via questionnaire and interview	CES-D	Depression associated negatively with medication adherence
Catz et al. [46]	72 patients with HIV; mean age 40 years; 56% white, 36% African American; cross-sectional design	Self-reporting via interview	CES-D	Depression associated negatively with medication adherence
Ciechanowski et al. [47]	367 patients with NIDDM and IDDM; mean age 61 years; 56% female; 86% white; cross-sectional; retrospective and prospective (both 6 months) designs	Prescription refills, self-report exercise, diet, glucose testing	Depression subscale of the Hopkins Symptom Checklist-90	Depression associated negatively with adherence to diet recommendations (diet type and amount) and medication, but not exercise or glucose testing
Ciechanowski et al. [48]	407 patients with type 1 and 2 diabetes; mean age 49 years; 53% female; 91% white; cross-sectional design	Self-report diet (amount, type), exercise, and blood sugar monitoring	Hopkins Symptoms Checklist-90 Revised	Depression associated negatively with adherence to diet (amount and type) and exercise, but not blood sugar monitoring
Cluley and Cochrane [49]	103 patients with asthma; mean age 42 years; 66% female; prospective design (8 weeks)	Electronic diskhalers	HADS and Structured Clinical Interview for DSM-III-R	Depression associated negatively with medication adherence
De-Nour and Czaczkes [50]	100 patients with ESRD; age 20–60+ years; 61% male; prospective design (3 years)	Physician report of interdialytic weight gain (i.e. diet recommendations for fluid intake)	Psychiatric interview	Depression associated negatively with diet recommendations

(cont.)

Table 17.1 (*cont.*)

Study	Sample/design information	Measure of adherence	Measure of depression	Results
Eaton *et al.* [51]	127 patients with IDDM; age 14–50+ years; 59% female retrospective design (1 year)	Self-report blood sugar checking and chart review of telephone appointment, office appointment and self-monitoring adherence	CES-D	Depression not associated with combined measure of behavioural adherence
Everett *et al.* [52]	42 patients with ESRD; mean age 47 years; 52% male; 69% African American; cross-sectional design	Interdialytic weight gain	CES-D	Depression associated negatively with fluid adherence
Frazier *et al.* [53]	241 renal transplant patients; mean age 42 years; 58% male; 91% white; cross-sectional design	Self-report of medication adherence, self-report of follow-up adherence (clinic attendance, reporting problems and laboratory values)	BDI	Depression associated negatively with medication and follow-up adherence, although effect not significant in a multivariate regression model
Gilbar and De-Nour [54]	53 cancer patients and 53 matched controls; mean age 31 years; 62% female; retrospective design (<1 year)	Drop-out of chemotherapy	Depression subscale of Brief Symptom Inventory	Depression associated positively with treatment drop-out
Glazer *et al.* [55]	46 patients with coronary heart disease; mean age 58 years; 74% male	Attendance at exercise sessions (cardiac rehabilitation)	BDI	Depression associated negatively with adherence to exercise sessions
Gordillo *et al.* [56]	366 HIV patients from Spain; 20–72 years; median age 35 years; 76% male; cross-sectional design	Self-report and pill count of medication (>90% vs. ≤90%)	BDI	Depression associated negatively with medication adherence, although effect not significant in a multivariate regression model
Graveley and Oseasohn [57]	249 male veterans with unspecified chronic illnesses; age 65–87 years; 54% white, 36% Hispanic, 7% African American, 3% Asian American; prospective design (2 weeks)	Pill count at home visits (>80% vs. ≤80%)	Zung Self-Rating Depression Scale	Depression associated negatively with medication adherence, although effect not significant in multivariate regression model

Study	Sample	Adherence measure	Depression measure	Findings
Guiry et al. [58]	264 post-MI patients; age ≤60 years; 79% male; prospective (1 year)	Self-report smoking cessation, weight loss, exercise	Unspecified semi-structured interview	Depression associated negatively with smoking cessation and exercise adherence, but not weight loss
Katz et al. [59]	56 dialysis patients; mean age 61 years; 46% female; cross-sectional design	Interdialytic weight gain (IWG); levels of serum sodium and potassium (all categorical), e.g. IWG < or ≥3.5 kg	Self-report of distress symptoms in past month, unstandardised	Distress not associated with dietary adherence for any of the three measures
Kiley et al. [60]	105 kidney transplant patients; mean age 42 years; 51% African American, 26% white, 20% Hispanic, 3% Asian American; retrospective design (mean duration 35 months)	Medical records of medication levels, weight gain prevention, appointment keeping (all categorical)	CES-D	Depression associated negatively with adherence to diet and medication measures, but not clinic visits
Kimmel et al. [61]	295 ESRD patients treated with haemodialysis; 42% with diabetes; mean age 55 years; 71% male; 90% African American, 6% white; prospective design (mean follow-up 26 months)	Behavioural measures of dialysis adherence (i.e. time dialysed, attendance)	Cognitive Depression Index of BDI	Measure of depressive symptoms associated negatively with total dialysis adherence; adherence predicted mortality risk, but controlling for depression did not attenuate association
Lebovits et al. [62]	51 breast cancer patients; mean age 53 years; 51% white; prospective design (26 weeks)	Patient interview and chart review of medication adherence (>90% vs. ≤90%)	Research Diagnostic Criteria via interview, SCL-90	Depressive symptoms associated negatively with medication adherence at week 26, but not at weeks 2, 4 or 13; depressive disorders were not related to adherence; depression not related to adherence in a multivariate regression model
McDonough et al. [63]	30 patients with head or neck cancer; mean age 62 years; 70% white; retrospective design (6 months)	Self-report measure of diet, medication use, physician appointments, smoking, alcohol consumption	BDI, BAI, PANAS	Positive affect associated positively with overall adherence, but depressive symptoms, negative mood and anxiety symptoms not associated; only anxiety predicted dietary adherence; nothing predicted adherence

(cont.)

Table 17.1 (cont.)

Study	Sample/design information	Measure of adherence	Measure of depression	Results
Mohr et al. [64]	85 patients with multiple sclerosis taking interferon beta-1b; 68%; female 85% white; 6% African American, 4% Hispanic; retrospective design (6 months)	Self-report question: 'Are you still taking Betaseron?'	3 self-report questions about depressive feelings, antidepressant medication and antidepressant counselling	New or increased depression associated negatively with medication adherence; antidepressant treatment (medication or counselling) associated with increased adherence to interferon beta-1b
Paterson et al. [65]	81 patients with HIV; median age 40 years (range 21–62 years); prospective design (median 6 months, range 3–15 months)	Medication Event Monitoring System (electronic pill caps)	BDI and chart review for history of depression	Depression associated negatively with medication adherence; medication adherence associated positively with virological failure, but depression not associated with virological failure
Rodriguez et al. [66]	12 'ideally adherent' and 12 'non-adherent' renal transplant patients in Puerto Rico; mean age 29 years; 63% male; retrospective design (time not reported)	Medical record review of patient's adherence to diet, appointments, medication and interdialytic weight gain	Medical record review of patient's psychosocial history conducted by transplant team social worker	Non-adherent patients significantly more likely to have history of depression
Schneider et al. [67]	50 patients with ESRD; mean age 56 years; 74% male; 78% white; retrospective (8 weeks)	Interdialytic weight gain (<3.0 kg or ≥3.0 kg) from medical chart review of preceding 8 weeks (24 measures)	BDI, Spielberger Trait Anxiety Scale	Threshold depression or anxiety not associated with dietary adherence
Singh et al. [68]	46 male HIV patients; median age 40 years; age 23–68 years; 65% white, 33% African American, 2% Hispanic; prospective design (1 year)	Prescription refills; biological assays to confirm medication consumption	BDI; POMS depression and anxiety factor scores	Depressive symptoms from the BDI not associated with medication adherence but POMS depression score associated negatively with adherence; POMS anxiety not predictive

Study	Sample characteristics	Adherence measure	Depression measure	Findings
Spire et al. [69]	445 patients with HIV; mean age 39 years; 78% male; ethnicity not reported; prospective design (4 months)	Self-report medication adherence	CES-D	Increased depression over time associated negatively with medication adherence in univariate (multivariate effect not reported)
Taal et al. [70]	86 patients with rheumatoid arthritis; mean age 60 years; 71% female; cross-sectional design	Self-report index of problems adhering to treatment recommendations derived via interview (i.e. joint protection, medication, physical therapy)	Dutch version of the Arthritis Impact Measurement Scales – depression subscale	Measure of depressive symptoms not related to problems with adhering to treatment recommendations
Tucker et al. [71]	1910 patients with HIV; 58% between ages 35–49 year; 78% male; 32% African American, 15% Hispanic; cross-sectional design	Medication adherence via interview	Short-form of the WHO Composite International Diagnostic Interview	Depression but not dysthymia associated negatively with medication adherence
Turner et al. [72]	5103 patients with HIV and substance dependence; 36% female; retrospective design (at least 60 days)	Prescription refills for anti-retroviral drugs	Prescription refill for antidepressant medication	Depression associated positively with medication adherence
Wang et al. [73]	496 patients with hypertension; 60% > 65 years old; 67% male; 95% white; cross-sectional design	Prescription refills	Modified version of the Brief Symptom Inventory	Depression associated negatively with medication adherence
Williams et al. [74]	40 ESRD patients, mean age 60 years; 56% female; 68% African American, 32% white; prospective design (12 weeks)*	Self-report via interview of adherence to exercise programme	BDI	Threshold depression not associated with exercise adherence
Wilson et al. [75]	184 NIDDM patients; mean age 58 years; 98% white; cross-sectional design	Self-report diet, exercise, glucose testing, medication taking	Composite of BDI and CES-D State–Trait Anxiety Inventory	Composite measure of depressive symptoms associated negatively with glucose testing adherence, but unrelated to diet, exercise or medication taking; anxiety associated negatively with diet and glucose testing

(cont.)

Table 17.1 (*cont.*)

Study	Sample/design information	Measure of adherence	Measure of depression	Results
Ziegelstein et al. [76]	204 post-MI patients; 30% with diabetes; mean age 64 years; 57% male; prospective design (4 months)	Self-report via telephone interview with Medical Outcomes Study Specific Adherence Scale (i.e. diet, medication exercise, stress, blood glucose checking, increasing social support)	BDI, SCID-III-R	Threshold depression, MDD and dysthymia associated negatively with diet, exercise, stress reduction and social support adherence; MDD and dysthymia linked with poor medication adherence; among diabetic patients, MDD and dysthymia linked with poorer diet adherence

*Only 22/40 patients completed the BDI.

BAI, Beck Anxiety Inventory; BDI, Beck Depression Inventory; BP = blood pressure; CAD, cardiovascular disease; CES-D, Center for Epidemiological Studies – Depression Scale; COPD, chronic obstructive pulmonary disease; DSM, *Diagnostic and Statistical Manual*; ESRD, end-stage renal disease; HADS, Hospital Anxiety and Depression Scale; HAM-D, Hamilton Rating Scale for Depression; HDL, high-density lipoproteins; HIV, human immunodeficiency virus; IDDM, insulin-dependent diabetes mellitus; LDL, low-density lipoproteins; MDD, major depressive disorder; MI, myocardial infarction; MMPI, Minnesota Multiphasic Personality Inventory; NIDDM, non-insulin-dependent diabetes mellitus; PANAS, Positive and Negative Affect Scale; POMS, Profile of Mood States; SCID, Structured Clinical Interview for DSM; SCL-90, Symptom Checklist-90; WHO, World Health Organization several of the stronger studies on this topic. These studies highlight the complexity of this topic, especially as it relates to the 'mediational hypothesis'.

Bosley *et al.* evaluated treatment adherence and depression among 102 patients with asthma [40] and 93 with chronic obstructive pulmonary disease (COPD) [41]. Strengths of these studies include the fact that electronic event monitoring was used to assess medication adherence and the Hospital Anxiety and Depression Scale (HADS) was used to assess depressive symptoms independent of anxiety. Prospective designs were used in both studies, with 12-week and 4-week periods in the asthma and COPD studies, respectively. The authors reported a negative association between depression and medication adherence in the asthma study but no association in the COPD study. They were not able to determine the cause for the mixed findings.

Another relatively strong methodological study was conducted by Kimmel *et al.* [61], who prospectively examined 295 end-stage renal disease (ESRD) patients over a mean follow-up period of 26 months. Adherence to dialysis was measured behaviourally, and depressive symptoms were measured via the BDI and the Cognitive Depression Index (CDI), a non-somatic version of the BDI. The BDI and the CDI were associated with poor adherence to dialysis treatment. Moreover, poor dialysis adherence predicted mortality risk. However, depression did not predict mortality. Thus, these data suggest that depression is associated negatively with adherence, but the data do not support the mediational hypothesis that depression affects mortality via treatment adherence.

Ciechanowski *et al.* [47] explored the impact of depressive symptoms on adherence to medical regimens (i.e. medication, exercise, diet, glucose self-monitoring) among 367 patients with diabetes who were seen in primary-care clinics of a large health-maintenance organisation. Medication adherence was measured retrospectively (previous six months) and prospectively (subsequent six months) by prescription refills from a centralised pharmacy database. Other adherence behaviours were measured cross-sectionally via self-report. Depressive symptoms were measured with the depression subscale of the Hopkins Symptom Checklist-90. Higher levels of depressive symptomatology were associated with poorer adherence to diet and medication regimens, but depression was not related to adherence to exercise or glucose self-monitoring. Importantly, depressive symptom severity was not associated with glycosylated haemoglobin levels, thereby failing to support a necessary condition of the mediational hypothesis.

Adherence to medical recommendations among 204 recent post-myocardial infarction (MI) patients was examined by Ziegelstein *et al.* [76]. Telephone interviews were used to assess adherence to several behaviours, including diet, exercise, medication, stress management, blood glucose checking for diabetics, and social support. Patients with above-threshold depressive symptoms (BDI > 10), major

Table 17.2 Association between depression and treatment adherence by disease category

Disease	Number of studies with negative correlations	Number of studies with positive correlations	Number of studies with null findings	Number of studies with mixed findings
Cancer	0	2	1	1
CAD	4	0	1	2
Diabetes	0	0	1	3
HIV	4	1	0	4
Pulmonary	1	0	1	1
Renal	4	0	3	2
Other	2	3	2	1

CAD, cardiovascular disease; HIV, human immunodeficiency virus.

depressive disorder (MDD) or dysthymia reported poorer adherence to a low-fat diet, regular exercise, reducing stress and increasing social support four months later. Those patients with MDD or dysthymia also reported adhering to the medication regimen to a lesser degree than those without depressive disorders. The use of several different approaches to the assessment of depression is a strength of this study. The finding that MDD may be associated more strongly with poor adherence than depressive symptomatology also appears true in between-study comparisons across Table 17.1.

Several studies have addressed adherence in patients infected with HIV. Turner *et al.* [72] studied 5103 patients who had HIV and substance dependence. Adherence was assessed by examining prescription refills for anti-retroviral drugs. Interestingly, these authors found that adherence was greater in patients who had been diagnosed with depression than in patients without depression. This finding may relate to the fact that most of the patients who were diagnosed with depression were receiving mental health services and receipt of mental health services was associated favourably with adherence. This evidence of an association between depression and use of mental health services shows the complexity of conducting research related to depression and adherence.

Table 17.2 summarises the 41 studies we have reviewed. Without considering the methodological quality of studies, we have simply identified studies as negative, positive, mixed or null (no association). We found that 37% reported the expected negative association between depression and adherence; 34% reported mixed associations (typically, depression was related negatively to some adherence behaviours but unrelated to others). Few studies (7%) reported positive associations, but 27% found no association between depression and adherence. Thus, depression appears to be associated negatively with adherence, but the relationship is less consistent than is typically assumed.

This conclusion of inconsistent relationships between depression and adherence contrasts somewhat with a meta-analysis of this literature. DiMatteo and colleagues [3] reviewed 12 studies published between 1968 and 1998. Six of the studies involved patients with ESRD or renal transplants, and the other six involved other medical diseases (cancer, angina, arthritis). No methodological criteria were set for inclusion of studies in the meta-analysis, and the effect sizes were not weighted according to the strength of the studies.

This meta-analysis concluded that the relationship between depression and adherence was consistent across studies and of moderate size (unweighted effect size of -0.27, $p < 0.001$); the odds that a patient would be non-adherent were three times greater for depressed patients than for non-depressed patients. The larger number of studies included in the present review, and in particular newer studies, may explain the differences in the findings.

Intervention studies

Four studies have moved beyond simply examining the correlation between depression and adherence to intervention approaches testing whether treatment of depression will result in improved levels of adherence [77–80]. In addition, these studies examined whether the changes in adherence were related to changes in health outcomes. These intervention studies are presented in Table 17.3. Goodnick *et al.* [77] conducted a 10-week open-label antidepressant intervention with 28 patients diagnosed with non-insulin-dependent diabetes mellitus (NIDDM) and MDD. All individuals were administered sertraline after a two-week single-blind placebo washout period. After the ten-week period, Hamilton rating scale for depression (HAM-D) and BDI scores were significantly reduced. Individuals with low baseline dietary adherence manifested significantly improved adherence during the period. Finally, 76% of patients with high baseline glycosylated haemoglobin levels showed significant reductions. These findings are suggestive of a link between depression and adherence, but the lack of a control group limits the conclusions that can be drawn.

Lustman and colleagues conducted two randomised controlled trials with diabetic patients. In the first trial [78], 68 patients with NIDDM or insulin-dependent diabetes mellitus (IDDM), 28 of whom had current MDD, took either nortriptyline or placebo for 8 weeks. Adherence to the medication and glucose self-monitoring regimen was measured with two electronic devices. Patients treated with nortriptyline experienced a significantly greater reduction in BDI scores than patients treated with placebo. Path analysis indicated that depression improvement had an independent beneficial effect on glycosylated haemoglobin levels; this association

Table 17.3 Intervention Studies on Depression and Adherence to Medical Regimens

Study	Sample/design information	Measure of adherence	Measure of depression	results
Goodnick et al. [77]	28 patients with NIDDM and MDD; mean age 54 years; 57% male; uncontrolled treatment study (10 weeks)	Unspecified dietary compliance	HAM-D, BDI	Individuals with low baseline dietary adherence and treated with sertraline showed significantly improved HAM-D and BDI scores and dietary adherence
Lustman et al. [78]	68 patients with NIDDM or IDDM; 30% diagnosed with MDD; mean age 49 years; 51% female; 88% white; prospective intervention study (2 months)	Electronic blister pacs (meds), electronic glucometers (i.e. measures blood glucose monitoring)	BDI	Nortriptyline led to reductions of depressive symptoms in depressed patients, but this improvement not associated with improved adherence in medication taking or glucose monitoring
Lustman et al. [79]	51 patients with NIDDM and diagnosis of MDD; mean age 55 years*; 60% female; 81% white; prospective intervention study (6-month follow-up)	Electronic glucometer	BDI	CBT led to greater reductions in depressive symptoms than in control group; blood glucose monitoring adherence declined in the CBT group compared with control group
Williams et al. [80]	417 patients with DM and MDD or dysthymia; mean age 71 years; 65% female; 77% white, 12% African American, 8% Hispanic; prospective intervention study (12 months follow-up)	Self-report measure of diet, exercise, glucose testing, foot care, medication adherence	SCL-90	Intervention (education, problem-solving treatment, or support for antidepressant management) led to reduction of depressive symptoms and to increase in weekly exercise days at 12-months' follow-up; intervention not associated with improved adherence in diet, glucose testing, medication taking or foot care; intervention did not lead to improvement in HA1$_c$ values

*All demographic data presented for study completers (42/51) only.

BDI, Beck Depression Inventory; CBT, cognitive–behavioural therapy; DM, diabetes mellitus, unspecified type; HA1$_c$, glycosylated haemoglobin; HAM-D, Hamilton Rating Scale for Depression; IDDM, insulin-dependent diabetes mellitus; MDD, major depressive disorder; NIDDM, non-insulin-dependent diabetes mellitus; SCL-90, Symptom Checklist-90.

was not mediated by improved adherence to blood glucose self-monitoring or medication taking.

In the second clinical trial, Lustman *et al.* [79] assessed the effects of cognitive–behavioural therapy (CBT) on depression among 51 patients with NIDDM. Patients were randomly assigned to receive ten weeks of individual CBT or to a control group that received no specific antidepressant treatment. Glucose self-monitoring was measured with an electronic device. Six months after treatment, 70% of patients in the CBT group compared with 33.3% of controls achieved a significant reduction in BDI scores. Mean glycosylated haemoglobin levels were significantly better in the CBT group than in the control group. However, a time-by-treatment group interaction indicated that over the ten-week treatment period, adherence with self-monitoring of blood glucose levels declined in the CBT group compared with the control group.

Williams *et al.* [80] studied 417 patients with diabetes and depression, recruited from primary-care clinics. Patients were assigned randomly to usual care or to receive a depression intervention that included education, problem-solving and/or antidepressant medication. Diabetes self-care behaviours were assessed by self-report, and the SCL-90 was used to assess changes in depression. Patients who were assigned to the intervention had less severe depression at 12 months than those in usual care; exercise increased in the intervention group but other aspects of self-care were not affected. Glycaemic control was not affected by the intervention, perhaps because most patients were well controlled at the start of the study.

Thus, in all of these intervention studies level of depression improved with treatment, and in several studies treatment of depression improved glycaemic control. However, changes in depression did not lead consistently to changes in adherence. Moreover, these studies provided very little support for the mediational model in which changes in adherence mediate the relationship between depression and outcome.

Conclusions

In conclusion, this review suggests that there is a negative relationship between depression and adherence, but this relationship appears less consistent than is typically assumed. Frequently, depression was related to some aspects of self-care behaviours but not to others. Moreover, the interventions studies suggest that treating depression does not consistently lead to improved adherence.

Research on depression and adherence is increasing rapidly. It is important that future research on this topic be designed with greater methodological sophistication. For example, objective measures of adherence should be used whenever possible. Self-reporting of adherence is particularly problematic in studies of the relationship between depression and adherence because individuals who are depressed may provide biased estimates of their behaviour, underestimating their actual degree of adherence. Assessing adherence is also difficult unless there are clear prescriptions for the behaviour; that is, it is hard to tell whether patients are adhering to a recommendation such as 'try to increase your physical activity'. Given that adherence to one aspect of the regimen is often unrelated to adherence to other aspects, it is important to include a variety of different self-care behaviours in this research.

A primary reason for interest in the relationship between depression and adherence is the belief that adherence mediates the effect of depression on health outcomes. Baron and Kenny [81] have proposed a methodological approach to studying mediators that should be applied to this area of research. In future studies of depression and medical outcomes, it would be very important to include assessments of adherence and then to conduct the appropriate statistical analyses to determine whether adherence is indeed mediating the effect of depression on outcomes. Research to date has found little evidence to support this mediational model.

As noted above, this field is beginning to move beyond correlational approaches to use randomised clinical trials to examine whether treatment of depression is related to improved outcomes and, if so, whether adherence mediates this relationship. To date, these trials have all been conducted within the area of diabetes. Diabetes may be a particularly difficult area for such research because the treatment regimen is complex and patients are encouraged to adhere to several different self-care behaviours (diet, exercise, medication, glucose monitoring). Additional randomised trials in other medical areas would be extremely helpful in advancing this area of study. Randomised trials could also be conducted in order to test strategies for improving adherence in depressed patients. For example, simplifying the regimen or providing adherence reminders may help to improve adherence in depressed patients. Researchers could then determine whether improved adherence was associated with improved medical outcomes.

Finally, we have argued previously [82] that the correlation between depression and adherence should not be interpreted as implying that depression causes poor adherence. In some situations, the direction of the relation may actually be reversed: the behaviours may be influencing the level of depression, rather than vice versa. Exercise and weight control may be two examples. There is a substantial literature showing that exercise and weight loss are related to improvements in mood. Moreover, changes in exercise or weight are also related to improved health. Given that the ultimate goal is to improve health outcomes, researchers should examine whether it is more effective to intervene on depression (and, thereby, improve adherence and consequently health outcomes) or to intervene on physical activity or weight control, which might impact on the levels of depression but should also have a more direct effect on improving health outcomes.

REFERENCES

1. W. Katon, Depression: Relationship to somatization and chronic medical illness. *J. Clin. Psychol.* **45** (1984), 4–11.

2. K. B. Wells, W. Rogers, M. A. Burnam, S. Greenfield, J. E. Ware, Jr, How the medical comorbidity of depressed patients differs across health care settings: results from the Medical Outcomes Study. *Am. J. Psychiatry* **148** (1991), 1688–96.

3. M. R. DiMatteo, H. D. Lepper, T. W. Croghan, Depression is a risk factor for noncompliance with medical treatment: meta-analysis of the effects of anxiety and depression on patient adherence. *Arch. Intern. Med.* **160** (2000), 2101–107.

4. R. B. Haynes, D. W. Taylor, D. L. Sackett, *Compliance in Health Care* (Baltimore, MD: Johns Hopkins University Press, 1979).

5. R. M. Kaplan, H. J. Simon, Compliance in medical care: reconsideration of self-predictions. *Ann. Behav. Med.* **12** (1990), 66–71.

6. J. M. Dunbar-Jacob, S. Sereika, J. Rohay, L. E. Burke, Electronic methods in assessing adherence to medical regimens. In *Technology and Methods in Behavioral Medicine*, ed. D. S. Krantz, A. Baum (Mahwah, NJ: Lawrence Erlbaum Associates, 1998), pp. 95–113.

7. J. M. Dunbar-Jacob, E. A. Schlenk, L. E. Burke, J. T. Matthews, Predictors of patient adherence: patient characteristics. In *The Handbook of Health Behavior Change*, 2nd edn, ed. S. A. Shumaker, E. B. Schron, J. K. Ockene, W. L. McBee (New York: Springer, 1998), pp. 491–511.

8. J. A. Trostle, The idealogy of adherence: an anthropological and historical perspective. In *Promoting Adherence to Medical Treatment in Chronic Childhood Illness: Concepts, Methods, and Interventions*, ed. D. Drotar (Mahwah, NJ: Lawrence Erlbaum Associates, 2000), pp. 37–55.

9. L. B. Myers, K. Midence, Concepts and issues in adherence. In *Adherence to Treatement in Medical Conditions*, ed. K. Midence (Amsterdam: Harwood Academics, 1998), pp. 1–24.

10. J. M. Dunbar-Jacob, L. E. Burke, S. Puczynski, Clinical assessment and management of adherence to medical regimens. In *Managing Chronic Illness: A Biopsychosocial Perspective*, ed. P. M. Nicassio, T. W. Smith (Washington, DC: American Psychological Association, 1995), pp. 313–49.

11. M. N. Gourevitch, W. Wasserman, M. S. Panero, P. A. Selwyn, Successful adherence to observed prophylaxis and treatment of tuberculosis among drug-users in a methadone program. *J. Addict. Dis.* **15** (1996), 93–104.

12. J. W. Mellors, Clinical implications of resistance and cross-resistance to HIV protease inhibitors. *Infect. Med.* Suppl (1997), 32–8.

13. A. L. Plough, Social and contextual factors in the analyses of mortality in end-stage renal disease: implications for health policy. *Am. J. Public Health* **72** (1992), 1293–5.

14. M. R. DiMatteo, Variations in patients' adherence to medical recommendations: a quantitative review of 50 years of research. *Med. Care* **42** (2004), 200–209.

15. L. J. Bauman, A patient-centered approach to adherence: risks for nonadherence. In *Promoting Adherence to Medical Treatment in Chronic Childhood Illness: Concepts, Methods and Interventions*, ed. D. Drotar (Mahwah, NJ: Lawrence Erlbaum Associates, 2000).

16. L. Warren, P. Hixenbaugh, Adherence and diabetes. In *Adherence to Treatment in Medical Conditions*, ed. L. B. Myers, K. Midence (Amsterdam: Harwood Academic, 1998), pp. 423–54.

17. J. Jakicic, R. R. Wing, C. Winters-Hart, Relationship of physical activity to eating behaviors and weight loss in women. *Med. Sci. Sports Exer.* **34** (2002), 1653–9.

18. L. C. Schafer, R. E. Glasgow, K. D. McCaul, M. Dreher, Adherence to IDDM regimens: relationship to psychosocial variables and metabolic control. *Diabet. Care* **6** (1893), 493–8.

19. R. J. Hill, P. S. Davies, The validity of self-reported energy intake as determined using the doubly labeled water technique. *Br. J. Nutr.* **85** (2001), 415–30.

20. M. Z. Vitolins, C. S. Rand, S. R. Rapp, P. M. Ribisl, M. Sevick, Measuring adherence to behavioral and medical interventions. *Control. Clin. Trials* **21**: Suppl 1 (2000), 188–94.

21. D. J. Ossip-Klein, G. Bigelow, S. R. Parker, S. Curry, Task force 1: classification and assessment of smoking behavior. *Health Psychol.* **5**. Suppl (1986), 3–11.

22. J. C. Coyne, Self-reported distress: analog or ersatz depression? *Psychol. Bull.* **116** (1994), 29–45.

23. American Psychiatric Association, *Diagnostic and Statistical Manual of Mental Disorders*, 4th edn (Washington, DC: American Psychiatric Association, 1994).

24. W. Coryell, H. S. Akiskal, A. C. Leon, *et al.*, The time course of nonchronic major depressive disorder: uniformity across episodes and samples. *Arch. Gen. Psychiatry* **51** (1994), 405–10.

25. A. T. Beck, C. H. Ward, M. Mendelson, J. Mock, J. Erbaugh, An inventory for measuring depression. *Arch. Gen. Psychiatry* **4** (1961), 53–63.

26. L. S. Radloff, The CES-D scale: a self-report depression scale for research in the general population. *Appl. Psychol. Meas.* **1** (1977), 385–401.

27. J. Rodin, J. Mancuso, J. Granger, E. Nelbach, Food cravings in relation to body mass index, restraint and estradiol levels: a repeated measures study in healthy women. *Appetite* **17** (1991), 177–85.

28. G. L. Flett, K. Vredenburg, L. Krames, The continuity of depression in clinical and nonclinical samples. *Psychol. Bull.* **121** (1997), 395–416.

29. R. L. Spitzer, J. Endicott, E. Robins, Research diagnostic criteria: Rationale and reliability. *Arch. Gen. Psychiatry* **35** (1978), 773–82.

30. L. N. Robins, J. E. Helzer, J. Croughan, K. S. Ratcliff, National institute of mental health diagnostic interview schedule. *Arch. Gen. Psychiatry* **38** (1981), 381–9.

31. M. B. First, R. L. Spitzer, M. Gibbon, J. B. W. Williams, *Structured Clincal Interview for DSM-IV Axis I Disorders*. Washington, DC: American Psychiatric Association, 1996.

32. G. Rodin, J. Craven, C. Littlefield, *Depression in the Medically Ill: An Integrated Approach* (New York: Brunner/Mazel, 1991).

33. K. A. Yonkers, J. Samson, *Mood Disorders Measures* (Washington, DC: American Psychiatric Association, 2000).

34. L. Smithline, Is depression a risk factor for cardiovascular disease? A critical review. Examination paper. Pittsburgh, PA: University of Pittsburgh, 1997.

35. D. G. Blazer, R. C. Kessler, K. A. McGonagle, M. S. Swartz, The prevalence and distribution of major depression in a national comorbidity survey. *Am. J. Psychiatry* **151** (1994), 979–86.

36. P. A. Ades, M. L. Waldmann, W. J. McCann, S. O. Weaver, Predictors of cardiac rehabilitation participation in older coronary patients. *Arch. Intern. Med.* **152** (1992), 1033–5.

37. S. K. Avants, A. Margolin, L. A. Warburton, K. A. Hawkins, J. Shi, Predictors of nonadherence to HIV-related medication regimens during methadone stabilization. *Am. J. Addict.* **10** (2001), 69–78.

38. A. Ayres, P. W. Hoon, J. B. Franzoni, *et al.*, Influence of mood and adjustment to cancer on compliance with chemotherapy among breast cancer patients. *J. Psychosom. Res.* **38** (1994), 393–402.

39. J. A. Blumenthal, S. Williams, A. G. Wallace, R. B. Williams, T. L. Needles, Physiological and psychological variables predict compliance to prescribed exercise therapy in patients recovering from myocardial infarction. *Psychosom. Med.* **44** (1982), 519–27.

40. C. M. Bosley, J. A. Fosbury, G. M. Cochrane, The psychological factors associated with poor compliance with treatment in asthma. *Eur. Respir. J.* **8** (1995), 899–904.

41. C. M. Bosley, Z. M. Corden, P. J. Rees, G. M. Cochrane, Psychological factors associated with use of home nebulized therapy for COPD. *Eur. Respir. J.* **9** (1996), 2346–50.

42. R. J. Botelho, R. Dudrak, Home assessment of adherence to long-term medication in the elderly. *J. Fam. Pract.* **35** (1992), 61–5.

43. R. M. Carney, K. E. Freedland, S. A. Eisen, M. W. Rich, A. S. Jaffe, Major depression and medication adherence in elderly patients with coronary artery disease. *Health Psychol.* **14** (1995), 88–90.

44. R. M. Carney, K. E. Freedland, S. A. Eisen, *et al.*, Adherence to prophylactic medication regimen in patients with symptomatic versus asymptomatic ischemic heart disease. *Behav. Med.* **24** (1998), 35–9.

45. M. P. Carrieri, M. A. Chesney, B. Spire, *et al.*, Failure to maintain adherence to HAART in a cohort of French HIV-positive injecting drug users. *Int. J. Behav. Med.* **10** (2003), 1–14.

46. S. L. Catz, J. A. Kelly, L. M. Bogart, E. G. Benotsch, T. L. McAuliffe, Patterns, correlates, and barriers to medication adherence among persons prescribed new treatments for HIV disease. *Health Psychol.* **19** (2000), 124–33.

47. P. S. Ciechanowski, W. J. Katon, J. O. Russo, Depression and diabetes: Impact of depressive symptoms on adherence, function, and costs. *Arch. Intern. Med.* **160** (2000), 3278–85.

48. P. S. Ciechanowski, W. J. Katon, J. E. Russo, I. B. Hirsch, The relationship of depressive symptoms to symptom reporting, self-care and glucose control in diabetes. *Gen. Hosp. Psychiatry* **25** (2003), 246–52.

49. S. Cluley, G. M. Cochrane, Psychological disorder in asthma is associated with poor control and poor adherence to inhaled steriods. *Respir. Med.* **95** (2001), 37–9.

50. A. K. De-Nour, J. W. Czaczkes, The influence of patient's personality on adjustment to chronic dialysis. *J. Nerv. Ment. Dis.* **162** (1976), 323–33.

51. W. W. Eaton, D. E. Larson, M. Mengel, R. Campbell, R. B. Montague, Psychosocial and psychologic influences on management and control of insulin-dependent diabetes. *Int. J. Psychiatr. Med.* **22** (1992), 105–17.

52. K. D. Everett, P. J. Brantley, C. Sletten, G. N. Jones, G. T. McKnight, The relation of stress and depression to interdialytic weight gain in hemodialysis patients. *Behav. Med.* **21** (1995), 25–30.

53. P. Frazier, K. Davis-Ali, K. E. Dahl, Correlates of noncompliance among renal transplant recipients. *Clin. Transpl.* **8** (1994), 550–57.

54. O. Gilbar, A. K. De-Nour, Adjustment to illness and dropout of chemotherapy. *J. Psychosom. Res.* **33** (1989), 1–5.

55. K. M. Glazer, C. F. Emery, D. J. Frid, R. E. Banyasz, Psychological predictors of adherence and outcomes among patients in cardiac rehabilitation. *J. Cardiopulm. Rehabil.* **22** (2002), 40–46.

56. V. Gordillo, J. delAmo, V. Soriano, J. Gonzalez-Lahoz, Sociodemographic and psychological variables influencing adherence to antiretroviral therapy. *AIDS* **13** (1999), 1763–9.

57. E. A. Graveley, C. S. Oseasohn, Multiple drug regimens: medication compliance among veterans 65 years and older. *Res. Nurs. Health* **14** (1991), 51–8.

58. E. Guiry, R. M. Controy, N. Hickey, R. Mulcahy, Psychological response to an acute coronary event and its effect on subsequent rehabilitation and lifestyle change. *Clin. Cardiol.* **10** (1987), 256–60.

59. R. C. Katz, J. Ashmore, E. Barboa, *et al.* Knowledge of disease and dietary compliance in patients with end-stage renal disease. *Psychol. Rep.* **82** (1998), 331–6.

60. D. J. Kiley, C. S. Lam, R. Pollak, A study of treatment compliance following kidney transplantation. *Transplantation* **55** (1993), 51–6.

61. P. L. Kimmel, R. A. Peterson, K. L. Weihs, *et al.*, Psychosocial factors, behavioral compliance and survival in urban hemodialysis patients. *Kidney Int.* **54** (1998), 245–54.

62. A. H. Lebovits, J. J. Strain, S. J. Schleifer, *et al.*, Patient noncompliance with self-administered chemotherapy. *Cancer* **65** (1990), 17–22.

63. E. M. McDonough, J. H. Boyd, M. A. Vavares, M. D. Maves, Relationship between psychological status and compliance in a sample of patients treated for cancer of the head and neck. *Head Neck* **18** (1996), 269–76.

64. D. C. Mohr, D. E. Goodking, W. Likosky, *et al.*, Treatment of depression improves adherence to interferon beta-1b therapy for multiple sclerosis. *Arch. Neurol.* **54** (1997), 531–3.

65. D. L. Paterson, S. Swindells, J. Mohr, *et al.*, Adherence to protease inhibitor therapy and outcomes in patients with HIV infection. *Ann. Intern. Med.* **133** (2000), 21–30.

66. A. Rodriguez, M. Diaz, A. Colon, E. A. Santiago-Delpin, Psychosocial profile of noncompliant transplant patients. *Transplant. Proc.* **23** (1991), 1807–809.

67. M. S. Schneider, R. Friend, P. Whitaker, N. K. Wadhwa, Fluid noncompliance and symptomatology in end-stage renal disease: Cognitive and emotional variables. *Health Psychol.* **10** (1991), 209–15.

68. N. Singh, C. Squier, C. Sivek, *et al.*, Determinants of compliance with antiretroviral therapy in patients with human immunodeficiency virus: prospective assessment with implications for enhancing compliance. *AIDS Care* **8** (1996), 261–9.

69. B. Spire, S. Duran, M. Souville, *et al.*, Adherence to highly active antiretroviral therapies (HAART) in HIV-infected patients: from a predictive to a dynamic approach. *Soc. Sci. Med.* **54** (2002), 1481–96.

70. E. Taal, J. J. Rasker, E. R. Seydel, O. Wiegman, Health status, adherence with health recommendations, self-efficacy and social support in patients with rheumatoid arthritis. *Patient Educ. Couns.* **20** (1993), 63–76.

71. J. S. Tucker, A. Burnam, C. D. Sherbourne, F. Y. Kung, A. L. Gifford, Substance use and mental health correlates of nonadherence to antiretroviral medications in a sample of patients with human immunodeficiency virus infection. *Am. J. Med.* **114** (2003), 573–80.

72. B. J. Turner, C. Laine, L. Cosler, W. W. Hauck, Relationship of gender, depression, and health care delivery with antiretroviral adherence in HIV-infected drug users. *J. Gen. Intern. Med.* **18** (2003), 248–57.

73. P. S. Wang, R. L. Bohn, E. Knight, *et al.*, Noncompliance with antihypertensive medications: the impact of depressive symptoms and psychosocial factors. *J. Gen. Intern. Med.* **17** (2002), 504–11.

74. A. Williams, R. Stephens, T. McKnight, S. Dodd, Factors affecting adherence of end-stage renal disease patients to an exercise programme. *Br. J. Sports Med.* **25** (1991), 90–3.

75. W. Wilson, V. Ary, A. Biglan, *et al.*, Psychosocial predictors of self-care behaviors (compliance) and glycemic control in non-insulin-dependent diabetes mellitus. *Diabetes Care* **9** (1986), 614–22.

76. R. C. Ziegelstein, J. A. Fauerbach, S. S. Stevens, *et al.*, Patients with depression are less likely to follow recommendations to reduce cardiac risk during recovery from a myocardial infarction. *Arch. Intern. Med.* **160** (2000), 1818–23.

77. P. J. Goodnick, A. Kumar, J. H. Henry, V. M. V. Buki, R. B. Goldberg, Sertraline in coexisting major depression and diabetes mellitus. *Psychopharmacol. Bull.* **33** (1997), 261–4.

78. P. J. Lustman, L. S. Griffith, R. E. Clouse, *et al.*, Effects of nortriptyline on depression and glycemic control in diabetes: results of a double-blind, placebo-controlled trial. *Psychosom. Med.* **59** (1997), 241–50.

79. P. J. Lustman, L. S. Griffith, K. E. Freedland, S. S. Kissel, R. E. Clouse, Cognitive behavior therapy for depression in type 2 diabetes mellitus: a randomized, controlled trial. *Ann. Intern. Med.* **129** (1998), 613–21.

80. J. W. Williams, W. Katon, E. Lin, *et al.*, The effectiveness of depression care management on diabetes-related outcomes in older patients. *Ann. Intern. Med.* **140** (2004), 1015–24.

81. R. M. Baron, D. A. Kenny, The moderator-mediator variable distinction in social psychological research: conceptual, strategic, and statistical considerations. *J. Pers. Soc. Psychol.* **51** (1986), 1173–82.

82. R. R. Wing, S. Phelan, D. F. Tate, The role of adherence in mediating the relationship between depression and health outcomes. *J. Psychosom. Res.* **53** (2002), 877–81.

Part 4

Conclusions

18

Integrating clinical with biobehavioural studies of depression and physical illness

Andrew Steptoe

Depression and health outcomes

The chapters in Part 2 of this book addressed the relationship between depression and specific conditions, including coronary heart disease (CHD), diabetes, cancer, chronic pain and obesity. There is also research linking depression and depressed mood with a number of other health outcomes, including acquired immunodeficiency syndrome (AIDS)-related mortality [1], hospitalisation and death in patients with end-stage renal disease [2], and death among patients with Parkinson's disease [3]. In some of these conditions, depression is associated with worse outcomes, but this is not always the case. As noted in Chapter 10, evidence linking depression with poor outcome in cancer is inconclusive, and Stage *et al.* [4] have reported in a small study of chronic obstructive pulmonary disease that depressive illness was associated with reduced rather than greater mortality. Some studies have suggested that insulin resistance (a risk factor for CHD and diabetes) is protective against depression [5,6].

There are two other common chronic conditions in which depression has been studied quite extensively, and these merit fuller discussion since they have not been the subject of separate chapters in this book. The first of these is stroke. Since the pathophysiology of many types of stroke closely resembles that of coronary artery disease, it is perhaps not surprising that associations between depression and future stroke have been identified. Results from the Baltimore Epidemiologic Catchment Area study showed that stroke was more than twice as likely in clinically depressed than non-depressed individuals after controlling for heart disease, hypertension, disability and smoking [7]. Similar results have been published from Wales [8]. In a more recent follow-up of the Multiple Risk Factor Intervention Trial cohort, greater depressive symptoms at the end of the trial predicted future stroke mortality after controlling for major risk factors, including age, race, education, smoking, blood

Depression and Physical Illness, ed. A. Steptoe.
Published by Cambridge University Press. © Cambridge University Press 2006.

pressure, cholesterol and non-fatal cardiovascular events [9]. It is notable that in both this study and the analysis from the Women's Health Initiative described in Chapter 3 [10], associations were observed between depression and stroke but not between depression and CHD.

The second condition is heart failure, since there is accumulating evidence from clinical studies that depression contributes to poor outcome and accelerated mortality in patients with congestive heart failure (CHF). For example, Jiang *et al.* [11] studied 374 CHF patients admitted to a single hospital and found that major depression was associated with more than doubling of mortality after one year, independently of age, New York Heart Association heart failure class, and baseline cardiac function. In a smaller study of clinically stable patients with heart failure in the UK, depressive symptoms predicted mortality after controlling for neuroticism, heart failure severity, gender and age [12]. Other studies have also indicated that depressive symptoms predict future death from CHF independently of clinical cardiological measures [13].

Depression and overall mortality risk

Studies of depression and specific health problems do not demonstrate unequivocally that depression is associated with worse health outcome overall. The associations between depression and increased risk for some conditions may be balanced by protective effects for other outcomes. One way of resolving this issue is to assess total morbidity or mortality in relation to depressive symptoms. There is a large literature on this topic, and studies published up to 2001 have been reviewed and meta-analysed. Schulz *et al.* [14] identified 61 studies, about a third of which were community studies. The majority of studies showed a positive association between depression and future mortality. In Cuijpers and Smit's [15] meta-analysis, the relative risk of dying was 1.81 (95% confidence interval [CI] 1.58 to 2.07) in depressed compared with non-depressed individuals. Interestingly, effects were comparable for clinical and subclinical depression. However, both reviews pointed out that confounding factors such as lifestyle and chronic illnesses were not controlled well in many investigations.

Since then, evidence has continued to accumulate. Ensinck *et al.* [16] reported on some 69 000 people from the Netherlands who were tracked for 15 years. Each person diagnosed with depression was matched with a non-depressed individual. A small positive association between depression and future mortality was recorded after adjustment for age, gender and socioeconomic status, but no data concerning lifestyle or pre-existing medical conditions were analysed. Two other studies reported positive associations between depression and total mortality after controlling for chronic illness and lifestyle factors [17,18]. By contrast, Everson-Rose *et al.* [19] analysed 7.5 years of follow-up in a national representative sample of adults in the USA, showing that the association between depression and increased mortality was no longer significant after baseline self-reported health and functional impairment were taken into account. Existing physical illness and disability can increase depressive symptoms, as is evident from many of the chapters in this book, and so the association between depression and future mortality may in some cases be due to existing physical pathology. This issue is difficult to resolve, since it is possible to overcontrol statistically in studies of depression and physical illness [20]. If biological and lifestyle factors are part of the pathway linking depression with health outcomes, then controlling for them eliminates part of what is being studied.

Causal and reciprocal processes

The research detailed in this book makes it clear that the relationships between depression and physical illness are complex. The role of depression in the development of physical illness and prognosis has become the subject of systematic scientific research only in recent decades, while the fact that many people suffering from illnesses or disability become depressed has been evident from clinical and personal experience for much longer. Many of the illnesses discussed in this book limit lifespan and curtail activities of daily living, impair social relationships and reduce sense of control, all of which can provoke depressed mood. The research on behavioural and biological processes described in Part 3 provides compelling evidence for the relevance of inflammatory, immune, neuroendocrine and behavioural processes. But only in the past few years have researchers moved beyond establishing cross-sectional associations to studying longitudinal processes.

The relationships between depression, illness and biological and behavioural processes are best represented as a system rather than in simple causal chains. Nevertheless, when teasing out the strands of this system, it is necessary to define distinct sequential links. The three main models underpinning understanding of depression in physical illness are outlined in Figure 18.1. The antecedent model proposes that clinical depression or depressed mood contributes to the aetiology and progression of physical illness, and that this relationship is mediated by biological and behavioural factors. The importance of the mediators will vary between health outcomes and stage of the illness process. For example, inflammatory processes stimulating vascular endothelial dysfunction may be relevant to CHD, while other types of inflammation contribute to disability and chronic pain. The evaluations of the literature on the development and prognosis of CHD (Chapters 3 and 4), physical disability (Chapter 6) and diabetes (Chapter 8) provide strong evidence for the antecedent causal model, while findings related to chronic fatigue (Chapter 9)

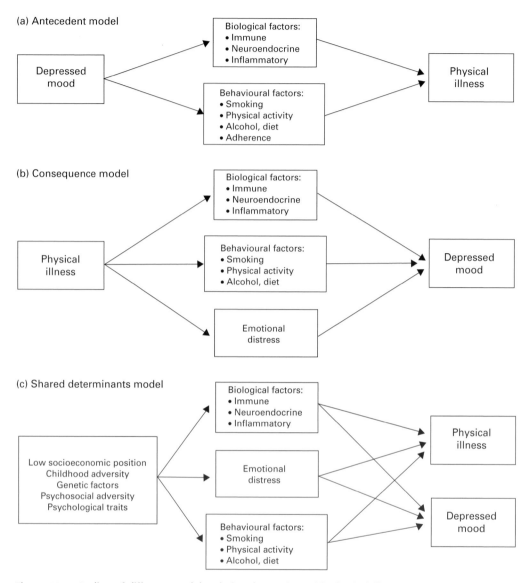

Figure 18.1 Outline of different models relating depression with physical illness.

and obesity (Chapter 11) are more equivocal, and the conclusion of the review of cancer is negative (Chapter 10).

There is also good evidence that the biological and behavioural factors discussed in Part 3 contribute to adverse health outcomes and are plausible mediators of depression effects. What has been demonstrated less clearly is that these factors mediate associations between depression and illness. For instance, Raynor and colleagues in Chapter 17 have provided a systematic analysis of the hypothesis that depression leads to poor adherence to treatment and medical advice, which in turn promotes disease progression and negative outcomes. The evidence for this sequence is far less impressive than some behavioural scientists and clinicians assume. Many studies have failed to show that depression predicts poor adherence, and there is even less support from either observational or intervention studies that adherence mediates associations between depression and health outcomes. Similarly, there is little direct evidence that smoking or physical inactivity are mediators (Chapters 15 and 16).

The second possibility outlined in Figure 18.1 is the consequence model, in which depressed mood arises as a result of physical illness. It is interesting that many of the same biological and behavioural factors could act as mediators of this process, just as they might operate in the reverse direction in the antecedent model. The fact that there are common mediators reflects either the reality of the situation or the possibility that research has not advanced sufficiently beyond the correlational to allow definitive conclusions about causal processes to be drawn.

Depression may arise in an individual with serious physical illness as an emotional response to diagnosis, treatment and the destruction of future life prospects. There are also more direct biological mediators. One biological pathway related to the consequence model is detailed by Dantzer and colleagues in Chapter 12, where they describe the impact of inflammation and cytokine release on depression, sleep disturbance and fatigue. The clinical manifestation of these processes is described in relation to chronic pain and fatigue in Chapters 7 and 9. Carney and Freedland in Chapter 5 point out that the depression experienced by patients following myocardial infarction may be qualitatively different from other forms of depression and may be stimulated partly by the acute inflammatory state that is present during acute coronary syndromes. Certainly, the risk factors for depression in cardiac patients differ from those observed generally [21]. One implication may be that depression in physically ill people needs distinctive treatment, since existing interventions may not target the relevant mechanisms. Different factors mediate the impact of illness on depressed mood in specific conditions. In stroke patients, for example, depression appears to arise from direct damage to certain regions of the brain, and particularly from lesions in the left frontal area and the basal ganglia [22].

The third model in Figure 18.3 is the shared determinants or common pathogenesis model. This argues that there are factors underlying increased risk for both depressed mood and illness, such that the relationship between the two has no causal significance. Stansfeld and Rasul in Chapter 2 detail how low socioeconomic background, poor educational attainment and childhood adversity contribute to risk of depression in later life; the same factors predict adverse physical health outcomes and biological and behavioural risk profiles. In Chapter 13, Goodyer outlines how early adversity affects both depression and hypothalamic-pituitary-adrenocortical (HPA) axis function, while Kassel and Hankin in Chapter 15 discuss links between early experience and smoking and possible shared genetic determinants of smoking and depression. Associations between early adversity and other health outcomes are increasingly being described [23,24]. Another shared determinant may be negative affectivity, a psychological trait that has been postulated to be an influence on many physical health problems [25,26] while also being a risk factor for depression. These shared processes make investigations even more complicated, and great pains are taken to discover whether associations between depression and physical illness are still significant after all potential confounders are taken into account.

Methodological problems

Numerous methodological issues have been discussed in this book that are significant in particular fields of clinical and basic research. But two overarching themes have emerged that are relevant across domains and warrant reiterating here.

The first is the issue of whether depression is regarded as a categorical diagnostic entity or as a continuous dimensional variable. It is generally agreed that there are gradations of depression. From the psychiatric perspective, there may exist a critical threshold of intensity and duration above which treatment is warranted, either because it is known to be efficacious or cost-effective with depression above this level or because there is serious concern about self-harm. The issue for studies of physical illness is whether relationships exist only with depression of a severity that is recognised psychiatrically, or whether lesser degrees of depression are important. A related question is whether dose–response associations are present.

There is good evidence from many of the contributions to this book that a dimensional approach to depression is valuable, in that associations exist between physical health problems and moderate or subclinical levels of depressed mood. However, evidence for dose–response effects is more elusive, and such associations have not been established definitively for many conditions. In the absence of this information, it is possible that depressed mood has to exceed a threshold in order to be relevant to physical illness, and that a categorical approach is still valid. Of course, the threshold may be different from the one that is relevant for psychiatric conditions and may not even be the same for different health outcomes.

The second general methodological issue raised in several chapters in this book is the confounding of depression and illness at the symptomatic level. This is particularly relevant to chronic fatigue, as pointed out by White in Chapter 9, but it also applies elsewhere. Many health problems are characterised by low energy levels and tiredness, and these phenomena are parts of depressive syndromes. More specific features of depression may also be present. For example, Musselman and colleagues in Chapter 8 detail the way in which diabetes is frequently accompanied by loss of libido and psychomotor retardation, while immune dysfunction and sleep disturbance are linked closely in depression (Chapter 14). Additionally, depressed people often exhibit reporting biases in relation to somatic symptoms, making it difficult to disentangle depression from illness and disability.

These issues are particularly problematic when definitions of health states depend on self-rated rather than objective indicators, and so provide an argument for the use of objective clinical, behavioural and biological markers wherever possible. It is arguable whether studies relating depressive symptoms with outcomes such as self-rated health can ever avoid this measurement confound. Methodological difficulties may also be exacerbated when depression is assessed by self-report questionnaire rather than by interview or observer ratings. There is an important message for researchers in this field to select study designs and assessments that eliminate these confounds as far as possible.

Depression and patient care in medical conditions

A central reason for studying depression in medical illness is to discover methods of improving patient care. One of the hopes of behavioural and psychosomatic medicine has been that psychological or lifestyle interventions will influence physical disease processes and prolong life. This shibboleth was present long before studies of depression became prominent. In the cardiovascular field, for example, there was great excitement at the evidence from the Recurrent Coronary Prevention Project that treating type A behaviour reduced risk of myocardial infarction [27], while Spiegel and colleagues' [28] study raised the possibility that supportive group therapy prolonged the life of women with breast cancer. Work on the adverse effects of depression in post-myocardial infarction patients (Chapter 4) led to the ambitious Enhancing Recovery in Coronary Heart Disease (ENRICHD) study described by Carney and Friedman in Chapter 5. The failure of this trial to demonstrate clear benefits to cardiovascular health might lead sceptics to doubt the wisdom of treating depression. This would be wrong for two reasons. First, a clinical trial should be viewed not in isolation but as part of a programme of treatment research. Lessons can be learned from unsuccessful trials, both in terms of how to do things better and through identification of subgroups of patients in whom favourable effects are observed [29]. The results of treating depression in other groups of medical patients suggest that physical health outcomes may be modified, as in some cases of diabetes and chronic pain (Chapters 7 and 8). Second, it is erroneous to prioritise the management of depression in physically ill people only if it has a demonstrable effect on survival or disease progression. The improvements in the psychological wellbeing and quality of life that may result from depression treatment are desirable aims in themselves.

Identification of depressive states in clinical medicine

A recurrent theme in this book is the lack of attention paid by physicians to the evaluation of the mental states of their physically ill patients. Creed and Dickens (Chapter 1) have described the high rates of depression present across the spectrum of physical illnesses, and in many medical specialties these problems are woefully underdiagnosed. In the past, it has been argued that convenient methods of assessment were not available to physicians, and that even if depression was identified specialists in non-psychiatric medicine were not well placed to do much about it. The situation has changed over recent years, with the development of brief, validated measures such as the seven-item depression scale from the Hospital Anxiety and Depression Scale (HADS) [30], the nine-item Patient Health Questionnaire (PHQ) [31] and even the two-item PHQ [32], which provide reasonably good data for screening depressive states. These can be supplemented if necessary by standardised psychiatric interviews, some of which (such as the Clinical Interview Schedule and the Depression Interview and Structured Hamilton) can be administered by non-psychiatric-trained personnel [33,34]. Access to psychological care has also improved through the implementation of integrated approaches to patient management and the creation of multidisciplinary teams in many branches of medicine.

However, it has to be said that clinical guidelines for the care of patients with many health problems still do not always provide clear recommendations about how to assess and manage depression. There is also the challenge of identifying depressive states that do not fulfil the criteria for psychiatric case status. It is evident from many chapters in this book that subclinical depressed mood is a major problem and diagnostic methods based on psychiatric models may not be sufficient.

Problems also surround decisions concerning the most judicious use of medical and mental health resources. Simon *et al.* in Chapter 10 argue that in the case of cancer, screening by questionnaire followed by clinical evaluation itself takes up considerable professional resources. If the yield of previously unidentified depressed patients is low, and if even fewer are prepared to accept psychological or psychiatric care, then other uses of scarce funding may be preferable.

Understanding the consequences of depressive states

Depression in physical illness has wide ramifications. Aside from the need for appropriate management of this distressing emotional state, it is important for clinical staff to understand its broader consequences. As has been emphasised in many chapters, depressed mood may have significant effects on the progression of disease and disability. What this means for the clinician is that two patients can be at an identical stage of illness as far as biological indicators or clinical manifestations are concerned, but one will show more rapid deterioration than the other by virtue of his or her emotional state. This factor may need to be taken into account in clinical decision-making. Depressive moods have a pronounced effect on the wellbeing of patients and their families. This means that physicians and nurses may be surprised at the mismatch between clinical indicators and a patient's symptomatic state and the patient's own sense health. There is also the possibility that more depressed people receive less optimal treatment and care than do non-depressed individuals [35], since the former may be perceived as tiresome, ungrateful, excessively complaining and less agreeable to help. The findings in Chapters 15–17 that depressed people are less physically active, smoke more, and may not always follow advice rigorously can lead to them being labelled as uncooperative and unwilling to help themselves. Additionally, some medical treatments may be terminated prematurely by patients who believe – sometimes with justification – that they are inducing depression (Chapter 12). These multiple effects of depressive states are often not recognised in primary or secondary clinical settings, leading to unsatisfactory medical care and loss of confidence that patients and clinical staff are engaged in a combined effort to treat disease and reduce disability.

Treatment issues

We are at an important stage in understanding how to treat depressive symptoms in medical patients. The effects of conventional cognitive–behavioural and pharmacological treatments have not been as great as expected in many conditions. Van Puymbroeck and colleagues in Chapter 7 point to studies in which cognitive–behavioural therapy (CBT) has had favourable effects on chronic pain without influencing depression, while the impact of antidepressant medication on depressive states in diabetic and post-myocardial infarction patients has been inconsistent (Chapters 5 and 8). Carney and Freedland in Chapter 5 speculate that the often elderly and medically ill people who survive an acute coronary event may find it difficult to engage with standard CBT, with its focus on automatic negative thoughts and core beliefs. Similar problems are apparent among cancer patients, many of whom are not prepared to engage with mental health issues (Chapter 10). At the same time, there is reason to suppose that mental healthcare methods can be adapted for these different settings, and some newer antidepressant mediations also look promising [22,36]. The knowledge that is accumulating about biological processes (Chapters 12–14) will stimulate further developments in treatments that may have effects on both psychological and biological outcomes. Other modalities, such as physical exercise training, may be useful in helping at least moderately depressed people, with the added benefit that they might also improve clinical risk profiles and help reduce disability (Chapters 6 and 16). The challenge will be how to integrate such methods into the clinical care of patients who do not primarily have psychological problems and who may consider attention to their mental state to be a distraction from the treatment of their physical condition.

REFERENCES

1. J. A. Cook, D. Grey, J. Burke, *et al.*, Depressive symptoms and AIDS-related mortality among a multisite cohort of HIV-positive women. *Am. J. Public Health* **94** (2004), 1133–40.

2. A. A. Lopes, J. Bragg, E. Young, *et al.*, Depression as a predictor of mortality and hospitalization among hemodialysis patients in the United States and Europe. *Kidney Int.* **62** (2002), 199–207.

3. T. A. Hughes, H. F. Ross, R. H. Mindham, E. G. Spokes, Mortality in Parkinson's disease and its association with dementia and depression. *Acta Neurol. Scand.* **110** (2004), 118–23.

4. K. B. Stage, T. Middelboe, C. Pisinger, Depression and chronic obstructive pulmonary disease (COPD): impact on survival. *Acta Psychiatr. Scand.* **111** (2005), 320–3.

5. B. A. Golomb, L. Tenkanen, T. Alikoski, *et al.*, Insulin sensitivity markers: predictors of accidents and suicides in Helsinki Heart Study screenees. *J. Clin. Epidemiol.* **55** (2002), 767–73.

6. D. A. Lawlor, G. D. Smith, S. Ebrahim, Association of insulin resistance with depression: cross sectional findings from the British Women's Heart and Health Study. *Br. Med. J.* **327** (2003), 1383–4.

7. S. L. Larson, P. L. Owens, D. Ford, W. Eaton, Depressive disorder, dysthymia, and risk of stroke: thirteen-year follow-up from the Baltimore epidemiologic catchment area study. *Stroke* **32** (2001), 1979–83.

8. M. May, P. McCarron, S. Stansfeld, *et al.*, Does psychological distress predict the risk of ischemic stroke and transient ischemic attack? The Caerphilly Study. *Stroke* **33** (2002), 7–12.

9. B. B. Gump, K. A. Matthews, L. E. Eberly, Y. F. Chang, Depressive symptoms and mortality in men: results from the Multiple Risk Factor Intervention Trial. *Stroke* **36** (2005), 98–102.

10. S. Wassertheil-Smoller, S. Shumaker, J. Ockene, *et al.*, Depression and cardiovascular sequelae in postmenopausal women: the Women's Health Initiative (WHI). *Arch. Intern. Med.* **164** (2004), 289–98.

11. W. Jiang, J. Alexander, E. Christopher, *et al.*, Relationship of depression to increased risk of mortality and rehospitalization in patients with congestive heart failure. *Arch. Intern. Med.* **161** (2001), 1849–56.

12. T. A. Murberg, G. Furze, Depressive symptoms and mortality in patients with congestive heart failure: a six-year follow-up study. *Med. Sci. Monit.* **10** (2004), CR643–8.

13. J. Junger, D. Schellberg, T. Muller-Tasch, *et al.*, Depression increasingly predicts mortality in the course of congestive heart failure. *Eur. J. Heart Fail.* **7** (2005), 261–7.

14. R. Schulz, R. A. Drayer, B. L. Rollman, Depression as a risk factor for non-suicide mortality in the elderly. *Biol. Psychiatry* **52** (2002), 205–25.

15. P. Cuijpers, F. Smit, Excess mortality in depression: a meta-analysis of community studies. *J. Affect. Disord.* **72** (2002), 227–36.

16. K. T. Ensinck, A. G. Schuurman, M. van den Akker, *et al.*, Is there an increased risk of dying after depression? *Am. J. Epidemiol.* **156** (2002), 1043–8.

17. K. Frojdh, A. Hakansson, I. Karlsson, A. Molarius, Deceased, disabled or depressed: a population-based 6-year follow-up study of elderly people with depression. *Soc. Psychiatry Psychiatr. Epidemiol.* **38** (2003), 557–62.

18. R. S. Wilson, J. L. Bienias, C. F. Mendes de Leon, D. A. Evans, D. A. Bennett, Negative affect and mortality in older persons. *Am. J. Epidemiol.* **158** (2003), 827–35.

19. S. A. Everson-Rose, J. S. House, R. P. Mero, Depressive symptoms and mortality risk in a national sample: confounding effects of health status. *Psychosom. Med.* **66** (2004), 823–30.

20. A. Steptoe, D. L. Whitehead, Depression, stress and coronary heart disease: the need for more complex models. *Heart* **91** (2005), 419–20.

21. C. M. Dickens, C. Percival, L. McGowan, *et al.*, The risk factors for depression in first myocardial infarction patients. *Psychol. Med.* **34** (2004), 1083–92.

22. R. G. Robinson, Poststroke depression: prevalence, diagnosis, treatment, and disease progression. *Biol. Psychiatry* **54** (2003), 376–87.

23. M. Dong, S. R. Dube, V. J. Felitti, W. H. Giles, R. F. Anda, Adverse childhood experiences and self-reported liver disease: new insights into the causal pathway. *Arch. Intern. Med.* **163** (2003), 1949–56.

24. M. Dong, W. H. Giles, V. J. Felitti, *et al.*, Insights into causal pathways for ischemic heart disease: adverse childhood experiences study. *Circulation* **110** (2004), 1761–6.

25. H. S. Friedman, S. Booth-Kewley, The 'disease-prone personality': A meta-analytic view of the construct. *Am. Psychol.* **42** (1987), 539–55.

26. J. Suls, J. Bunde, Anger, anxiety, and depression as risk factors for cardiovascular disease: the problems and implications of overlapping affective dispositions. *Psychol. Bull.* **131** (2005), 260–300.

27. M. Friedman, C. E. Thoresen, J. J. Gill, *et al.*, Feasibility of altering type A behavior pattern after myocardial infarction: Recurrent Coronary Prevention Project Study – methods, baseline results and preliminary findings. *Circulation* **66** (1982), 83–92.

28. D. Spiegel, J. R. Bloom, H. C. Kraemer, E. Gottheil, Effect of psychosocial treatment on survival of patients with metastatic breast cancer. *Lancet* **2** (1989), 888–91.

29. N. Schneiderman, P. G. Saab, D. J. Catellier, *et al.*, Psychosocial treatment within sex by ethnicity subgroups in the Enhancing Recovery in Coronary Heart Disease clinical trial. *Psychosom. Med.* **66** (2004), 475–83.

30. C. Herrmann, International experiences with the Hospital Anxiety and Depression Scale: a review of validation data and clinical results. *J. Psychosom. Res.* **42** (1997), 17–41.

31. K. Kroenke, R. L. Spitzer, J. B. Williams, The PHQ-9: validity of a brief depression severity measure. *J. Gen. Intern. Med.* **16** (2001), 606–13.

32. K. Kroenke, R. L. Spitzer, J. B. Williams, The Patient Health Questionnaire-2: validity of a two-item depression screener. *Med. Care* **41** (2003), 1284–92.

33. K. E. Freedland, J. A. Skala, R. M. Carney, *et al.*, The Depression Interview and Structured Hamilton (DISH): rationale, development, characteristics, and clinical validity. *Psychosom. Med.* **64** (2002), 897–905.

34. G. Lewis, A. J. Pelosi, R. Araya, G. Dunn, Measuring psychiatric disorder in the community: a standardized assessment for use by lay interviewers. *Psychol. Med.* **22** (1992), 465–86.

35. B. G. Druss, D. W. Bradford, R. A. Rosenheck, M. J. Radford, H. M. Krumholz, Mental disorders and use of cardiovascular procedures after myocardial infarction. *J. Am. Med. Assoc.* **283** (2000), 506–11.

36. C. L. Raison, A. H. Miller, Depression in cancer: new developments regarding diagnosis and treatment. *Biol. Psychiatry* **54** (2003), 283–94.

Index